Equitation Science

Equitation Science

Second Edition

Paul McGreevy
University of Sydney
New South Wales, Australia

Janne Winther Christensen
Aarhus University
Denmark

Uta König von Borstel
University of Giessen
Giessen, Germany

Andrew McLean
Australian Equine Behaviour Centre
Victoria, Australia

WILEY Blackwell

Registered Office(s)
John Wiley & Sons, Inc., 111 River Street, Hoboken, NJ 07030, USA
John Wiley & Sons Ltd, The Atrium, Southern Gate, Chichester, West Sussex, PO19 8SQ, UK

Editorial Office
9600 Garsington Road, Oxford, OX4 2DQ, UK

For details of our global editorial offices, customer services, and more information about Wiley products visit us at www.wiley.com.

Wiley also publishes its books in a variety of electronic formats and by print-on-demand. Some content that appears in standard print versions of this book may not be available in other formats.

Library of Congress Cataloging-in-Publication Data

Names: McGreevy, Paul, 1964– author.
Title: Equitation science / Paul McGreevy, University of Sydney, Sydney, New South Wales, Australia, Janne Winther Christensen, Aarhus University, Denmark, Uta König von Borstel, University of Giessen, Giessen, Germany, Andrew McLean, Australian Equine Behaviour Centre, Victoria, Australia.
Description: 2nd edition. | Hoboken, NJ : Wiley, [2018] | Revised edition of: Equitation science / Paul McGreevy and Andrew McLean. 2010. | Includes bibliographical references and index. |
Identifiers: LCCN 2017055296 (print) | LCCN 2017055987 (ebook) | ISBN 9781119241447 (pdf) | ISBN 9781119241386 (epub) | ISBN 9781119241416 (paper)
Subjects: LCSH: Horses–Training. | Horsemanship. | Horses–Psychology.
Classification: LCC SF287 (ebook) | LCC SF287 .M4426 2018 (print) | DDC 636.1/0835–dc23
LC record available at https://lccn.loc.gov/2017055296

Cover Design: Wiley
Cover Image: © John Lund/Gettyimages

Set in 10/12pt Warnock by SPi Global, Pondicherry, India
Printed and bound by CPI Group (UK) Ltd, Croydon, CR0 4YY

C9781119241416_270324

Contents

Preface

This is a book for horse-industry personnel, and indeed everyone who spends time with horses and ponies. It will help to ensure that humane, proficient horsemanship becomes more prevalent.

Many equine scientists, veterinarians, ethologists and behaviour therapists share the view that the current lack of science in equitation contributes to the prevalence of undesirable equine behaviours with human-related causes. The number of horses worldwide is large and growing. As a consequence, there are increasing numbers of horse-owners, many of whom are new to horse-keeping, with little knowledge of how to train their animals. This has led to a rise in the number of associated horse-welfare problems culminating in high wastage rates. Such problems reflect the uninformed practices, poor training techniques, inappropriate use of training equipment and, in some cases, inhumane handling of horses. In addition, horse-related injuries are a major public-health concern, with most fatal injuries occurring while the rider is mounted. Death rates from horse-related injuries are in the vicinity of one death per million head of population and in terms of injuries, horse-riding is more dangerous than motorcycle riding. Improving riders' understanding of horse behaviour and subsequently reducing the number of 'conflict behaviours' horses develop will reduce the prevalence of such accidents. Furthermore, the increasing profile of 'Natural Horsemanship' and 'horse whisperers' has made horse-industry personnel question some traditional practices, prompting them to consider how novel techniques operate and

to question how the language relating to horse-training and riding relates to what is known through psychology, ethology and veterinary science. This book will help them in these endeavours.

This second edition contains updated information on research results that have emerged since the publication of the first version. Since publication of the first edition, equitation science has become an established scientific discipline that aims to provide an understanding of the behavioural mechanisms that underpin the human–horse interface. Equitation science is the measurement and interpretation of interactions between horses and their riders. While many horse-training systems focus on a purely ethological approach with scant attention paid to learning processes, we have attempted to redress this to give a full account of the interactions of both ethological and learning processes (known in behavioural science as learning theory). Compared to the first edition, the focus of this book has shifted to include a broader description of the range of training systems that variously align with learning theory. Because horse-training relies so heavily on the use of tactile pressures, our book attempts to describe the optimal use and pitfalls of these interactions and the relative potential of combined reinforcement through the inclusion of positive reinforcement.

The objective measurement of variables is important, so this book explains, from first principles, traditional and novel techniques to reveal what works, what does not, and why. Most importantly, it also explores the welfare consequences of training and competing with horses under different disciplines.

Equitation science has an extremely promising future since it is more humble, global, accessible and accurate, and less denominational, commercial, open to interpretation and misinterpretation than traditional interpretations of horse-training. Because of this, it has the potential to be the most enduring framework to inform every facet of horse–human interactions.

The authors offer unique perspectives by being able to combine tertiary qualifications in veterinary medicine (PM), ethology (PM, JWC, UvB), zoology (AM & JWC), comparative cognition (AM), animal welfare (PM, JWC, UvB), animal breeding and genetics (UvB), and stress biology (JWC & UvB), with significant experience in animal-training (AM, PM, UvB), elite equestrian competition (AM), clinical behaviour modification (AM & PM) and coaching (AM & PM).

Acknowledgements

We wish to acknowledge the tremendous support we have received over many years from our colleagues in academe and the horse industry. Early attempts to apply learning theory to horse training were made by AM (Horse Training the McLean Way) and PM (Why does my horse…?). Since then, the emerging discipline of equitation science developed rapidly following discussions between Debbie Goodwin, Natalie Waran and PM at the Havemeyer Foundation Workshop on Horse Behaviour and Welfare in Iceland in 2002.

The first workshop on equitation science was held at the Royal (Dick) School of Veterinary Studies, University of Edinburgh in 2004, where AM gave practical demonstrations of the application of 'learning theory' in-hand and under-saddle. As a result of the interest of approximately 30 equine scientists at this workshop, it was decided to launch the first symposium in equitation science at the Australian Equine Behaviour Centre the following year. Since then, the annual conferences of the International Society of Equitation Science (ISES) have attracted an increasing number of delegates from all over the world.

The formation of the ISES is a great step forward for horses and is a direct result of the growing worldwide interest in this area by equine scientists and equestrian professionals alike. The equestrians we wish to acknowledge include Portland Jones, Manuela McLean, Jody Hartstone, Anjanette Harten, Warwick McLean and Nicki Stuart.

For their help with the first edition, we wish to thank Bob Boakes, Hilary Clayton, Ruth Coleman, Debbie Goodwin, Carol Hall, Camie Heleski, Machteld van Dierendonck, Katherine Houpt, Kathalijne Visser, Jan Ladewig, Leo Jeffcott, Daniel Mills, Jack Murphy, Nicki Stuart, Julie Taylor, Natalie Waran, Amanda Warren-Smith and Mari Zetterquist-Blokhuis; all of whom reviewed at least one chapter each. Robert Corken assisted with checking citations. Lynn Cole gave invaluable advice on each chapter. Nicki Stuart displayed extraordinary patience and diplomacy as the project manager of the current text. We warmly acknowledge the contributions of Marc Pierard, Carol Hall, Lesley Hawson, Alison Averis, Kathalijne Visser and Charlotte Nevison to the current descriptions of research methodologies and of Cristina Wilkins to the overview on the effects of head and neck positions. JWC would further like to thank the Danish Center for Animal Welfare (Videnscenter for Dyrevelfaerd) and the KUSTOS Foundation of 1881 for funding, and Jens Malmkvist and Susan Kjærgaard for comments and support. UK would like to thank Thórvaldur Árnason for kindly reviewing content related to gaited horses. The illustrations are largely the work of an outstanding equestrian illustrator, Samantha Elmhurst.

Photographs were supplied by Manuela McLean, Andrew McLean, Elke Hartmann, Julie Wilson, Julie Taylor, Christine Hauschildt, Amelia Martin, Minna Tallberg, Philippe Karl, Sandy Hannan, Amanda Warren-Smith, Greg Jones, Jenny Carroll, Pierre Malou, Sandra Jorgensen, Christine Hauschildt, David Faloun, Georgia Bruce, Roz Neave, Susan Kjaergard, Portland Jones, Sophie Warren,

Carol Willcocks, Becky Whay, Cristina Wilkins Eric Palmer, Don and Sandy Bonem, Dagmar Heller, Diana Krischke, Sandra Kuhnke, Klaus Ohneberg, Philipp Seifert, Niels Stappenbeck, Kasia Olczak, Kristina Leth and Nanna Luthersson. While we have made every possible effort to contact the rights owners of other images used in this book, there have been cases where it has not been possible to trace the relevant parties. If you believe that you are the owner of an image or images used in this book and we have not contacted you prior to publication, please contact us via the publisher.

Disclaimer:

The book is not a manual and is not intended to endorse any specific training system, discipline or apparatus.

About the Companion Website

This book is accompanied by a companion website:

www.wiley.com/go/mcgreevy/equitation

The website includes:

- Powerpoint slides with downloadable figures

1

Introduction – The Fascination with Horses and Learning

Introduction

Everyone who spends time with horses will from time-to-time become fascinated by their behaviour and learning abilities. One does not have to search for long to find reports of extraordinary learning performance in individual horses; examples range from 'Clever Hans', the horse that appeared to be able to count and read but, even more interestingly, was responding to very subtle cues from human bystanders; to reports of horses being able to open box doors and gates (Figure 1.1), to everyday accounts of circus and sports horses performing precise movements in response to small cues from their trainers or riders (Figure 1.2).

Humans have been fascinated by animal learning for centuries and, since the 1800s, scientists from various fields have investigated the mammalian and avian brain to understand how animals of different species learn and adapt to their environments. The best-studied species are rodents and birds, primarily because these species are easy to study and to keep in a laboratory. Despite the evolutionary differences between these species, remarkable similarities exist in the way they learn. This has resulted in the development of 'learning theory', a set of principles that apply to all animals and explain how animals learn. Learning theory has revolutionised the way humans think about animal training, and learning theories are applied with great success in the training

of, for example, dogs, marine and other zoo animals (Figure 1.3). Indeed, it is difficult to find a modern training manual for these animals that does not use learning theory as a basis. Learning theory establishes clear guidelines and training protocols for correct training practices and methods of behaviour modification. It is truly fascinating, easy to relate to and simple to understand. Throughout this book, we will repeatedly refer to 'learning theory' as simply a comprehensive term for 'the ways in which animals learn'.

Similarly, more and more horse-trainers use and teach learning theory and understand the opportunities it can offer trainers in every discipline. Like all other animals, horses learn in predictable and straightforward ways. However, traditional horse-training differs fundamentally from the food-based training methods used for marine mammals, exotic carnivores and most companion animals, because it largely relies on what is termed 'negative (subtraction) reinforcement'. During their early training, horses learn that the correct response results in the reduction of pressure from the bit via the reins when they *stop* or *slow*. Pressure from the rider's legs or spurs is reduced when the horse moves forward. To be effective and humane, the application of pressure must be subtle and its removal immediate once the horse complies. This reliance on pressure and the release of pressure underlines the need to ensure that training programmes are effective and humane. Science can and

Equitation Science, Second Edition. Paul McGreevy, Janne Winther Christensen, Uta König von Borstel and Andrew McLean.
© 2018 John Wiley & Sons Ltd. Published 2018 by John Wiley & Sons Ltd.
Companion website: www.wiley.com/go/mcgreevy/equitation

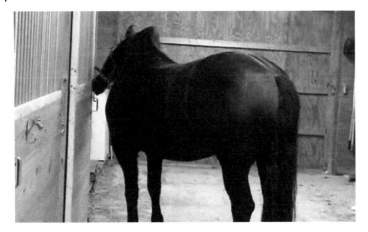

Figure 1.1 'Horses on the run': In 2013, the story about Mariska hit the world press after her owner posted a YouTube video showing how Mariska could open not only her own box door but also make her way to open the doors of the other horses' boxes. (Photo courtesy of Sandy and Don Bonem.)

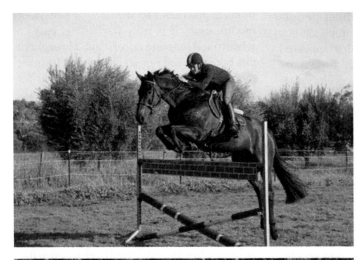

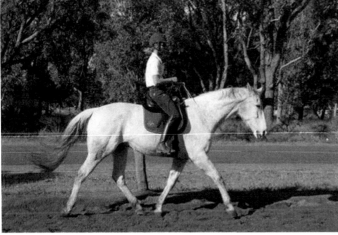

Figure 1.2 Horses can learn to respond to and differentiate between light tactile cues from their riders, regardless of the type of gear used. (Photo courtesy of Dr. Portland Jones and Sophie Warren.)

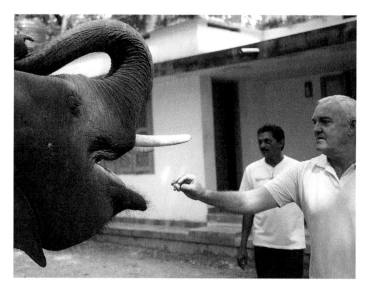

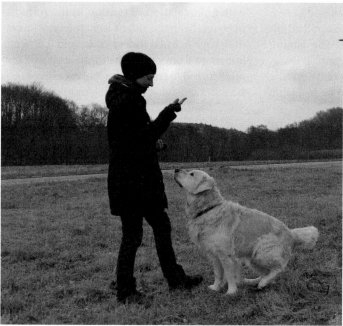

Figure 1.3 Modern training manuals for many species are based on learning theory.

should step in to measure, analyse and interpret what we do with and to horses.

Understanding the rules of learning can help horse-trainers work with their horses in a way that maintains the horse's welfare as paramount. Learning theory is not necessarily an ethical theory but it helps us train horses in a way that makes it as easy as possible for the horse to respond and succeed during training. Furthermore, it allows us to avoid behavioural side effects such as fear or aggression, caused by inappropriate training.

Veterinary epidemiologists, whose job it is to describe the spread and impact of disorders, often talk about wastage within a population. This is the percentage of animals or, in the case of working animals, the percentage of potential

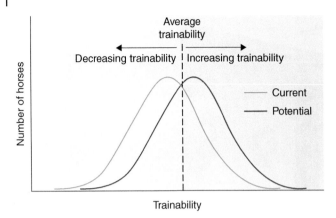

Average trainability

Decreasing trainability | Increasing trainability

—— Current
—— Potential

Number of horses

Trainability

Figure 1.4 Theoretical normal distributions to show how the numbers of horses that cope with training can be increased by using more enlightened approaches. (Reproduced from *Equine Behavior*, copyright Elsevier 2004.)

working days lost through illness or disease. Problem behaviours are the cause of much of this wastage, and in the world of the riding horse it is more significant than many of us would like to imagine (Hothersall and Casey, 2012). A global improvement in application of learning theory, particularly the timing and consistency of pressure and release, could lead to a significant increase in the number of horses considered to be trainable (Figure 1.4).

Horses are being confused on a very regular basis by less-than-ideal handling and become unusable or, worse, dangerous as a result (Hawson *et al.*, 2010a). For example, Buckley (2007) reporting on 50 out of 84 Pony Club horses, noted that this focal sub-set of owners reported a total of 251 misbehaviour days during a 12-month period. Importantly, on more than half of these days, this misbehaviour was classified as dangerous enough to cause potential injury to horse and/or rider. Horse-riding is generally considered to be more dangerous than motorcycle riding, skiing, football and rugby (Ball *et al.*, 2007). In Australia, horse-related injuries and death exceed those caused by any other non-human species (domestic or otherwise) (AIHW National Injury Surveillance Unit, 2005).

Among non-racehorses, previous studies indicate that up to 66% of euthanasia in horses between 2 and 7 years of age was not because of health disorders (Ödberg and Bouissou, 1999). The implication is that they were culled for behavioural reasons. Clearly, this level of behavioural wastage is unacceptably high. The likelihood is that many such horses are mistrusted or labelled troublesome. With their reputation for being dangerous preceding them, they are met with an escalation of tension in the reins or pressure from the rider's legs, the very forces they have learned to fear and avoid. Difficult horses go from one home to the next and are often forced to trial new ways of escaping pressure and satisfying competing motivations.

The Scientific Approach

Science is sometimes accused of objectifying animals, but the emergence of animal welfare science has already created changes in legislation that have improved animal wellbeing. It has shown us how modern diets may prompt obsessive–compulsive disorders; how weaning can affect social relations among animals; and how the behaviour of a breed can be a product of its shape.

It is the rigour of the scientific approach that ensures that we arrive as closely as possible to the truth about horses. The scientific method sometimes seems tedious because of its insistence in dismantling the elements of the questions piece by piece and its tactic in not setting out to prove a hypothesis but to disprove the null hypothesis (the non-existence of it). It is rather like the legal notion of innocent until proven guilty. Similarly, in science it is empty until proven full. An important tenet in behaviour science is Lloyd Morgan's canon, which dictates that in no case should an animal activity be interpreted in terms of higher psychological processes if it can be reasonably interpreted in terms of processes that stand lower in the scale of psychological evolution and development. Occam's razor (The Law of Parsimony) is a more general maxim that decrees that in making explanations, you should not make more assumptions than the minimum needed, so if a phenomenon can be explained in terms of simple rather than more complex ways, it is more likely to be correct. The more assumptions you have to make, the more unlikely an explanation is. This principle underpins all scientific theory building. It is easy to make rash assumptions about horse behaviour, intent and purpose.

Those with concerns about applying a scientific approach to equitation seem to fear the *construction* of equitation as a science, which is certainly not our intent. Equitation science represents the scientific *study* of equitation; it does not seek to turn equitation into a science. Scientific measuring of variables is important because it allows riding and training techniques to be compared so as to demonstrate what works and what does not. Equitation science will also allow us to measure the welfare consequences of doing the wrong thing. The *physical* interactions between humans and their horses are readily available for study. For welfare reasons, understanding these interactions correctly is crucial because, on the one hand, excessive pressure is often being used to signal to horses and, on the other, we cannot expect horses to know what we require of them without at least some cues.

In all other sports, technologies such as kinematic analysis and pressure-detecting devices have been able to refine human technique. If we accept that horses work best when riders have good technique, we can see that, as sentient beings, they are more deserving of these advances than any piece of sporting apparatus. Like all animals, horses learn most effectively when the training methods are appropriate. Inappropriate training practices can also have a negative impact on a horse's welfare and can lead to conflict behaviours that jeopardise the safety of riders

and trainers. Equitation science gives us a way of measuring and interpreting interactions between horses and their riders.

Equitation science has the potential to address a series of important problems. First, it elucidates the role of negative reinforcement and habituation in the learning processes of horses on which we ride and compete. Second, it addresses the need to measure rider interventions that may compromise horse welfare, which will assist the administrating body of equestrian sport, the Fédération Equestre Internationale (FEI), in determining what practices and interventions are acceptable on welfare grounds. For example, devices such as whips and spurs are still used routinely by some trainers. Indeed, at elite levels, spurs and double bridles (which are more severe in their action than regular single bits) are mandatory. Third, and perhaps most important, equitation science will educate current and aspiring riders in how best to apply the core principles of learning theory.

By improving riders' and coaches' basic appreciation of the science that underpins their work, we have been able to engage them in improvements that occupy the cutting edge of equitation. For a scientific horse-training manual, readers are directed to *Academic Horse Training: Equitation Science in Practice* (McLean and McLean, 2008) (www.esi-education.com).

In some sectors of horse-training, such as the sport of dressage, the cues and signals used to elicit alterations in the mobility and posture of horses are known as 'aids'. This word is antique in origin, derived from the French verb 'aider', meaning 'to help'. The notion that cues in any way offer assistance to horses is anthropocentric and has been abandoned in our text because it nourishes the notion of the 'benevolent' horse, the horse that is a willing partner. Horse-trainers should respectfully recognise that training is an act of equine exploitation rather than equine enlightenment, and modern equitation must take full account of the cognitive processes of the horse.

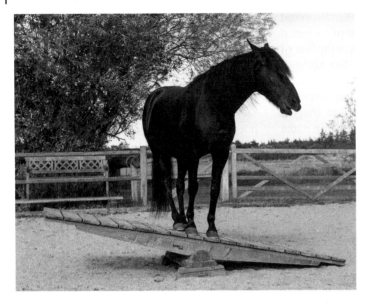

Figure 1.5 Equitation science is for everyone who spends time with horses and ponies. The training techniques presented in this book apply to all types of horses and all disciplines. Regardless of whether you are an international competition rider, a horse-trainer or a leisure rider, knowing how to use learning theory is the key to all good training and good horse welfare. (Photo courtesy of Dagmar Heller.)

Any system of riding that aligns with learning theory will result in subtle signalling and therefore, by implication and necessity, an independent seat. Our contention is that *stop* responses to the bit and *go* responses to the rider's legs are the foundations that underpin all advanced riding techniques. It would be good to see a return to traditional coaching protocols that required novice riders to learn to balance before picking up the reins. This would avoid them delivering conflicting signals.

This book is essentially an introductory text because there is much still to discover about the way mechanisms of horse-training align with more than a century of studies of learning in laboratory animals. There is also room for considerable caution because there is no laboratory equivalent for the ridden horse – you cannot ride a rat. Without restraining a rat, you cannot easily apply and then release pressure, and the horse probably provides the best model for studies of negative reinforcement. This possibility represents one of the most exciting aspects of equitation science.

The aim of this book is twofold: we partly aim to describe learning theory and give examples of how learning theory can be applied to practical horse-training. We also aim to provide an overview of the current state-of-the-art of scientific studies relating to equitation.

The purpose of this book is not to sell or publicise a particular training method, but to communicate the principles of learning theory and the science of equitation (Figure 1.5). It should be noted that just because a training method can be explained through learning theory does not necessarily mean that it is ethical or safe. Training is essentially an exploitative event and it is always the responsibility of the trainer to prioritise the horse's welfare and safety above any training goal.

2

Ethology and Cognition

Introduction

Ethology is primarily the scientific study of adaptive behaviour in animals, as it evolved in a natural environment; applied ethology is the study of animal behaviour in the human domain. Equine ethology is, strictly speaking, limited to the study of horse behaviour in free-ranging contexts (Figure 2.1). Cognition, on the other hand, is mechanisms by which animals acquire, process, store, and act on information from the environment. The study of cognition covers many topics, such as perception, learning, memory and communication. We will explore equine cognition later in this chapter, but let us first look at the horse's natural or innate behaviours (i.e. its ethology).

It is useful to think of a horse in terms of the way it fits into its social group, the domestic setting and its interactions with humans, including the work we require of it. These can be encapsulated by the term *umwelt* (from the German word for 'environment' or 'surrounding world' (von Uexküll, 1957)). Every organism reshapes its own umwelt when it interacts with the world. *Umwelt* is a useful concept as it explains how invasions into a horse's world can have effects in other domains. Physiologically, we can think of a single stressful facet of the horse's world as lowering the threshold at which other events become frustrating (Figure 2.2). Therefore, a horse that is in an inappropriate social group

may be less responsive during training and, equally, a horse that has encountered inconsistent training may be more likely to be stressed by marginally frustrating aspects of its world when not being ridden.

The biological constraints on what a horse can physically do clearly set limits to what it can be trained to do. Its cardiovascular characteristics affect its stamina and ability to take in oxygen and expel carbon dioxide (Evans *et al.*, 2006). Its musculoskeletal attributes affect its ability to contract and extend its scope over obstacles. In addition, its perception and visual acuity affect its ability to judge the position of hazards (Hall, 2007).

Beyond these physical constraints, there are also cognitive restraints that apply to the horse's ability to process and remember information. These are limitations to learning and, therefore, limitations on training that we will consider in this chapter. It is interesting to reflect upon strategies that have facilitated survival. They include a horse's ability in making associations between stimuli and weakness in generalising among stimuli. Clearly, on an individual level, such cognitive characteristics can have a critical impact on the success of our work with horses. Even with the most outstanding training programmes, with perfect timing and consistency, these constraints may have considerable impact on performance in competition.

Equitation Science, Second Edition. Paul McGreevy, Janne Winther Christensen, Uta König von Borstel and Andrew McLean.
© 2018 John Wiley & Sons Ltd. Published 2018 by John Wiley & Sons Ltd.
Companion website: www.wiley.com/go/mcgreevy/equitation

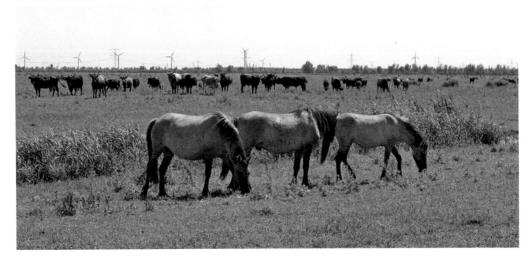

Figure 2.1 Feral horses and herds that receive minimal management, such as these Konik horses in Oostvaarders Plassen, the Netherlands, provide critical information on normal horse behaviour.

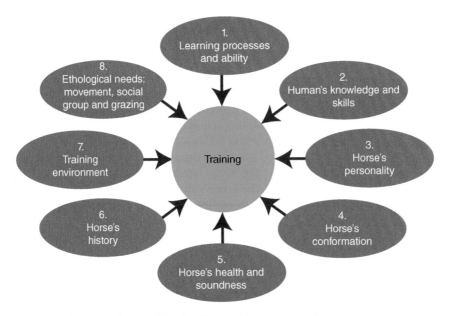

Figure 2.2 Success in horse-training is influenced by many variables.

The Horse in a Domesticated Niche

While humans have been interacting with horses for many millennia through hunting, it is only relatively recently that horses have become beasts of burden and been used for transport, war, agriculture and, more recently, sport and leisure. Direct evidence suggests that horses were domesticated at around the end of the second millennium BC (Levine, 2005), although some sources suggest a much earlier onset of domestication. However, genetic analyses suggest that domestication in the horse was not a single event, but rather took place at several separate locations (Jansen *et al.*, 2002). Since the beginnings of domestication, various techniques for horse-training have been developed and passed on to subsequent generations orally or through literature. The oldest preserved written treatise on horse-training stems from Xenophon [translated by Morgan, 1962]. All these techniques are underpinned and constrained by the biology of the horse. Many, but not all, of these training systems align with contemporary learning theory (Boot and McGreevy, 2013). When it comes to getting the most out of horses in sport and work, we need to be well acquainted with their behaviour. Effective and humane training *always* takes account of the animal's ethology, but training systems, however successful, can only ever partially align with the animal's ethogram (behavioural repertoire).

The word 'wild' is deliberately avoided here, as there are no longer any examples of truly wild horses. Most free-ranging horses are feral horses (i.e. descendants of domesticated horses that escaped from intensive human management). An exception is the Przewalski horse (*Equus przewalski*). These horses were, until recently, considered a separate species from domestic horses (*Equus caballus*) due to anatomical and genetic differences. However, genetic differences are due to chromosome fusion (i.e. the same genetic material is present, only arranged in a different number of chromosomes). Przewalski horses became extinct in their natural habitat in the 1950s (Mohr, 1971), but from a small nucleus of 13 foundation animals (one of which was a hybrid with the domestic horse), they survive today in captivity and in successfully re-introduced free-ranging populations (e.g. in Mongolia) (Boyd and Bandi, 2002; King, 2002). The survival story of Przewalski horses is an extraordinary one, and we are indeed fortunate to be able to study them in a variety of contexts. It is likely that since domestication, selective breeding has altered their fear threshold, but the hyper-reactive tendencies of the horse have not been completely eradicated.

Nevertheless, it has been proposed that the major cognitive change that occurred during selective breeding over the millennia was the capacity for habituation, including the tolerance of the nearby presence of potential predators (such as humans or dogs). Indeed, the driving force of domestication is thought to be selection for tameness (Trut *et al.*, 2009). While tameness involves innate changes of reactions to humans, it is likely in part also comprised of increased habituation abilities. The domestic horse habituates readily to a wide array of environmental and social stimuli (Miller, 1995). Such an ability to habituate to threatening stimuli may have been maladaptive for the wild horse but has been selected for in the domestic horse.

Perception

The laboratory challenges we design for horses to test learning are constrained by the subject's ability to perceive. For example, when we give horses visual learning tasks, their performance depends upon the features of their visual system. A horse's ability to look at the ground when grazing and simultaneously scan the horizon for potential predators (Harman *et al.*, 1999) may limit its ability to focus attention on a single object (Lea and Kiley-Worthington, 1996). A horse must lower its head to observe stimuli on the ground because doing so projects the image onto the most sensitive area of the retina (Harman *et al.*, 1999). The need for visual surveillance and the necessity to respond in ways that afford the horse a better view of potential threats are attributes that often provide troublesome intrusions in ridden work (Hall, 2007). In terms of vision, horses are classed as dichromats because they have two types of cone photopigment. Consequently, the colours they most easily discriminate are yellow, orange and then blue (Grzimek, 1952; Hall *et al.*, 2005).

Horses have evolved to spend approximately 60% of their time grazing so their eyes are at a set height above the ground, but it is a mistake to assume that all horses perceive the world in the same way. Studies of ganglion cell distribution suggest that skull shape may affect visual acuity (Evans and McGreevy, 2006) (Figure 2.3). Equally, the height of stimuli above the ground (Hall *et al.*, 2003)

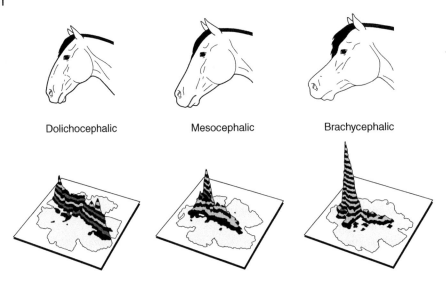

Dolichocephalic   Mesocephalic   Brachycephalic

Figure 2.3 Retinal ganglion cell-density maps from horses of three breeds with the dorsal part of the retina in the background, ventral in the foreground, nasal to the left and temporal to the right. Each shaded band represents 400 cells/mm². Studies of the retinae of horses with different skull shapes have shown that (at least some of) the neural tissue of morphologically diverse breeds differs. Brachycephalic horses, such as Arabians, are thought to have lower acuity in their peripheral vision field and a central field with higher acuity.

and relative to the height of the observing animal's head will affect the way in which stimuli are perceived. So, ponies and horses cannot be expected to perceive the same stimuli in the same way, and experimental tests with visual stimuli should take account of the head and neck position of subjects. In addition, individual horses, like humans, may possess different levels of visual acuity, which can be expected to impact their reactivity to visual stimuli.

Although horses have limited ability to focus on objects that are close to them, they have good distance vision and a very extensive visual field (Harman *et al.*, 1999). This is important as it allows them to scan the horizon for potential threats. However, they rarely need to see close up with high acuity and because the eye's proximity to objects is generally limited by the length of the nose (Wouters and De Moor, 1979), very close objects are felt via the skin and vibrissae of the muzzle. Within the retina of the horse there is an area of maximal sensitivity (similar to the fovea of the human eye) termed the visual streak and it is only in this area that the horse has any real visual acuity (Ehrenhofer

et al., 2002). In the more peripheral areas of the retina, the structure suggests that the horse is particularly sensitive to subtle changes in light and stimulus motion (Ehrenhofer *et al.*, 2002).

Heffner and Heffner (1983; 1984; 1986; 1992) have explored the horse's ability to discriminate between sounds of variable frequency and intensity. They report that sounds need to be louder for horses than for humans and indicate that equine hearing is more ultrasonic than the human counterpart (50 Hz–33.5 kHz for horses compared with 20 Hz–20 kHz for humans).

There is also intriguing evidence of horses' ability to recognise individuals cross-modally, from both their appearance and the sounds of their voices. Horses were shown a familiar conspecific and then heard the played-back call of a different affiliated conspecific. They indicated that the incongruent combination violated their learned associations by responding faster and looking for longer in the direction of the call than when the call matched the herd member they had just been shown (Proops *et al.*, 2009). The impact of the special features of equine hearing on training may be limited in some equestrian codes where the use of the voice by trainers and riders is either not encouraged or actively forbidden. Some interesting exceptions are the use of the voice in driving, to cue transitions on the lunge and in other codes of horsemanship.

Trainers usually report that horses are quick to acquire these cues, so it is worth bearing in mind that, if they can be used with consistency, auditory signals are humane. It is fascinating to note that in 360 BC Xenophon [translated by Morgan, 1962] regarded it as orthodox to calm down a horse with a chirrup, a smooching noise made with the lips alone, and to rouse it by clucking the tongue against the roof of the mouth. Without using terms that have their origins in modern learning theory, he also noted that these behavioural outcomes were the product of classical associations with operant techniques, so swapping the learned cues would also swap the effects: 'Still, if from the first, you should cluck when caressing and chirrup when punishing, the horse would learn to start up at the chirrup and calm down at a cluck.'

Generally, ears that are constantly pricked forward are associated with fearful behaviour, and the horse flickers its ears loosely forward and back when it is ridden and relaxed (McLean and McLean, 2008). It is important to note that many riding guidelines (e.g. German National Equestrian Federation, 2012) describe ear movements (especially alternate pinnae flicking caudally) as evidence that the horse is attending to the rider's signals (Figure 2.4), an aspect that is commonly evaluated in dressage tests. However, in a study in which riders were asked to tense their bodies, pretending to be nervous, horses reacted with predominantly backwards pointing, rather than flicking pinnae, compared to control situations (von Borstel, 2008), perhaps providing some evidence that horses' ears indeed provide information on their direction of attentional focus. A more in-depth assessment of the significance of ear movements in the ridden horse may assist dressage judges of the future

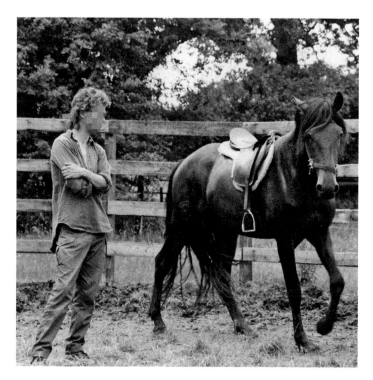

Figure 2.4 Ears moving independently are typically regarded as a sign of attentiveness.

if they are to score a given performance for behavioural legacies of inhumane training.

In general, there is a great deal still to be discovered about equine perception. While vision has received the most attention in studies of equine perception, it has been pointed out that 'senses probably of more crucial importance to the horse's environment have been neglected' (Saslow, 2002; Nielsen *et al.*, 2015). For example, olfaction is critical in interactions between horses, but has been the focus of remarkably few studies (Christensen and Rundgren, 2008). The same is true for tactile perception, despite its importance in equitation (Ahrendt *et al.*, 2015). Tactile sensitivity is determined by different types of mechanoreceptors in the skin, ranging from receptors that can detect finest pressures of less than 1 g to nociceptors that are activated at very high pressures sending signals of pain to the brain (Woolf and Ma, 2007; Maricich *et al.*, 2009). Distribution of these receptors determines tactile sensitivity, and there are considerable, individual differences in horses' responses to standardised tactile stimuli (König von Borstel and Krauskopf, 2016). Sensitivity of the skin of the ventral thorax (the sides, where the rider's legs make contact) and the mouth has a profound impact on a horse's response to training cues from the legs and reins. Likely, from a training perspective, there is an optimal level of tactile sensitivity, such that neither overly sensitive horses perform best with conventional training techniques (as they easily suffer from pain or discomfort due to tack or rider interactions), nor highly insensitive horses perform best as they may be more likely to react to pressure by ignoring it rather than by attempting to evade it through a learned response. Surprisingly, no relationships between tactile sensitivity and various aspects of trainability, such as the horses' reactions to rider cues, could be detected (König von Borstel and Krauskopf, 2016). However, this may well be due to the weaknesses of the traditional evaluation system for trainability and other personality traits (König von Borstel *et al.*, 2013). rather

than to a true lack of relationships between tactile sensitivity and trainability.

Breed and individual differences may be in part due to cushioning effects of thicker layers of skin tissue and subcutaneous fat but it is also possible that different patterns of mechanoreceptors are responsible for differences in sensitivity.

The Equid Ethogram

We do well to study the horse's social behaviour repertoire (its social ethogram) when considering how to be effective and remain safe while handling these animals. The agonistic ethogram of the bachelor band (all-male groups found in free-ranging herds) has been described in detail and includes a total of 49 basic behaviours, 3 complex behavioural sequences and 5 distinct vocalisations (McDonnell and Haviland, 1995).

Like humans, horses are highly social animals. This explains why horses kept in isolation are more likely to show separation-related behaviours and stereotypies than those kept in group-housing conditions (Cooper and McGreevy, 2002; Hartmann *et al.*, 2012). Companionship is important to horses. The instinct for togetherness is so strong that grooming each other at the base of the neck can have relaxing effects. Feh and de Mazières (1993) showed that grooming and stroking horses just in front of the withers (Figure 2.5) causes a significant lowering of heart rate compared with other regions. Apparently, this serves to strengthen familial bonds. It would be interesting to explore how much of the heart-rate response to wither scratching is learned and how much is innate.

Given that all aspects of behaviour are subject to natural selection, ethology is not merely the study of innate behaviours but also the study of how selection, both natural and artificial, has influenced learning processes and capabilities. Natural selection will, for example, have influenced whether an animal learns well individually, or learns by observing conspecifics, or both. It will have influenced such variables as relative attention

(a)

(b)

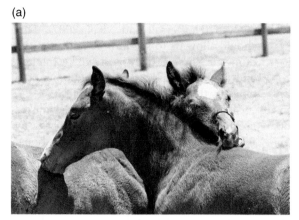
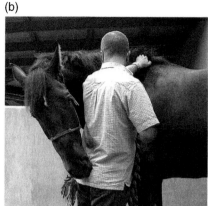

Figure 2.5 (a) Horses allogrooming and (b) human grooming a horse's withers.

devoted to learning new food-finding techniques versus scanning for predators.

The predisposition of an individual horse to learning and training reflects interactions between the ethology of the horse and the selection of breeds, maternal behaviour, weaning protocols, nutrition, housing, early handling, subsequent training and numerous individual differences. The complexity of the unique background that emerges for each horse from these influences explains why an identically rigid structure and timeframe of training can never be imposed on all horses effectively, although the need for fundamental responses (including *stop*, *go* and *turn*) is universal and learning theory can be optimally applied to all horses. Fundamental differences between horses lie in the time needed to train a specific quality. Good trainers recognise this and customise their interventions with each horse accordingly (Podhajsky, 1966). That said, to be effective, the mechanisms used in each custom-built approach should be applied with absolute adherence to the principles of learning theory.

Therefore, equine ethology informs us not only about communication but also about equine behavioural needs and preferences, learning processes and motivation. It helps us to predict some of the ways horses *out* of their natural environment (i.e. in the domestic context) might react and cope with various challenges, and how behaviourally flexible,

compliant and adaptive they may be. As such, equine ethology underpins enlightened and effective training but, despite the efforts of some marketing teams, it cannot be used to label a training system or philosophy *per se* without misrepresenting ethology itself.

Cognition: Memory and Learning

While horses show considerable performance in how quickly they can learn certain things, their performance is nowhere near the levels achieved by some primates and dolphins. These species rapidly learn to apply certain rules to novel problems and can often solve novel problems at first attempt (Leslie, 1996). Rule-learning is likely to be more adaptive for a cooperative predator than a grazing animal for which food procurement relies more on memory than higher mental abilities such as planning. In addition, the extra neural circuitry for higher mental abilities requires extra brain tissue which, as Deacon (1990) showed, is significantly more expensive energy-wise than any other tissue in the body. Evolutionary theory decrees that, like its physical abilities, an animal's mental abilities would be the result of the adaptive forces that it faced, particularly in procuring food, over the eons of its evolution (McLean, 2001).

Free-ranging horses occupy a home-range that they learn to exploit for resources and safety. By using different parts of the range, they can capitalise on the available food and water resources, even by using different terrains at different times of year (Olsen, 1996; Linklater *et al.*, 2000). The capacity of horses to return to bountiful grazing spots is a critical contributor to their success in foraging. Horses choose the richest patches when they have recent experience of them, but when they do not have such experience, they adopt a strategy of dynamic averaging that allows them to choose their feeding sites according to the long-term average richness of the available sites (Devenport *et al.*, 2005) (Figure 2.6).

Horses' knowledge of the range facilitates their escape from predators and even biting insects (Linklater *et al.*, 2000). Their daily treks allow them to become familiar with tiny landscape changes, especially visual ones (Hall, 2007) that are avoided or otherwise investigated if they appear innocuous from afar. Horses require considerable spatial representation abilities to migrate when seasonal ecological conditions demand, to be able to navigate between patches of preferred grazing in their home range (Howery *et al.*, 1999) and travel up to 25 km to drink (Stoffel-Willame and Stoffel-Willame, 1999). How free-ranging horses use this to structure their home ranges and form cognitive maps (Tolman, 1948) warrants further investigation (Leblanc and Duncan, 2007), and this is

best studied in the niche for which they have evolved (Hothersall and Nicol, 2007). This should allow us to see how cognition in the domestic horse is truly illustrated, exploited and at times frustrated by conditions provided by the domestic environment.

Clearly, memory and learning mechanisms are intimately entwined. Nerve fibres grow by following genetically determined positional cues towards the general target with which they synapse. Then, fine-tuning of the pattern and density of projections is accomplished by the horse's experience. Relationships between synapses are constantly being remodelled through increases or decreases in the size and strength of associations that also lead to the formation of new pathways. Working memory, declarative memory and procedural memory are well understood as is the process of long-term potentiation, which increases synaptic strength and strengthens pathways (Kandel *et al.*, 2000). What is less clear is the extent of the working memory in horses and if it relates to long-term potentiation in the same way as it does in humans.

Memory

A memory is a set of encoded neural connections. The encoding can take place in several parts of the brain and the neural connections can be widespread. The horse's memory is

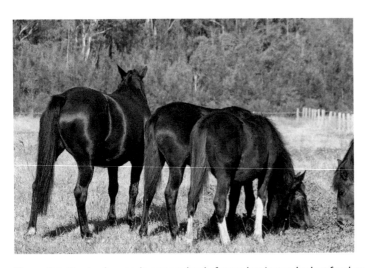

Figure 2.6 Grazing horses do not randomly forage but instead select food on the basis of sight, smell, taste and previous experience of that pasture.

excellent and in some respects may be superior to human memory. While our memory can be altered by our recall, contexts and reasoning abilities, the memory of the horse appears more stable, perhaps because it is unclouded by reflection or projection (McLean, 2001), or perhaps we just have yet to design methodologies that reveal that horses are capable of these (Goodwin, 2007). Hanggi and Ingersoll (2009) showed that horses could remember stimulus categorisation tasks without practice for up to 10 years, and horses were also able to apply the previously learned concepts immediately to novel stimuli. However, thinking, analysing and reflecting can corrupt memory. Humans are continuously reflecting (i.e. thinking without 'doing') on some of our memories, retrieving them from storage when we think or tell a story, then later re-storing them. Importantly, after this process of reflection, the memories are stored a little differently. They are altered by the contexts in which we reflect on them (physical, emotional, perceptual aspects of the moments of reflection). Our elaborate prefrontal cortex, the characteristics of which are uniquely human (Bermond, 1997), is responsible for this reflective ability (Kandel

et al., 2000). The absence of tissues with the unique cellular characteristics of the human prefrontal cortex (Kandel *et al.*, 2000; Premack, 2007) and the stability of equine working memory currently suggest that such reflection does not occur in horses.

Learning

As with all species, learning in the horse relates directly to survival requirements and it is generally accepted that it is appropriate to discuss issues of cognition, learning and memory without resorting to the term 'intelligence' (Linklater, 2007). Intelligence aside, the complexity of learning can be mapped-out in accordance with a hierarchy of learning abilities from habituation to conceptualisation (Table 2.1).

Every horseperson knows that the horse is acutely aware of changes in its visual environment. To the detriment of training, the horse appears to remember far better than the rider 'what happened where'. For example, riders may occasionally notice that the horse goes better on one part of the circle than elsewhere and, gradually, if training is correct, the length of this sector increases. The horse makes associations between the

Table 2.1 Hierarchy of learning abilities.

Level	Learning
1) Habituation	Learning not to respond to a repeated stimulus that has no consequences
2) Classical conditioning	Making responses to a new stimulus that has been repeatedly paired with an established effective stimulus
3) Operant conditioning	Learning to repeat a voluntary response for reinforcement or not to repeat a voluntary response to avoid punishment
4) Chaining responses	Learning a sequence of responses to obtain a reinforcement at the end of the sequence
5) Concurrent discriminations	Learning to make an operant response to only one set of stimuli from more than one set of stimuli applied concurrently
6) Concept learning	Discrimination learning based on some common characteristic shared by a number of stimuli
7) Conjunctive, disjunctive and conditional concepts	Learning of concepts that emerge from the relationship between stimuli such as 'A and B' (conjunctive), 'A or B' (disjunctive) and 'If A, then B' (conditional)
8) Bi-conditional concepts	Logical reasoning, such as 'Option A is likely if,' and only if, 'Option B is present'

Source: Adapted from Thomas (1986) and Murphy and Arkins (2007).

behaviour it is currently doing and where it is doing it. This context-specific (or place-dependent) learning can be a very useful tool in training (Chapter 8, Training). For example, some behaviours that are hard to train should be trained in the same place until some reliability emerges. On the other hand, context-specific learning can be a hindrance if, through classical conditioning, the horse learns to exacerbate flight-response behaviours in certain places or contexts. The horse learns tense and fearful responses more rapidly and more indelibly than other responses (McLean, 2004). Sometimes it takes just one or two episodes of a flight response to cause repetition in the same contexts. Fear memories can be suppressed with error-free practice, but when circumstances are the same, the response can return with alarming speed and accuracy. This is known as spontaneous recovery. For this reason, it is an essential principle that flight response behaviours (Figure 2.7) should be properly identified and training schemes should generally be tailored to avoid them.

At the same time, it is acknowledged that horses may detect subtle differences in the behaviour of a nervous human and respond with increased preparedness. von Borstel (2008) and Keeling *et al.* (2009) have shown how a nervous human can affect a horse's reactions or responses. They demonstrated how variations in equine heart rate followed very similar heart-rate activity patterns for both trainers and riders. The relationship between these patterns persisted when some individuals were told in advance that an umbrella would be opened suddenly as they rode or led a horse past an experimenter with the umbrella. Although the umbrella was not actually opened, the person's anticipation of fear responses significantly increased the heart rate in both the person riding or leading and the horse when compared with control conditions. Thus, horses appear to be able to detect subtle changes in a rider's emotional state and react to them with changes in their own level of arousal. Since an appropriate level of arousal is important for optimal learning performance (Starling *et al.* 2013), it

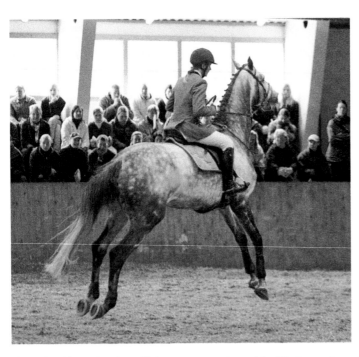

Figure 2.7 Horse showing a flight response under-saddle. (Photo courtesy of Minna Tallberg.)

is important to keep in mind the potential effects a nervous human might have on the horse and its learning performance.

As mammals, horses have brain characteristics that suggest their learning mechanisms may be similar to those of humans (Hahn, 2004). Like humans, they are proficient at trial-and-error learning (learning to perform a reaction through reward), classical conditioning (learning associations between events) and habituation (learning to ignore aversive stimuli that do not hurt). Beyond these basic learning mechanisms, horses can also learn to generalise stimuli (Christensen *et al.*, 2011c), and they may even be able to learn to categorise objects based on similar physical characteristics (Hanggi, 1999), and in a few studies a proportion of, but not all, horses showed simple forms of concept learning (Sappington and Goldman, 1994). However, cognitive research to date has produced limited empirical evidence that horses can develop abstract concepts (Nicol, 2002). Indeed, there is no peer-reviewed published evidence that horses possess significant higher mental abilities beyond simple concept learning (Level 6 in Table 2.1). What horsepeople erroneously consider examples of reasoning in their horses turn out to be excellent examples of trial-and-error learning. The pony that fiddles with the gate latch and learns to open it is a typical example. It has a high learning ability, but does not offer an example of reasoning.

The biological relevance of tasks we have tended to give horses in learning studies has been questioned many times (Bekoff, 1995; McLean, 2001; Nicol, 2002) and although early results from Haag *et al.* (1980) indicated a good correlation between learning for appetitive and aversive outcomes, later results failed to show this (Visser *et al.*, 2003; Christensen *et al.*, 2012). More recently, interest in research on negative reinforcement in horses appears to have increased (Warren-Smith and McGreevy, 2007; Innes and McBride, 2008; Hendriksen *et al.*, 2011). However, technology for measuring tactile pressure as it applies to horses is still in its infancy (Ahrendt *et al.*, 2015). Clearly, if equine learning research is to make the results more applicable to equestrian techniques, consistent, easily applied methods of delivering and measuring aversive events, however mild, must be developed. The need for technological advances in this domain has been addressed (McGreevy, 2007) so that we can effectively study learning in the unridden horse. In addition, we must acknowledge that lack of learning performance in the experimental situation may not necessarily reflect lack of learning ability (Lefebvre and Helder, 1997). Furthermore, the insufficient use of discrete subtle signals in equitation generally reflects the inability of trainers to deliver these rather than any shortcoming in terms of learning or perception by the horse (Creighton, 2007).

There has been considerable research into the mental characteristics of horses. Much of this has centred on testing their abilities in negotiating mazes (Kratzer *et al.*, 1977; Haag *et al.*, 1980; McCall *et al.*, 1981), discriminating various visual stimuli (McCall, 1990; Hanggi, 1999) and acquiring and implementing 'rules' to solve problems (Hanggi, 2003). Researchers have used food rewards as well as avoidance-learning paradigms and, in general, it has been shown that younger horses learn faster, are more interested in novel stimuli than older horses (Mader and Price, 1982; Houpt *et al.*, 1982) and are more investigative in trial-and-error learning (Lindberg *et al.*, 1999). This may simply reflect the fact that older horses must 'unlearn' associations and have had more life experience to discriminate between relevant and irrelevant cues. It has also been shown that female horses tend to outperform males in certain rule-learning tests (Sappington *et al.*, 1997) as well as tests with combinations of barriers (spatial detour tests) (Wolff and Hausberger, 1996). Finally, horses managed in small groups at pasture learn faster than those housed singly in stalls (Rivera *et al.*, 2002; Søndergaard and Ladewig, 2004).

If establishing relevant tests and gathering together a group of standardised subjects is difficult, then so is extrapolation from a study to other contexts. Although links between learning ability and training ability have been explored in numerous equine studies (Fiske and Potter, 1979; Wolff and Hausberger, 1996), poor correlations exist between any individual horse's performance in different learning tasks.

We must exercise caution when interpreting the results of learning studies published to date. Studies of learning in horses must be carefully designed because horses are easily and inadvertently influenced by humans nearby. For example, Clever Hans (Pfungst, 1965), who was trained to 'count' and 'calculate' by tapping the ground with his hoof to provide his answers, was inadvertently trained to stop counting when he reached the right number. His owner and countless spectators convinced themselves that Hans could indeed count and calculate, even though they were unwittingly sending him the visual cues (such as looking at his hoof and titling their heads) to stop counting as he reached the right number (Figure 2.8). This story reminds us that horses can moderate their behaviour because of operator effect, especially if those operators have been training them. This suggests that horses should be isolated from personnel when they are being tested, with observations ideally being made from video recordings. They should not, however, be isolated from conspecifics, since this can induce fearfulness in the horse (Lansade *et al.*, 2004).

Flannery (1997) described horses making higher-order discriminations based on matching shapes that allowed them to generalise this learning under several different conditions. Beyond that, attempts to demonstrate concept formation by horses remain rare in the literature and are so far confined to the conceptual categorisation of objects by size (among objects) (Hanggi, 1999), shape (Sappington and Goldmann, 1994), open or closed centres (among two- and three-dimensional objects) (Hanggi, 2003) and hard and soft materials (Watt and McDonnell, 2001). A concept is the 'idea of a class of objects'. Lea (1984) argues that a concept represents an idea, such as common functional properties, rather than physical attributes, which is

perhaps why some horses adopt a flight response when they first encounter a donkey or even a small pony, defaulting to categorise quadrupeds as potential predators. Concept formation, especially in animals that have no language, is a topic of enormous theoretical interest. The relevance of these tasks to the horse's behavioural repertoire merits detailed consideration (McCall, 2007). When concept learning in the three highest levels of learning in Thomas's hierarchy (Levels 6–8 in Table 2.1) is described in horses, the reporting authors note that horses take some time to grasp the concept (McLean and McGreevy, 2004), but having done so, their responses become more rapid and accurate (Creighton, 2007). So, rather than concept learning, this may be what is called learning to learn, the horses having overcome novelty and having learned the salience of various elements in the experimental apparatus.

Certainly, a horse's motor laterality (its left- or right-leg preference) could affect learning, for instance, in a maze with left and right turns (Murphy and Arkins, 2007). Therefore, controlling for or standardising the experimental group for these variables may be as important as standardising the group's prior exposure to learning opportunities, including conspecifics (Søndergaard and Ladewig, 2004), prior training (Le Scolan *et al.*, 1997) and regular handling (which generally is already biased in most cultures to the left side by convention) (McGreevy and Rogers, 2005).

Perseveration is the term used to describe the behaviours of animals that continue to offer a trained response, even when it no longer yields rewards. It is recognised as a feature of stereotypic birds and rodents (Garner and Mason, 2002), but more recently has been reported in horses (Hemmings *et al.*, 2007; Hausberger *et al.*, 2007a; Roberts *et al.*, 2015). The equine studies in this domain have positively reinforced subjects for pressing levers, so there is a need for caution when applying these findings to the ridden horse that is trained almost exclusively with negative reinforcement.

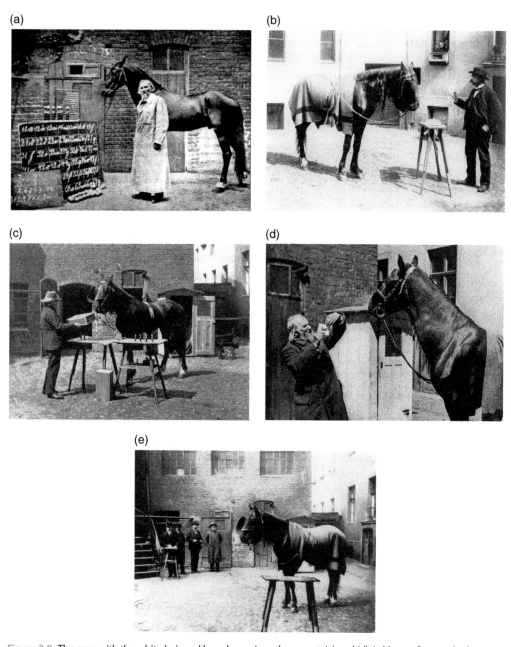

Figure 2.8 The man with the white hair and beard, wearing a long coat, (a) and (d), is Mr von Osten, who became famous for claiming that his horse, Clever Hans, had been successfully trained to count, perform mathematical calculations and read. von Osten never accepted the criticism of this claim. Instead he helped some of his admirers, (b) and (c), to train and test successors to Clever Hans, as shown in this set of photographs from 1912. In (e), von Osten is on the right of the four onlookers and wearing the hat that, unknown to him, was probably critical in training Clever Hans, since it would have amplified the inadvertent visual cue of head tilting.

Anecdotally, however, riders do not seem to pick up on any critical differences between stereotypers and other horses with respect to training. Perhaps riders simply fail to notice those horses that are somehow resistant to extinction under a negative-reinforcement training paradigm. Nevertheless, this area merits detailed investigation.

Equine Cognition in Equitation

The personality of a horse is a topic characterised by poorly defined terms but, nevertheless, it is of tremendous importance to riders (Hennessy *et al.*, 2007). For example, it has been found that less-reactive horses perform significantly better in some experimental tasks, possibly because the apparatus itself or other environmental influences may distract more-reactive horses, compromising their performance (Clarke *et al.*, 1996; Christensen *et al.*, 2012). In addition, social ranking appears unrelated to learning ability in visual-discrimination tasks, simple maze tasks and avoidance-learning tests. Differences in performance between individual horses are much more likely to reflect differences in motivation rather than in so-called learning ability (McLean and McLean, 2008). For example, a less-reactive but highly food-motivated horse may show poor performance in avoidance learning but may be impressive in tasks that involve food rewards, and vice versa. Therefore, it can be concluded that characteristics such as fearfulness and motivation have a significant influence on success or failure in both laboratory and real-life situations (Christensen *et al.*, 2012).

Aside from the above constraints, perhaps the most important aspect of equine cognition for horse-trainers concerns the presence of higher mental abilities. Because of the unique characteristics of the mental life of humans, many people expect to find similar abilities in animals. If insufficient thought is given to the ramifications of cognitive differences between humans (whose competencies are domain general and serve numerous goals) and horses (whose competencies are mainly adaptations of a few specific goals), significant mistakes can be made. Thus, misunderstanding a horse's cognitive abilities has important implications not only for its training programme but also for its welfare. There are negative welfare implications in both *overestimating* and *underestimating* mental abilities in animals.

Historically, underestimating an animal's cognitive capacities was a typical viewpoint that elevated mankind above the animal kingdom. Animals such as horses had no intrinsic moral value because they were unable to reason and apparently had no soul. This anthropocentric view gave implicit approval to the abuse of animals. Nowadays, the pendulum has swung the other way and some argue that a closer analysis of the dissimilarities between human and non-human animals is needed to prevent us from confusing similarity with equivalence (Premack, 2007). Until this analysis is fully applied to all aspects of equine and human cognition (including teaching conspecifics, short-term memory, causal reasoning, planning, deception, transitive inference and language), the current prevalent tendency will be for most horsepeople to overestimate the mental abilities of horses. The dangers here are subtle but no less anthropocentric. To suggest, as some lay authors such as Skipper (1999) have, that horses have similar mental abilities to humans, is to suggest that there is something more desirable about our own mental abilities. Furthermore, such expectations encourage the use of delayed punishment, which is often justified on the grounds that 'the horse knows what it did wrong'. Overestimating equine cognitive abilities can give tacit approval to poor timing of signals and reinforcement ('the horse knows what I am asking for, it's just being stubborn!'). This can encourage punishments (Figure 2.9) that bear little or no relation to the original (incorrect) response and so, from a learning standpoint, are useless and detrimental (Chapter 6, Associative Learning (Aversive stimuli), which describes the uses and abuses of punishment).

In the light of our cultural connection with the horse, it is hardly surprising that humans tend to err on the side of overestimating higher mental abilities in horses. To most humans, the horse is a rare mixture of benevolence, beauty and power. So important was the horse to Western civilisation in the past two millennia that most older European cities are adorned with many statues of horses, primarily as the carriers of human leaders (Endenburg, 1999). Horses fought in our wars, toiled for us and helped us build much of

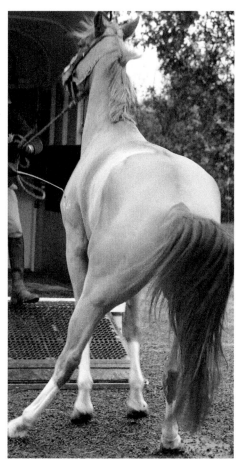

Figure 2.9 The notion of the horse being 'stubborn' encourages punishment.

detail in Chapter 9, Horses in Sport and Work, which sets out the ethological, learning and cognitive challenges of various sports and forms of work involving horses. Although many breeds present a genetic predisposition to develop certain skills, representatives of these breeds have refined these skills over an extensive period of structured, guided practice and feedback. Thus, some horses may develop skills in a particular type of sport or work and may exhibit what might be regarded as expertise (Helton *et al.*, 2009). Similarly, it is worth pointing out that there are some situations where acknowledging horses' superior sensory abilities allows them to communicate these and influence the rider's decisions. Examples are endurance-riding over unfamiliar land or trail-riding where hazards (e.g. bogs, weak bridges and predators) may be undetected by the rider to the detriment of the safety of both participants (Figure 2.10).

Social Learning

Animals can acquire new behaviour through both individual and social learning. Individual learning refers to behaviour acquired from the individual's own experience, while social learning refers to situations where the behaviour is acquired after observation of a conspecific (Heyes, 1994). True social learning may require reasoning and insight to allow exact imitation (Nicol, 1996). It requires animals to see and remember a behaviour sequence, mentally transpose it to their own repertoire, and then perform it. Social learning of novel behaviour (copying a novel act) has long been considered indicative of some degree of higher mental ability, so when considering the transfer of information between animals, we must distinguish between social facilitation, stimulus enhancement and true social learning. In social facilitation, innate behaviours are initiated or increased in rate or frequency by the presence of another animal carrying out those behaviours. For social animals, this synchronisation of behaviour can be adaptive (i.e. when one animal eats,

the Old World as well as the New. Nowadays, it fulfils our dreams, and still fires our imaginations. Horses are not just pleasure vehicles – much more is expected of them. A horse may be our best friend, our only friend, our child or our partner. The Swiss psychologist Carl Jung (1968) believed that the image of the horse is a powerful symbol in the human psyche: how could such a big, powerful beast, so capable of rebellion, be typically so tolerant, gentle, forgiving and even what onlookers may perceive as being patriotic? Most likely, the answer partly lies in the horse's cognitive characteristics and the ways it learns.

It is important to acknowledge that different equestrian pursuits place different demands on horses. This is explored in some

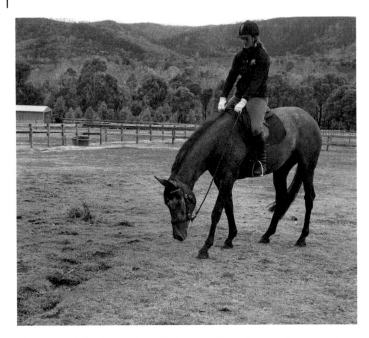

Figure 2.10 It is adaptive for naïve horses to investigate water or marshy ground.

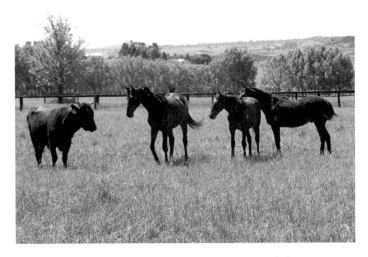

Figure 2.11 Strength in numbers facilitates investigative behaviour.

others are compelled to do so; when one lies down, others may follow) (Figure 2.11).

Stimulus (or local) enhancement is the ethological term that describes the ability of one animal (the demonstrator) to draw the attention of another animal (the observer) to a particular stimulus (or location). A common example arises when a horse rattles a bucket while feeding from it and arouses the attention of neighbouring horses. The noise has enhanced the current salience of the bucket stimulus but any subsequent learning is based on individual trial-and-error learning (Figure 2.12). Social learning is said to have occurred when a naïve individual (the observer) acquires a new behaviour after observing a more knowledgeable conspecific (the demonstrator). The new behaviour should be retained in the subsequent absence of the demonstrator.

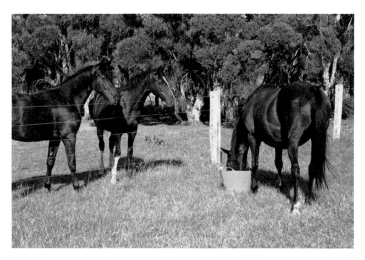

Figure 2.12 The relevance of a bucket to a naïve horse may be enhanced by observation of feeding.

If the environment is unpredictable, individual learning can be dangerous because the animal is bound to make mistakes, whereas social learning allows animals to acquire locally adaptive information from conspecifics without having to pay some of the costs associated with individual learning (Kendal *et al.*, 2005). The opportunity for social transmission of adaptive behaviour patterns from experienced group members to younger or less experienced individuals is one major benefit of group formation (Krause and Ruxton, 2002). Social transmission of dietary preferences and acquisition of foraging skills by birds and mammals have been shown in numerous studies. Well-known examples include potato-washing by Japanese macaques and food-well-opening by pigeons (reviewed by Galef and Giraldeau, 2001; Nicol, 2006; and others).

It makes sense for offspring to learn from their parents and for social animals to learn from one another, for example, what food is safe to consume or, in the case of predators, how to dispatch prey. As social animals with excellent vision, we might predict that horses would use observations to improve their biological fitness. It could also be predicted that they should be able to learn from pre-trained conspecifics; for example, young farm horses were traditionally harnessed alongside a steady mature plough horse to be taught verbal driving commands. However, this effect may be explained through individual learning in combination with the calming effect of the experienced horse. While horses seem good at responding to socially enhanced stimuli, empirical evidence of social learning is limited. Controlled studies have provided some evidence that stimulus enhancement may result from the behaviour of demonstrator horses as they approach and interact with the experimental apparatus that delivers food, causing observer horses to approach the apparatus more quickly than control horses (Clarke *et al.*, 1996). However, early studies have failed to demonstrate that the opportunity to observe a trained conspecific enhances observer horses' ability to perform an operant task (Lindberg *et al.*, 1999) or make a choice between two feeding sites (Baer *et al.*, 1983; Baker and Crawford, 1986; Clarke *et al.*, 1996). These early studies were criticised for not taking into account the social relationship between demonstrator and observer, because studies in other species have demonstrated that animals do not observe all conspecifics with the same enthusiasm. For example, chickens pay particular attention to the feeding strategy of dominant members of the group (Nicol, 2006).

More recent research on horses has taken these factors into account, by ensuring that the demonstrator horse was socially higher ranking than observer horses, and attempting to optimise the experimental design so that demonstrator and observer horses were free to interact during the demonstrations (Ahrendt *et al.*, 2012), or through attempting to increase the motivation in observer horses (Rørvang *et al.*, 2015b). In spite of these potential improvements, Ahrendt *et al.* (2012) and Rørvang *et al.* (2015b) found no effect of prior demonstrations on observer horses' ability to perform an operant task (opening a box for food) (Ahrendt *et al.*, 2012) and a spatial task (navigating around a fence to approach a food bucket) (Rørvang *et al.*, 2015b). In contrast, Krüger *et al.* (2014a) reported that young horses copied novel behaviour of familiar, dominant demonstrators, but not of younger, subordinate or unfamiliar demonstrators. However, some horses required a very large number of demonstrations, and some horses did not use the same technique as the demonstrator horse, leaving the question open for debate, as to how much stimulus enhancement combined with individual trial-and-error learning was involved with the successful horses, rather than true social learning. Transfer of information may occur more reliably and more independently of social relationships between horses in fear-eliciting situations, where a calm demonstrator appears to reduce fear reactions in naïve horses

(Christensen *et al.*, 2008a; Rørvang *et al.*, 2015a). These situations may reflect a more biologically relevant situation compared to the operant tasks that are traditionally used in social learning studies. Therefore, these studies have also challenged the notion that stereotypies can be acquired by mimicry. The fact that often several stereotyping horses can be found within the same barn is more likely the result of the affected horses being exposed to the same husbandry conditions that frustrate their behavioural needs for social contact and continued feeding.

Future studies on social learning should focus on the role of the dam as tutor to her foal, because vertical transmission of information seems the most likely form of social learning in a social species (Figure 2.13). Houpt *et al.* (1982) reported no evidence of foals learning a spatial task from their dams. However, foals that were exposed in the first five days of life to humans as they groomed and fed their mothers during a short period (total of 1.25 hours) approached and initiated physical interactions with humans sooner than those subjected to forced handling of the foal itself that included imprinting and haltering (Henry *et al.*, 2005). Similarly, foals that were exposed to usually fear-inducing situations together with their habituated mother for 10 minutes per week in the first 8 weeks post-partum, reacted significantly

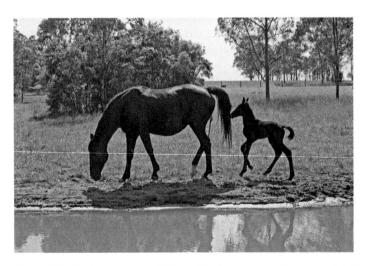

Figure 2.13 The transmission of information from mare to foal merits detailed scrutiny.

less than control foals to both the training stimuli and novel fear-inducing stimuli when tested at 5 months of age (Christensen, 2016). Studies of this sort may help us to explore how innate behavioural reactions can be modulated through an appropriate maternal environment.

Ethological Challenges

Like all sentient animals, the horse does whatever it can to reduce pain and discomfort. This underpins the basic responses of the ridden horse but equally explains the importance of pathologies in the emergence of behavioural responses that can cause problems. Physical causes of such behavioural responses should always be ruled out before any behavioural therapy is embraced. For example, undiagnosed pelvic or vertebral disorders can easily lead to poor performance in horses (Haussler *et al.*, 1999). The effect of disorders such as 'cold-back syndrome' and the relationship between dental problems and behaviour under-saddle should also be more thoroughly explored (McGreevy, 2004).

Ethological challenges include interventions that generate both social and environmental stressors (Figure 2.14). Although horses may subsequently investigate them, they are inherently cautious of new stimuli (neophobia), which is why jumping unfamiliar and unnatural obstacles initially presents an appreciable challenge to most horses. Examples of *social* challenges include leaving the social group, taking the lead in the company of established leaders, being forced to stay at the rear, being close to aggressive conspecifics, walking abreast rather than trekking in a line, and ignoring displays by other horses. Enforced proximity to conspecifics can cause one horse to tread on another in ways that seldom occur in the free-ranging state. During steeple chasing, for example, when horses are clustered, vision is limited and the race becomes hazardous. Furthermore, as jockeys well know, when galloping horses are too closely spaced, they may be prompted by conspecifics to jump when they are not close enough to the obstacle to clear it safely.

Even when riding alone, we may demand responses from the horse that naturally arise only in social contexts that are far removed from the manège. The elevated steps required in higher levels of dressage, for instance, may be appropriate when horses greet one another but may be ethologically discordant in the absence of a conspecific or a startling object. Examples of *environmental* challenges include leaving the home range, deviating from an obvious track and traversing, rather than avoiding, obstacles. Other examples of the ways in which equitation provides environmental challenges to horses that run counter to their ethology appear in Table 2.2.

(a)

(b)

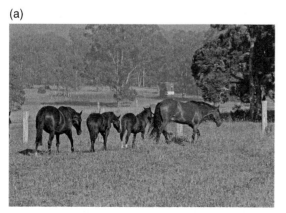
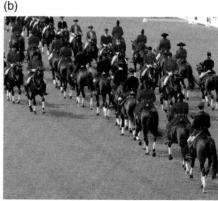

Figure 2.14 (a) Horses following one another. (b) Horses being ridden towards each other in a formal exercise. (Photo courtesy of Julie Wilson.)

Table 2.2 Some examples of regular equitation that represent environmental challenges to horses by running counter to their ethology.

In-hand	Under-saddle	Comfort
• Lungeing • Entering small spaces, including trailers • Proximity to humans • Standing on moving platforms • Approaching frightening objects	• Walking, rather than running, through unfamiliar creekbeds • Passing under overhanging elements • Approaching erratically moving/sounding unfamiliar objects • Maintaining speed while travelling from light to dark areas or across uneven terrain or downhill (head is usually lowered to assist detection of the safest path) • Maintaining a fixed postural outline while changing gait • Advancing when familiar conspecifics are emitting fearful signals • Walking backwards for more than a body length (i.e. entering any unfamiliar cul-de-sac that would require reversing)	• Not rolling when hot and standing in water • Walking on stony ground • Standing square for extended periods • The presence of a bit • Sweaty head covered with a bridle and trunk covered with a girth, saddle and saddle cloth • Wearing blankets

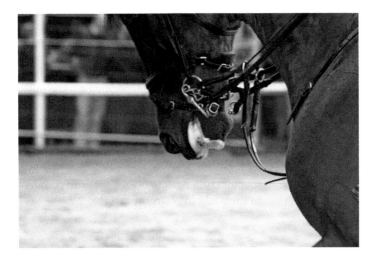

Figure 2.15 A horse being hyperflexed under-saddle (Rollkur).

Riding brings both social and environmental challenges and is a useful example of the way we overcome and suppress horses' adaptive responses and thus ignore their preferences. For example, free-ranging horses rarely maintain a rounded posture while changing gait. The current debate surrounding hyperflexion (Rollkur) (Figure 2.15) highlights the extent to which riders can force a horse to maintain an abnormal posture to sometimes gain a competitive advantage (Kienapfel *et al.*, 2014; Lashley *et al.*, 2014).

Responses to physical discomfort under-saddle generally have more to do with physiology than ethology. Here, the most obvious sources of *physical* discomfort are the bit, the rider's leg/spur, the whip and the girth. This is important because there seems to be an implied assumption that the relationship between human and horse in-hand is identical to the relationship when mounted. It is by no means certain that horses connect pressure in the mouth with the rider. They have not evolved to expect that another animal can apply pressure to the inside of the buccal cavity via a piece of metal. This cognitive aspect may account for the apparent tolerance (or habituation) horses show when allowing heavy-handed riders to mount them time after time. It is therefore unnecessary and inappropriate to complicate a rider's interventions by giving them anthropomorphic labels, such as *asking* (e.g. asking the horse to lower its head), *encouraging* (e.g. using the inside leg to encourage forward movement) and *supporting* (e.g. applying the outside rein to support the impulsion). It may be the intention to use common words in everyday usage to convey an attitude of cooperation rather than supremacy, but the abiding problem with the use of an anthropomorphic framework to explain rider–horse interactions is that it can disguise and justify abuse of horses that offer undesirable responses, even though these may have been accidentally induced/trained by humans. So, most horses benefit when science provides mechanistic explanations of equitation, even though some horsepeople argue that this is undermining the bond they share with their horses (McGreevy, 2007).

The Role of Ethology in Horse-Training

The complexities of the equine sociogram are explored elegantly elsewhere (Tyler, 1972; Houpt and Keiper, 1982; Keiper and Sambraus, 1986; McDonnell and Haviland, 1995; van Dierendonck *et al.*, 1995), but there remain some elements that are relevant to equitation (Hall and Heleski, 2017). When riding in company, agonistic responses between horses that derive from unfamiliarity or previous aggressive encounters can be extremely dangerous. Riders can be seriously injured by horses kicking. Equally, sexual advances by stallions can injure riders of oestrous mares and, for that reason, owners of stallions and oestrous mares are encouraged to avoid taking them to shows and events. This may be part of the reason why

the owners of competition mares look to hormonal and other medical treatments to suppress oestrous behaviour.

Aggression is not the only unwelcome influence from the equid ethogram in equitation. Social responses include the tendency to remain in the company of the herd. This provokes a suite of responses that can be described as separation anxiety (McGreevy and McLean, 2005). Horses may refuse to leave the stableyard, refuse to lead on the trail or over obstacles and bolt back to their group when turning for home. Instead of fighting these tendencies, it is preferable to focus on getting affected horses under stimulus control and to capitalise on the inclination to return to the herd (e.g. to train negotiating certain obstacles by following affiliated conspecifics) (Figure 2.16).

When free-ranging horses travel, they generally do so in company by trekking or, far less commonly, by being herded (McDonnell and Haviland, 1995). This explains why ridden horses travel well in single file. Experience shows that certain individuals prefer to take the lead, but how this relates to social rank is far from clear. The racing industry could profitably invest in research that explores the social interactions between unfamiliar horses during a race, since this may partly explain why some individuals fail to reach the potential suggested by their cardiovascular and pulmonary attributes.

Social Organisation

Wild and feral horses typically live in either bachelor bands (all stallions not currently living with a harem), or in harems with one stallion keeping his group of mares and foals together. Social relationships between horses in a group are not as straightforward as they were once thought to be, with a clear linear hierarchy. Indeed, there are great difficulties in determining social hierarchies among groups of horses. We can measure the relative ease with which one horse can displace another from resources, but the outcomes of such interactions usually depend on the resource in question as well as the context

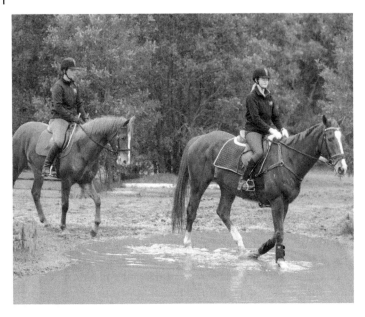

Figure 2.16 One horse following another into water.

(e.g. how vulnerable or protected a horse is in the given situation, say, by barn design) and, hence, reflect the current motivation of the individual to access or retain that resource (Weeks *et al.*, 2000). Even if we confine ourselves to a study of food-related displacements, motivation can change from one hour to the next. For example, a horse is less likely to defend a feed bucket after it has recently sated its appetite. Furthermore, hierarchies are often not simply linear because coalitions among horses within an established social group mean that the presence of key affiliates affects the ability of individuals to retain and access resources (McGreevy, 2004).

If, when handling horses on the ground, we are to correctly exploit the social organisation of horses, it is important to recognise that in the equestrian context, when practitioners claim to be imposing their rank, this always involves the application and withdrawal of aversive stimuli and, therefore, cannot be considered outside the framework of learning theory (McGreevy, 2007). There is distaste among some authors (e.g. Goodwin, 1999) for the term 'alpha', since this implies non-negotiable and permanent status. This resistance is also found in dog-training circles, and

accounts for the alternative notion of leadership having gained traction.

Leadership and its attributes have been extensively studied across mammalian species and decision-making processes about where to go and what to do have also recently been empirically assessed in horses (Hartmann *et al.*, 2017). The focus has been on studying group movements (e.g. moving between foraging places or to shelters), and results across a number of studies suggest that leadership, in contrast to the traditional dogma, is not unique to the highest-ranked or oldest horse but that any horse in the group can act as leader. Bourjade *et al.* (2009; 2015) found shared leadership in groups of Przewalski horses, where several individuals could depart from the group simultaneously. The authors concluded that the decision-making process prior to movement was partially shared and was largely based on pre-departure behaviour displayed by several horses (e.g. moving away without foraging, staying at the periphery of the group, following an individual that is moving away, and joining a peripheral individual). Results from Andrieu *et al.* (2015) and Krüger *et al.* (2014a) indicate that high-ranked horses were followed significantly more often than subordinates but this was not supported by Briard *et al.* (2015), who posited that collective movements depend more on the motivations of the followers than the characteristics of the one individual acting as leader (i.e. that the latter acts as the trigger but that effectively the collective decision has already been taken by group members). Furthermore, some authors reported that socially bonded horses, as evaluated by nearest-neighbour recordings, were more likely to move together (Wells and von Goldschmidt-Rothschild, 1997; Briard *et al.*, 2015), whereas Krueger *et al.* (2014b) assessed social bonds through an analysis of agonistic and affiliative interactions and found no such correlation.

The concept of humans as leaders of horses has gained currency in equestrian contexts, but this brings its own set of problems. In a study that involved school horses (used to being handled and ridden on a regular basis by different riders) as well as privately owned horses (used to being ridden and handled by just one person on a regular basis for about 1 hour per day) and mounted police horses (used to being ridden and handled by just one person on a regular basis for several hours per day), there were hardly any differences in stress responses and fear reactivity to novel objects when school horses or privately owned horses were ridden by familiar rather than unfamiliar riders. Only with the mounted police horses were differences observed between rides by the familiar compared to unfamiliar riders (König von Borstel and Krienert, 2012) and while significant, these differences were only mild. These findings suggest that for bonding between horses and humans to affect ridden work, it requires engagement with the horse on a nearly daily basis for several hours per day (as is the case with mounted police horses and their riders) – much more time than the average person will typically be able to invest into the horse–human relationship. Whether the observed effects were indeed a sign of trust in or acceptance of leadership by the familiar rider, or rather the general effect of stress due to the novelty of the unfamiliar rider remains unclear. Notwithstanding the rather blurred definition of leadership and with the exception of the above study, with all the restrictions that apply to its interpretation, there is no evidence in the scientific literature of such phenomena occurring. Furthermore, those who subscribe to the notion of leadership do not explain how leadership qualities can be developed. Rather, they describe operant techniques that condition some useful responses.

Horses will typically find conspecifics more salient than humans as leaders and, for that matter, companions. Analogues drawn between human–horse interactions and elements of the equine ethogram are tenuous. For example, it is suggested that simply being behind a horse and driving it forward (as in long-reining) is analogous to the herding behaviour of stallions (Zeitler-Feicht, 2004). This assumption is very difficult to test, but convincing evidence would include behavioural analogues in horses driven by humans of the responses herd members typically make when driven by a familiar stallion. Such findings are thwarted by the fact that, when long-reining horses, humans do not make snaking neck movements or bite threats. Equally, when a horse directs other horses, it never uses pressure cues in the mouth. The analogues are elusive. Perhaps humans should simply accept that we are food-bearers and companions, and when we are not giving care and companionship, we are trainers. Conspecifics, including dams, can condition members of their social group (Figure 2.17) and this activity may facilitate some later outcome, but it is unlikely that training is the intention. Although there is clearly some overlap between care-giving, companionship and training, it makes sense to compartmentalise them. To do so helps us to approach each set of activities with clearer expectations of likely outcomes.

The Role of Communication in Horse-Training

There is an appealing notion that we can apply equine social strategies to human–horse interactions, but data and scientific rigour are lacking in this domain. When there is social

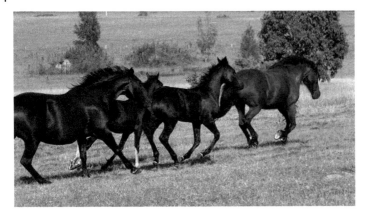

Figure 2.17 It is interesting to speculate on whether horses train one another.

conflict among horses, it is often submission signals that switch off aggression (McGreevy, 2004) and determine the outcome. These signals may be very subtle: indeed, so subtle that they are the subject of considerable debate among equine ethologists (Goodwin, 1999). Horses have rod-dominant photoreceptors arranged in a visual streak, giving tremendous peripheral vision, which contrasts with the cone-dominant trichromatic *area centralis* of humans (Evans and McGreevy, 2006). They can detect minute cues from animals (and not just horses) around them. It seems likely that most human signals are not necessarily interpreted as surrogate equine signals (Roberts and Browning, 1998). How crude are the signals from a human to an equine observer? With no tail, fixed ears, a short, inflexible neck and only two legs, we can hardly expect horses to regard us as equine. The chance that we can mimic equine signalling with any subtlety seems remote. Perhaps this is partly why humans rarely claim an ability to issue putative appeasement signals to horses and why agonistic advances from humans prevail. Humans who fall into the trap of assuming they can communicate eloquently with horses may fail to recognise the aversiveness of some of their behaviour. Ultimately, however, any search for equine analogues of human interactions with a horse becomes virtually irrelevant when the human gets on the horse's back. This point is based simply on the observation that horses mount conspecifics far more occasionally and far more briefly, in play and

sex, and, in feral horses, being mounted by another species is associated with predation. When we ride horses, we should not expect all the learned associations, affiliative and otherwise, based on the equid social ethogram to apply. That said, responses trained in-hand can reliably transfer to the ridden context.

The extent to which horse–horse status translates to horse–human contexts seems minimal and is highly unlikely when humans behave in ways that are not analogous to elements of the equine social ethogram. It is also unlikely that horses see humans as horses (McGreevy and McLean, 2007; McGreevy *et al.*, 2009a). We do not and may never know precisely how horses perceive and interpret their world.

Despite this, most 'New-Age' training methods assume that the interactions between horses and humans are analogues of the social relationships existing between horses. Such methods claim that dominance, submission and leadership behaviours account for the quality of horse–human interactions and are apparently understood by the horse (Parelli, 1995; Roberts, 1997). At first glance, this may seem plausible, but equine scientists familiar with learning theory do not find this argument convincing. Consider, for example, a horse's licking and chewing behaviour, which has been subject to various interpretations. One popular interpretation of licking and chewing in horses during chasing (Figure 2.18a) is that it corresponds to the submissive snapping behaviour of foals

(a)

(b)

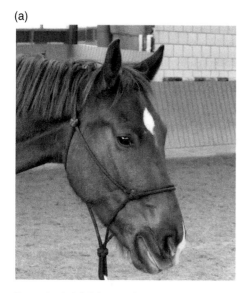
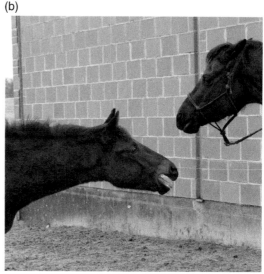

Figure 2.18 Adult horses showing licking and chewing (a) in response to a stressor, such as chasing, adopt a different posture, and mimic, typically with lowered head and only slightly opened mouth, compared to foals showing the snapping response (b) towards an adult horse displaying threats. In the latter case, the foal's head is typically extended horizontally, with the mouth wide open and the corner of the mouth pulled backwards and upwards. To date there is limited scientific evidence that the two different behaviour patterns share a common biological background. (Photos courtesy of Philipp Seifert.)

shown towards adult horses (Figure 2.18b). However, the snapping response by foals is only shown when adult horses are close enough to the foal to allow bodily contact, while licking and chewing is shown in various contexts, and often when there is a rather large distance between horse and trainer. Furthermore, demeanour and posture differ considerably between licking and chewing in adult horses and snapping in foals (Figures 2.18). It is unclear why the demeanour of this behaviour should change considerably as the horse matures, if the meaning is to remain the same. Licking and chewing are also commonly seen in horses after they have been exposed to a fearful stimulus (König von Borstel *et al.*, 2010a). Thus, a much more plausible explanation of the licking and chewing seen in adult horses after a stressful experience may be that stress leads to activation of the sympathetic nervous system and a corresponding decrease in parasympathetic activity, leading to a shut-down of the gastro-intestinal system and diminished saliva production. The sanctuary provided by the outcome of the escape response may trigger the switch from the sympathetic nervous system to the parasympathetic nervous system with the associated return of saliva production. Therefore, a chased horse may simply suffer from a dry mouth and try to relieve that state by licking and chewing motions (König von Borstel *et al.*, 2010a).

Horses do not do things for us because they sense strong human leadership. They learn to respond because their human trainers have rewarded the correct responses (i.e. they have reinforced certain responses). As a trainer, you need only to reinforce the correct response, clearly and consistently; you do not need to stand tall and puff your chest out. Your demeanour does not matter. Even if it did, you would want to train your horse to react consistently to cues rather than to your demeanour. Such training has important safety reasons, as you will probably want your horse to reliably react to cues if you are, for example, injured or ill and therefore unable to show off impressively, or if a child is handling your horse. It is perhaps for this reason that the importance of correct application of learning theory appears to be particularly well recognised among disabled riders and horse owners. What does matter is what behaviours you reinforce in the horse. For example, the horse that does not load into the float/trailer does not refuse to load because he does not trust or respect you or because he sees your leadership as weak. The horse refuses because it is fearful of the trailer or because its training to lead forward has not been sufficiently generalised to include leading into a trailer. The horse, therefore, remains more under the control of environmental cues than it is under the control of your signals in this context.

A horse's environment is full of competing stimuli and, in this case, the contest for control is between the aversiveness of the trailer and the conditioning of the lead forward signal. The horse that refuses to load into the trailer is clearly not under the control of the lead forward signals. Thoroughly attending to reversing this situation in combination with appropriate habituation results in horses loading successfully because leading signals outcompete the trailer for salience. That said, it does not provide any justification for beating horses to drive them into a trailer, a practice that would be entirely counter-productive. since most horses make an association between the trailer and the beating and so learn to avoid all trailers.

Any consideration of human–horse interactions can be blurred by terms that only vaguely relate to equine ethology. From an objective point of view, we should also be cautious in ascribing terms such as 'trust' and 'respect' to horse–human interactions, because these terms have little relevance in a scientific interpretation (Figure 2.19). Such qualities (Table 2.3) are impossible to identify or measure. We may sense that they exist, but if they cannot be clearly measured or defined, their usefulness as components of systematic training will remain questionable.

Applying elements of the horse's social repertoire in a bid to bond with them rarely has an impact on ridden work. Allogrooming may be an exception. Head-rubbing by horses on people (most often after the horse has developed a layer of sweat under its bridle) should not be reinforced because buckles on bridles can easily damage human skin. Horses quickly learn that head-rubbing on humans is fruitless if their trainers step away when this behaviour is directed at them. Riders who wish to relieve the itchiness of sweat on their horses should remove the

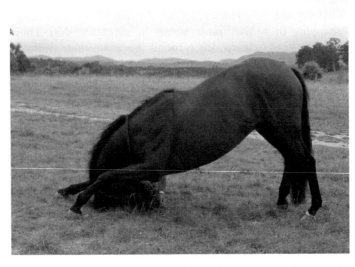

Figure 2.19 There is no convincing evidence that horses showing trained postural responses are offering either submission or respect.

Table 2.3 Common attributes and elusive terms assigned to horses with plausible scientific interpretations.

Term	Scientific interpretation	Likely extent of horse being under stimulus control of the rider	Likely extent of horse being under stimulus control of the environment
Honest	Well-trained	+++*	++*
Genuine	Predictable (low flexibility in responses to the same stimuli)	+++	++
Bomb-proof	Unreactive	++++	+
Thorough 'gentleman'	Calm and well-trained	+++	++
Perfect manners	Well-trained	+++	+
Forward going	Reactive	++	+++
Dirty (stop at a jump)	Unreliable *go* response	++	+++
Cheeky	Poorly trained	+	++++
Naughty	Poorly trained	+	++++
Sharp	Sensitive	++++	+
Prefers the company of other horses	Likely to stall when leaving conspecifics	+	++++
Not for a novice rider	Reactive, with a tendency to show flight responses and to be unresponsive to rein signals	++	+++
Keen	Tendency to show flight responses	++	+++
Bold	Tendency to traverse unfamiliar obstacles without stalling	++++	+
Lazy	Unresponsive to leg pressures	+	++++
Stubborn	Fearful, in pain and/or poorly trained	+	++++
Intelligent	Easily trained	Depends on the horse's motivation and the skill of the trainer	

* On a scale from 1 to 4, one plus means 'unlikely' and four pluses means 'highly likely'.

bridle and scratch the horse only when it keeps its head still. Stopping the scratching whenever the horse moves is a form of negative punishment (Chapter 5, Associative Learning (Attractive stimuli)). Equally, riders can scratch horses to reward them, because horses are motivated to relieve an itch or to experience calming social interaction.

It has been suggested that humans can enter the social 'hierarchy' of groups of horses by mimicking their behaviour, most notably through their signals (Roberts, 1997; Sighieri *et al.*, 2003). This approach, based on the controversial premise that a herd is organised by social status established by means of ritualised conflict, has grown in popularity, but it lacks scientific rigour. Consider round-pen training, for example. The chief appeal of this approach lies in the notion that it is possible to manage unhandled horses without coercion by mimicking behaviours from the equid social ethogram. The merits of this type of hands-off training are purported to be that it is humane and carries with it little risk of learned helplessness. But round-pen training does involve coercion. For unhandled horses, being approached and touched by humans seems to lie on the same continuum of aversive interactions as being whipped: they are all interactions worth avoiding

(McGreevy, 2004). Round-pen training may be ineffective insofar as achieving anything useful in human–horse interactions. Indeed, it has been proposed that horses might simply learn to avoid being chased (Krueger, 2007), in other words, by negative reinforcement. In some circumstances (with fearful horses, for example), round-pen training can be inhumane. It can precipitate chronic stress if horses are conditioned into constant states of hyper-reactivity and, therefore, may increase behavioural wastage in the form of loss of usefulness and commercial value – a downward trend that can lead to euthanasia or the abattoir. Furthermore, rewards in round-pens often take the form of rubbing, typically on the forehead. Although this intervention may indeed serve as an effective reward, it lacks ethological salience, given that allogrooming of the forehead by conspecifics is far rarer than wither-scratching. Interestingly, an investigation of responses to round-pen training states that grooming as a reward (Figure 2.20) appeared to have no significant

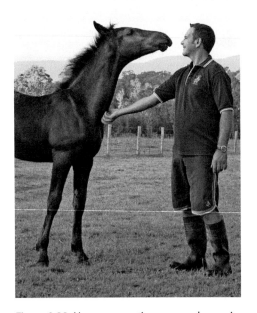

Figure 2.20 Humans sometimes groom horses in areas that are usually not groomed by other horses.

effect on the horse's tendency to follow trainers in the round-pen itself (Krueger, 2007). In other words, the following response was not placed under stimulus control (Chapter 5, Associative Learning (Attractive stimuli)).

An array of questions is launched by the philosophy of human-as-leader: What if, despite embracing the notion wholeheartedly, trainers cannot persuade their horses to comply? Does that mean the *horse* has better and more consistent leadership characteristics? If the horse fails to follow the trainer into a trailer, does that simply mean the human was perceived as a poor leader? What aspect of the human's leadership was lacking? How can this be studied scientifically? Are there negative welfare implications for the horse that does not recognise any human as leader? If a third party successfully leads the horse, using a correct application of negative or positive reinforcement, is he or she showing subliminal leadership?

We might expect horses that genuinely regard certain humans as leaders to seek out the company of the human leaders and forsake their conspecific affiliates. However, there is currently insufficient evidence that horses in a paddock approach humans for reasons other than mere curiosity or because they have been conditioned to do so. Indeed, considering that after 'successful' round-pen training, horses show no increase in their tendency to follow trainers outside the round-pen, it leads us to question the utility of such a potentially detrimental technique.

If horses are deprived of equine company (which is a common mistake seen in rearing orphan or home-bred single, rather than stud-bred, multiple foals), they may engage with humans as play partners. Equine play involves biting, rearing, boxing and kicking (McDonnell and Haviland, 1995). It is never safe to encourage these responses in horses of any age or size.

Ethological Solutions

Purely ethological solutions for horse-training are limited (McGreevy and McLean, 2006), as they are confined to the evolutionary adaptive behaviour of the animal that humans can capitalise upon or modify (social facilitation, stimulus enhancement and group behaviours such as trekking). However, horses did not evolve to carry people and so when we ride them, ethology has little further to offer. In contrast, learning theory provides greater possibilities to alter behaviour through the non-associative processes of habituation and sensitisation, and associative modalities, such as operant and classical conditioning.

It has been suggested that a trainer's interactions with horses should be based on three elements fundamental to the equilibrium of the herd: flight, herd instinct and 'hierarchy' (Sighieri *et al.*, 2003). However, this approach overlooks the importance of foraging, coalitions, kinship and affiliation, as well as the reality of the effects of conditioning on all innate responses. Ethologically sound solutions should not depend on a notion of the horse's benevolence – that the horse is 'wanting to be with' or 'wanting to please' the trainer.

The importance of habituation, sensitisation, operant and classical conditioning should never be underestimated because they facilitate efficient learning and underpin training techniques. They are informed by learning theory and supported by ethology. All training systems use a blend of these processes, yet there are fundamental gaps in the understanding and acceptance of their place in equestrian coaching (Warren-Smith and McGreevy, 2006). Studying equine ethology demands consideration of how natural selection shaped horse behaviour and the learning capacity of the horse. Training philosophies that embrace learning theory can be ethological in the sense that they might take into account the types of stimuli horses are most likely to respond to and the types of reinforcers that are most rewarding (from our knowledge of ethology).

Instinctive responses predicted by ethology can facilitate horse-handling without the need for deliberate training. However, these are adaptive mechanisms that evolved for group cohesion, and they can and do act upon behaviours that are themselves subject to conditioning.

Labelling training systems as forms of ethology (e.g. for a short period in the UK, Natural Horsemanship was marketed under the brand 'Equine Ethology') denies the importance of learning theory and implies that we must 'speak the language of horse'. This may be a beguiling idea, but it is ultimately an illusion. The illusions of horse-owners are generally harmless unless they create unrealistic expectations. Learning theory can and should be used to explain all training techniques, no matter how elaborately they are camouflaged. As noted previously, most round-pen techniques (e.g. Roberts, 1997) are based as much on negative reinforcement as the physical pressure/release systems used in the ridden horse (McGreevy and McLean, 2007). Similarly, advance-and-retreat techniques (e.g. Blackshaw *et al.*, 1983) are examples of negative reinforcement plus habituation in that the trainer's retreat is made just before the horse initiates a flight response.

Environmental Enrichment

Social behaviour, dietary requirements, physiology, personality and genetics all influence the way a confined animal behaves in its enclosure. Equally, the environment we provide for any domestic animal affects its behaviour and, therefore, its welfare. However, as the context and purpose of confinement change, so do our perceptions of what amounts to appropriate space and what that space must contain (Webster, 1994). Paddocks of adequate size reduce the amount of time spent standing passively (Jørgensen and Bøe, 2007). In horses, locomotion is integrated with grazing and, because horses seldom take more than two mouthfuls in one spot before stepping to the next, large areas may be traversed in a single grazing bout (Archer, 1971; Houpt and Wolski, 1982; Fraser, 1992; Francis-Smith and Wood-Gush, 1997). Unless they are disturbed by a threat or displaced by a conspecific, foraging horses look up only when moving from one patch to another and then only long enough to help locate the next suitable food source (via olfaction and vision).

As the horse moves forward while grazing, its forelegs move alternately, with the hindlimbs following in diagonal couplets. GPS-based and accelerometer-based measurements show that domestic horses travel daily distances of 2–10 km in conventional pasture and free-stall systems, but clearly this will depend on the size of the available premises (Hampson *et al.*, 2010), the quality of the pasture and aspects of facility design, such as enclosure shape and allocation of other resources (e.g. water and shelter). Facilities specially designed to encourage locomotion, so-called 'activity barns' with automated feeding or the 'paddock trail' system (c. 13 km) (Küllmar and König von Borstel, 2015) may further increase the distances travelled, although only rarely are these comparable with distances covered by feral horses (average of 18 km daily) (Hampson *et al.*, 2010). When stabling and isolation prevent horses from moving and playing, the motivation to perform these behaviours increases (Mal *et al.*, 1991; Houpt *et al.*, 2001; Christensen *et al.*, 2002; McGreevy, 2004; Chaya *et al.*, 2006). Clearly, this affects work in-hand and under-saddle. Too much concentrated food and insufficient exercise can lead to hyper-reactivity (Figure 2.21) and muscular disorders, within a matter of 24 hours, so all good horse-keepers

appreciate the need to reduce food intake in anticipation of reduced exercise. Confinement to a stable becomes more rapidly excessive if horses are maintained on full rations and not exercised at least once a day.

As horses spend most of their time not being ridden, their maintenance environment is a prime consideration in horse management. However, the behavioural relevance of this is frequently overlooked. There are several areas for consideration in improving a suboptimal environment, including:

1) *Environmental enrichment.* The main aim of this method of enrichment is to create an environment that mimics the horse's natural habitat and allows it to express its natural adaptive behaviours and so reduce frustration. Behavioural enrichment that requires an extremely diverse environment plus a large amount of space can be impractical, so the behavioural relevance of enrichment methods is paramount. Also, there must be limits on the extent to which full behavioural repertoires (within the equid ethogram) can be accommodated. We have to acknowledge that allowing a horse to 'express all its natural behaviours' is not entirely feasible. If it were, we would have to let them express their natural reproductive behaviours

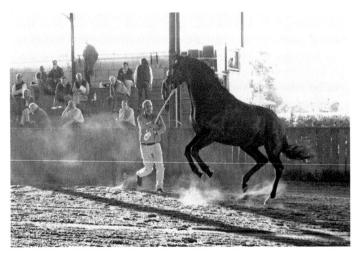

Figure 2.21 Behaviours described as exuberance can reflect previous confinement. (Photo courtesy of Sandy Hannan.)

and fears. With domestic horses, it is arguable that riding can offer a form of behavioural enrichment. Riding in environments that are more complex than a familiar arena, such as on reasonably familiar trails, may be akin to the treks free-ranging horses take within their home range. The risks of not doing so can result in horses for which riding outside the arena presents abnormal stimuli (Appleby, 1997) such that they become unsafe to ride. Riding out also appears to help horses to develop mental maps.

2) *Companions.* Like all social species, horses require companions (Figure 2.22). However, many are housed individually, effectively preventing almost any social behaviour. This social isolation is likely to lead to frustration and suffering for the animals. Placing animals in groups is one of the most easily achieved forms of environmental enrichment, but this is often not implemented because of the prospect of fighting and injury at the time of mixing. However, compared to single-housed horses, group-housed horses are overall not at higher risk of injuries requiring surgical care (König von Borstel *et al.*, 2016a; Hartmann *et al.*, 2012), while single-housed horses are at higher risk of displaying unwelcome behaviours such as overt aggression, fearfulness or stereotypies (König von Borstel *et al.*, 2016b). However, it is not sufficient to assume that any horse will provide the right sort of company. Optimal stable management includes taking the time to establish which horses socialise appropriately as neighbours.

(a)

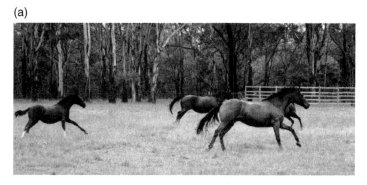

(b)

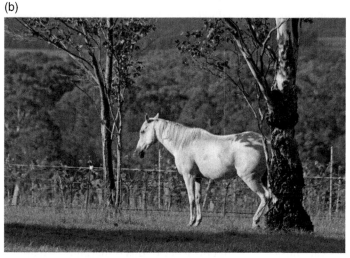

Figure 2.22 (a) A well-established social group provides important enrichment in domestic contexts. (b) Even at pasture, isolated horses may have compromised welfare.

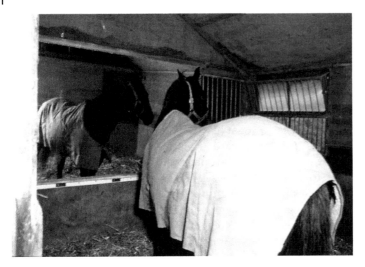

Figure 2.23 The value of ethologically relevant visual stimuli for stabled horses is becoming better understood.

3) *Artificial appliances.* Various devices have been designed for confined animals. Although these may have little similarity to anything that horses are likely to encounter in their natural environment, nonetheless, they may provide some enrichment, at least while they are novel and thus offer options to show explorative behaviour. Examples are plastic bottles suspended from the roof of the stable. Inexpensive items are preferred because they can lose their appeal completely as the horses become habituated to them. The less likely outcome is that these appliances can become the focus of abnormal behaviour patterns such as repetitive, invariant and apparently functionless interactions (i.e. stereotypies).

While some yard managers insist that a quiet stable block is beneficial because it allows horses to rest, others play radios in a bid to keep horses mentally occupied. The efficacy of this approach remains unclear since studies have failed to show either an effect of music on ponies during isolation or any preference for one style of music over another (Houpt *et al.*, 2000). This contrasts with studies of dairy cattle, which have shown that classical music facilitated milk flow when compared with rock (Albright and Arave, 1997).

Cooper *et al.* (2000) reported beneficial effects of providing a mirror for isolated horses, especially for those that showed stereotypic weaving (Figure 2.23). The apparent presence of a conspecific seems to be an effective stimulus for these horses and even a poster of a horse may be sufficient to have a similar effect (Mills, 2005). However, the effect of tactile social contact between horses should not be underestimated and mirrors and posters should not be used as substitutes for real social contact between horses.

4) *Foraging enrichment.* Concentrate feeds do not represent a natural diet for horses. The use of concentrated rations means that horses consume their daily ration very rapidly. This has at least two major disadvantages: it reduces the total oral activity per day and increases the risk of gastric ulceration. These consequences are probably linked in that reduced oral activity is thought to result in reduced saliva production and increased physiological stress responses, both of which compromise the stomach lining (Waters *et al.*, 2002). It seems likely that there is also a deleterious effect on performance, but evidence of this is marginal to date.

Increasing the variety of forage provided to stabled horses allows natural patch-foraging behaviour, and has been shown to reduce the performance of established stereotypies (Goodwin *et al.*, 2002). Thorne *et al.* (2005) report that offering multiple forages can help to normalise feeding behaviour. There is also evidence that offering multiple concentrate diets that vary only in flavour (viz., molasses, garlic, mint or herbs) can prompt stabled horses to show natural patch-foraging behaviour on concentrates (Goodwin *et al.*, 2005).

5) *Control of the environment.* The lack of control of the environment is often pinpointed as a cause of frustration and stress in confined animals. The absence of an ability to travel through time mentally may prevent horses from looking forward to better times ahead and ruminating on the past (McLean, 2003; 2004; Mendl and Paul, 2008). However, it does not mean that sub-optimal environments, including those of the past, do not affect welfare (Mendl and Paul, 2008). When the animal cannot control variables, such as feeding time or the lighting schedule, and when it cannot escape from events it finds unpleasant, it often behaves in ways that suggest frustration. Animals that have learned (as in so-called shuttle-box experiments) that rewards and punishments are continually interchanged at random tend to stop responding. They become withdrawn from their environment and exhibit what is termed learned helplessness. They have lost control of their environment. Learning that there is no escape from aversive stimuli differs from habituation (Hall *et al.*, 2007). Clearly, horses in training are vulnerable to this outcome because the pressures that underpin negative reinforcement may be excessive and sustained, even when horses have responded appropriately. When animals learn that resistance is futile, they typically become apathetic (Webster, 1994). The lack of active behavioural responses in such animals increases the need for physiological measures that characterise the state of learned helplessness.

Giving horses control of their own environment can be a very successful method of enrichment. Operant devices can be used to assess horses' preference for environmental conditions such as illumination (Houpt and Houpt, 1992), shelter, by means of a blanket (Mejdell *et al.*, 2016), or paddock turnout (Lee *et al.*, 2011). Another application of such operant devices is in consumer-demand studies, where custom-built devices are operated by the horse (as the consumer) to measure the strength of their desire to obtain certain resources, for example, social contact (Søndergaard *et al.*, 2011). The work that horses put into using these devices reflects, at least in part, the value they place on each resource. Training horses to use switches of this sort can also allow them access to resources in commercial, rather than experimental, contexts. Commercial systems that allow group-housed horses to access feeding stations with automated feeding programmes, including individualised access to pasture, are now well established in some parts of Europe. This technology allows horses to receive small amounts of concentrates throughout the whole day rather than in a few, distinct meals, which suits their digestive physiology better, while at the same time not unduly increasing workload for barn managers (König von Borstel *et al.*, 2010b). If larger amounts of concentrate feeds are required at all in a horse's diet, preference should be given to such housing systems, where available.

Ethologists are likely to contribute significantly to welfare by further explaining human impact on domestic horses while they work and rest. It is generally accepted that signals given to highly trained horses are elegant in their subtlety (Loch, 1977; Sivewright, 1984; McGreevy and McLean, 2007). The development of cognitive ethology and the application of learning theory to equitation may allow us to plot the emergence of the subtle signals given to horses as they progress through training and, thus, detect the transition between operant and classical conditioning.

Once we can distinguish between operant and classically conditioned cues, we will have all the mechanistic data that explain human–horse interactions in the context of the ridden horse. This will allow conceptual investigations of the unique characteristics of elite horses and riders (including talent, flair and intuition) that transcend scientific analysis. Although elite riders will always be those who learn the fastest and get the best from their horses with a minimum of apparent effort, the use of the mechanistic data from the studies of the horse–rider interface will be valuable from an educational perspective, since it will allow novice riders to mimic elite riders and catalyse their ascendance from novice to advanced horses.

By measuring the pressures and weight distribution of riders and saddles on the horse's spine while in motion, we will also be able to relate lameness and performance problems to asymmetry (McGreevy and Rogers, 2005). An additional welfare benefit is that we will be able to measure the thresholds of tolerance of flexion and hyperflexion in naïve horses and trained horses from a variety of disciplines. This will and has greatly informed the welfare debate surrounding controversial training techniques such as Rollkur (McGreevy, 2007).

Ethology helps us to describe a ridden or otherwise trained horse's responses as clearly as possible. This is the first step to measuring when they occur, what triggers them and

what can be done to reduce the likelihood of conflict behaviour. The differences in the ethological and cognitive challenges of various forms of horse use appear in Chapter 9, Horses in Sport and Work.

Individual Differences: The Role of Conformation, Personality and Laterality

It takes about five years to train a horse to Grand Prix level. The elements of dressage are difficult for horses to learn and the learning must be accompanied by significant physical development. Some horses find some aspects of dressage more difficult than others. Certain types of conformation lend themselves to collection and an analysis of croup to wither ratio covers the most important principles. For classical dressage, where there is an emphasis on collection, a short back and a higher wither-height to croup-height ratio are preferred (Figure 2.24). Compared with the modern performance breeds (especially the Thoroughbred), the baroque breeds, such as the Lusitanians, Andalusians, Friesians and Lippizaners, are naturally more upstanding in the forequarters and, thus, more easily collected.

There is evidence that selecting for small heads and long legs may inadvertently lead to a population bias to graze with one leg in advance of the other and morphological

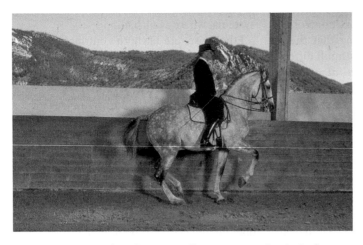

Figure 2.24 Baroque breeds are naturally more upstanding in the forequarters than many modern breeds and are, thus, more easily collected. (Photo courtesy of Cadmos Verlag and Philippe Karl.)

asymmetry because individuals with these morphological attributes are compelled to reach relatively farther than others for food on the ground (van Heel *et al.*, 2006). This lead preference may compromise balance in performance horses (McGreevy and Rogers, 2005).

Even without the involvement of social learning, the influence of parents should not be overlooked, since the influence of the sire has been found to have a significant effect on the training of leading (Warren-Smith *et al.*, 2005a) as well as on spatial tasks (Wolff and Hausberger, 1996). The inheritance of desirable, and indeed dangerous, qualities merits further scientific scrutiny. For example, evidence is accumulating that reactivity to novel or sudden stimuli has comparably high heritabilities of 5–40% (König von Borstel, 2013), and reactions to handling or veterinary inspections are

likewise characterised by moderate heritabilities (Oki *et al.*, 2007) that allow for genetic selection for these traits.

The individual differences that characterise equine personality have been dubbed 'horsonality' (Visser, 2002). They include features such as fearfulness and trainability. In addition, laterality (Figure 2.25) is of growing interest to equitation scientists as the impact of left- and right-hemispheric dominance and consequent motor preferences becomes more clearly understood. In humans, the right cerebral hemisphere has been associated with emotional responses, including negative effects (nervousness, distress, fear, hostility) (Wittling and Roschmann, 1993), while in rodents, left-paw preference and leftward turning behaviour have been associated with heightened physiological stress responses (LaHoste *et al.*, 1998; Neveu

(a)

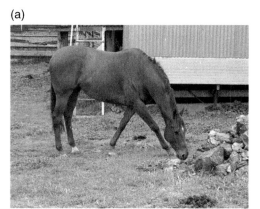

(b)

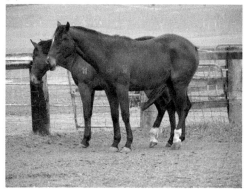

(c)

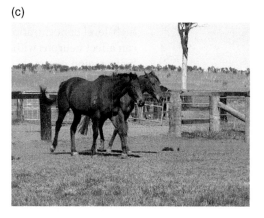

Figure 2.25 Studies of grazing horses (McGreevy *et al.*, 2007) have examined the preference for many lateralised behaviours, including standing (a), flexing (b) and moving relative to conspecifics (c).

and Moya, 1997), suggesting that right-brain dominance and speed of arousal may be correlated in these animals. Arousal responses are important in horses because they may indicate what type of work best suits an individual. For example, many forms of equitation demand low reactivity (e.g. to be safe in traffic), while with others, such as racehorses, this aspect is of lesser importance.

Fortunately, it is becoming clear that performance in avoidance-learning tests can be measured early in life and that early detection of this quality in yearlings gives a reliable prediction for life and is more consistent than responses in reward-based (positive reinforcement) tests (Visser *et al.*, 2003). Given the links between laterality and emotionality mentioned above, it may be that, in selecting for differing flight responses, breeders have unwittingly influenced the lateralisation of breeds.

Horses graze from a stationary position, moving the head and neck in an arc limited on one side by the presence of the advanced forelimb (McGreevy *et al.*, 2007). After each step, grazing follows an arc medial to the advanced limb. There is no evidence that the head/neck position is a result of one or other eye being preferred for surveillance. Although the forelegs alternate in leading during grazing, the time some horses spend with the left leg advanced is generally longer than that for the right (Figure 2.26). This manifests as a significant directional bias to graze with the left foreleg in advance of the right (McGreevy

and Rogers, 2005; Kuhnke and König von Borstel, 2016a). If advancing a forelimb when grazing reflects greater mobility on that side of the midline, then it is possible that the brains of left-preferent animals are right-hemisphere dominant. However, a counter argument is that the non-advanced limb is the more critical for survival because it supports more weight, reflects greater agility on the weight-bearing side of the animal and is arguably better positioned to launch the animal into a flight response and a more dominant left turn (owing to the abduction of the right foreleg in the stance phase) (McLean and McLean, 2008). However, contrary to expectations, there seems to be no clear relationship between the advanced foreleg during grazing and the laterality during ridden work (Kuhnke and König von Borstel, 2016b). Indeed, various measurements of laterality such as the preferred foreleg during grazing or during feeding from a bucket, the preferred eye for inspecting novel objects, lateral displacement of the hindquarters in relation to the median plane, and rein tension patterns during riding, show limited or no relationship among each other. The only known measurement of laterality taken in unmounted horses that has some predictive qualities for laterality during riding is the displacement of hindquarters relative to the median plane (Figure 2.27).

Fearfulness in horses affects the frequency of eating and drinking, defaecation, locomotion and contact with herd-mates (McCann *et al.*, 1988). In addition, fearfulness may interfere with learning, because prolonged high-level concentrations of stress hormones can affect neurons within the hippocampus, a brain region central to learning and memory (Sapolsky, 2004). Exclusive selection for speed, as prevalent in racing breeds, may have led to heightened flight responses compared to other horses, such as Warmbloods, draughthorses and ponies. Also, based on genetic linkage or pleiotropy (one gene influencing several traits simultaneously), selection for specific characteristics may inadvertently also influence traits such as emotionality. For example, selection for good show-jumping abilities appears to have led to horses with lower fear reactivity and higher speed of

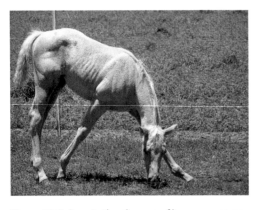

Figure 2.26 Even in the absence of lameness, some foals lock in a strong preference for an unbalanced grazing stance before weaning.

habituation compared to horses of dressage or non-specialised lines of the same breed (König von Borstel *et al.*, 2010a). Breed differences in the fear reactivity of horses and their tendency to be especially sensitive and thus easily sent into conflict are of great interest to those studying, working and competing with horses.

Conclusions

To apply learning theory correctly, we must identify an individual horse's physical limits, and most important, the motivational state of the horse so that we can predict its responses and capture or redirect them as appropriate. Horsemanship depends on both detailed knowledge of functional patterns of equine behaviour and the flexibility to correctly apply learning theory. All good trainers display both attributes to some extent.

Take-Home Messages

- Equitation presents significant ethological challenges.
- Training must reflect the physical abilities and learning capacity of the horse.
- Any ability humans may have to relate to horses using equine communication cues is of no use once they mount to ride.
- A rider often runs into difficulties when he or she assumes that the horse knows what the rider wants to achieve.

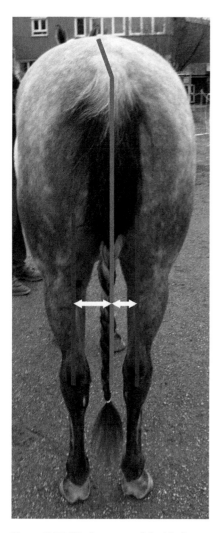

Figure 2.27 Displacement of the hindquarters (red) relative to the median plane (blue) may have some predictive qualities for laterality during riding. (Photo courtesy of Sandra Kuhnke.)

Areas for Further Research

- Personality characteristics of elite horses should be measured and characterised more fully to be able to better understand what makes an elite horse and, possibly, to predict early on which horses are most suited to various activities.
- Further exploration of personality and laterality tests as predictors of different aspects of reactivity and suitability for certain sports and work may reduce behavioural wastage.

- Further studies on social learning that focus on designing biologically relevant test situations in which horses are more likely to show social learning, such as the dam as tutor to her foal, or in general required learning contexts or qualities of the (equine or human) demonstrators.
- Further study of the relationship between behaviour under-saddle and disorders such as 'cold-back syndrome' and dental problems will reduce the application of equine behaviour therapy to horses with clinical pathologies.

3

Anthropomorphism and the Human–Horse Relationship

Introduction

Assigning human characteristics to animals and other non-human agents (i.e. anthropomorphism) has been identified by many scholars (Hume, 1757; Darwin, 1872; Freud, 1930). Until fairly recently, anthropomorphism has been a common approach used to describe horse behaviour; it is unhelpful at best and may promote poor welfare at worst, particularly when it comes to describing problem behaviours as having some malevolent component. In addition, it may be very dangerous to expect that a horse will act like a human friend (Figure 3.1). Regardless of the quality of the human–horse relationship, a horse is likely to react with an innate fear response if frightened above a certain threshold. Such unexpected fear reactions are a major cause of horse–human accidents (Keeling *et al.*, 1999).

Debate still surrounds the validity of anthropomorphism in scientific discourse, but there is something inherently appealing about attributing human characteristics to non-human agents. When the computer crashes, we may playfully ascribe malevolent intentions to it, but when we do this with an animal, it can colour our interactions with that animal.

The cognitive boundaries between humans and animals are unclear; consequently, the boundaries of anthropomorphism are also unclear. We might say that a horse is naughty, but we must question whether our notion of human naughtiness can possibly apply to horses (Figure 3.2). We should also question whether the so-called naughty behaviour was a response that had been inadvertently reinforced. Perhaps the naughty horse is merely confused and the naughtiness is an expression of the horse's conflict behaviour or frustration. The problem that then arises is what are we going to do about it? Do we have the right to punish the naughty horse?

Horses are commonly described using terms such as brave, loyal, dependable, naughty, bad, nasty, malicious, bad-tempered, that he hates, loves, regrets, is compassionate, and has a will to win, as well as benevolent with a will to please. While it is understandable, it can be very inaccurate to describe a horse's behaviour and character as mental states (e.g. the horse is crazy) rather than to simply describe what you observe directly and know to be true. For example, a horse that kicks out at the farrier and then runs a few steps is more likely to be successfully rehabilitated if the trainer simply identifies the origin of the flight response and the particular loss of control than if the horse is labelled malevolent. Clearly, there can be serious welfare problems in attributing human characteristics to horses, because of the potential consequences for them.

Teleological explanations of the horse's behaviour that imply purposeful deliberate mental states are also tempting but similarly misleading. The horse that bucks or rears may not necessarily do so to injure or even

Equitation Science, Second Edition. Paul McGreevy, Janne Winther Christensen,
Uta König von Borstel and Andrew McLean.
© 2018 John Wiley & Sons Ltd. Published 2018 by John Wiley & Sons Ltd.
Companion website: www.wiley.com/go/mcgreevy/equitation

(a)

(b)

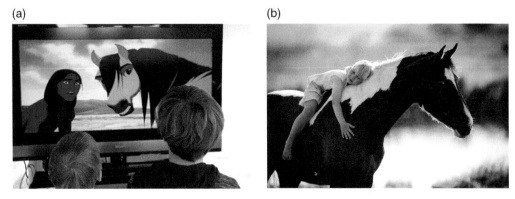

Figure 3.1 Horses star in numerous movies and comics and are often assigned human characteristics (a). This may contribute to an anthropomorphic view on horse behaviour and indirectly to horse–human accidents when children anticipate human-like reactions from horses (b) (*Source:* http://www.123rf.com)

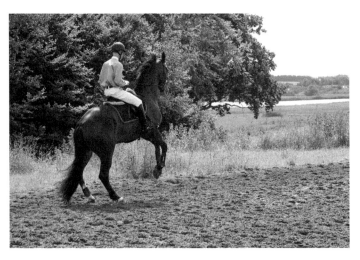

Figure 3.2 Horse misbehaviour – naughty or confused? Terms such as naughty inappropriately shift the blame from the rider to the horse. (Photo courtesy of Julie Taylor/ EponaTV.)

dislodge the rider; instead, these counter-predator responses may be simply triggered by certain sensations and events. Teleological explanations can lead to assumptions that are difficult to verify, or are perhaps simply convenient oversimplifications. For example, 'My horse behaved badly because he was paying me back for my being late to feed him last night'; or he is 'thinking of ways to get out of work'. Attributing human thought processes to animals may be the most inappropriate way of describing cognitive processes. For instance, when the horse is given a spell (extended rest) after a period of work, one hears that it 'gives him time to think about what he has learned'. The unique effect of human language on human thought processes provides reason for caution in attributing the same processes to other species. For this reason, the term higher-order linguistic thought (HOLT) was coined and considered to be a uniquely human capability (Rolls, 2000).

Anthropocentrism

The doctrine of the human-centred universe is pivotal to the anthropomorphic mindset and makes a number of assumptions. One of the most detrimental is assuming that the horse *knows* and, if this is so, he must *know* the difference between right and wrong, so punishing him when his response is incorrect is an appropriate human intervention. However, punishment only tells the horse what it *should not do*, and not what it *should do*, and the use of punishment during training has a long list of negative side-effects (Chapter 6, Associative Learning (Aversive stimuli)).

It is often suggested that one of the main reasons horses comply with riders' requests is their willingness to please (Warren-Smith and McGreevy, 2008a). Although appealing to some horse-owners, the chief problem with this approach revolves around the higher cognitive skills required to do this. Also, it is questionable whether horses are motivated to please other horses, let alone humans, or indeed, that human expressions of pleasure can even be correctly interpreted by horses. Why should a horse wish to bring pleasure to its rider by jumping a fence when its species-specific response is simply to avoid it?

Beyond mere compliance lies the implicit assumption that horses may actively cooperate with riders to achieve shared goals (e.g. in play) (Goodwin and Hughes, 2005). True cooperation would demand very complex cognitive skills, as the horse would have to know the outcome and want it for some reason (Figure 3.3). For example, to be considered 'cooperative', a racehorse would have to know that it is racing, presumably over a certain distance, and recognise the critical importance and benefits of being in the lead when running past the finishing post. One of the dangers in adopting a teleological and anthropomorphic framework to explain horse motivation is that a rider may assume that a horse knows what the rider wants. This can lead the rider to give unclear cues and become angry and perhaps feel disappointed when these fail to produce the desired outcome.

How did Anthropomorphism come About?

Anthropomorphism has an appeal to many humans when interpreting animal behaviour, because it by-passes dry descriptors. Epley *et al.* (2007) suggest that at least two dimensions of similarity must be present for anthropomorphism to occur: similarity in both morphology and motion. Children as young as 9 months seem able to attribute intentions to an action when performed by a human-like hand but not when performed by a wooden rod (Woodward, 1999). Furthermore, if robots are given human-like faces and bodies, they are anthropomorphised more readily, and when products are designed with human features, they are more successful in the marketplace (Epley *et al.*, 2007).

Anthropomorphic behaviours include regarding the pet as a family member or best

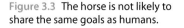

Figure 3.3 The horse is not likely to share the same goals as humans.

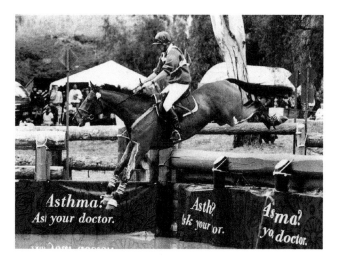

friend, assigning a human role, such as baby, to the pet, taking on a specific maternal or paternal role (Greenebaum, 2004), and even dressing the pet in human clothing and celebrating its birthdays (Archer, 1997). Data from a US pet hospital (Gardyn, 2002) revealed that between 1995 and 2001 there was a 28% increase in pet owners describing themselves as the father or mother of their pets. Commercial interests have been quick to capitalise on this behaviour, so pet owners can now send their pets to day care, weight-loss holidays and spas, massage and home-opathic therapies, as well as taking them to cafés and restaurants and away on holidays (Duvall-Antonacopoulos and Pychyl, 2008). The vast array of colours and styles of horse rugs/covers and equipment available is testimony to the horse-owner's participation in this response (Figure 3.4).

What Purpose does Anthropomorphism Serve?

Epley *et al.* (2007) proposed that anthropomorphism satisfies a desire to feel effective in one's environment and to increase a sense of social connection – it should increase as a function of these two motivational states. They suggested that anthropomorphism has an important function in humans by reducing uncertainty and increasing understanding of one's environment, and the tendency positively correlates with loneliness. In such states of isolation, a lonely person is likely to see a pet as thoughtful and consecrated, but less likely to see it as vengeful or deceitful

(Epley *et al.*, 2007). Their research also reports that developmental influences, such as the quality of social relationships and feelings of attachment to animals or detachment from other humans, also increase the likelihood of anthropomorphism. Surveys by Beck and Madresh (2008) revealed that relationships between humans and their pets were more secure than human–human relationships on every measure. In addition, relationships with pets affect other aspects of the pet-owner's life, perhaps by buffering the experience of negative human social interactions.

Using a scale for anthropomorphism designed by Albert and Bulcroft (1988), studies by Duvall-Antonacopoulos and Pychyl (2008) revealed that on a scale of increased anthropomorphism:

- women scored higher than men;
- unmarried people scored higher than people in married or *de facto* relationships;
- people without children at home scored higher than those with children at home;
- people without university degrees scored higher than those with degrees;
- people with less family support scored higher than those with greater family support.

Anthropomorphism can, thus, be seen as an adaptive human behaviour. Surprisingly, however, the studies showed a small but significant positive correlation between a person's stress level and the tendency to anthropomorphise pets.

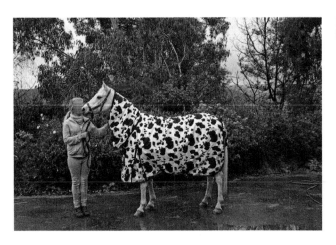

Figure 3.4 The pet horse: a projected image of ourselves?

The Dangers of Anthropomorphism

Fisher (1990) has argued that the mistakes or fallacies of anthropomorphism are neither well defined nor fallacious. He claims that the charge of anthropomorphism oversimplifies a complex issue and, worse, it inhibits examination of vital issues in an empirical sense. Human language provides unclear boundaries of anthropomorphic possibilities. For example, a racehorse might be trying hard to be in front of other horses, thus allowing it to win the race, but it probably has no idea of the consequences of winning. It is even more inappropriate to describe it as courageous. Fisher distinguishes between making descriptive mistakes where we misinterpret behaviour (such as a stallion's bared teeth being mistaken for smiling and affection) or anthropomorphism resulting from inaccuracy (what might not be anthropomorphism when describing a chimpanzee's behaviour could well be when describing a worm's). Thus, caution is required in laying charges of anthropomorphism.

Dennett (1996) cautions us against assuming without proof that animals have insight into their innate behaviours. To do so 'is to ignore the null hypothesis in an unacceptable way – if we are asking a scientific question'. Scientifically, such a view is unnecessarily complex and it is incorrect to assume without proof that animals have 'a stream of reflective consciousness something like our own' that accompanies apparently clever activities (Dennett, 1996).

Anthropomorphism remains an important cautionary beacon for horse-trainers. For example, Midkiff (1996) illustrated the benevolent and anthropomorphic viewpoint: 'One of the most compelling reasons women love horses is the promise and reality of unconditional love.' However, anthropomorphism also allows for the malevolent notion. For example, Schramm (1986), writing about difficult horses, describes some as 'depraved'. The notion of the malevolent horse is commonplace in the horse world, even though such anthropomorphism provides a great danger in diagnosing and treating behaviour problems and training issues in general that may compromise the welfare of the horse. It can encourage punishments that bear little or no relation to the original (incorrect) response.

When humans have expectations that animals 'understand' what is required, they are likely to give inappropriate signals to the animals, such as delayed, inconsistent or meaningless reinforcements, resulting in deleterious behavioural changes. These changes are manifest in conflict behaviours, such as redirected, ambivalent and displacement behaviours, stereotypies and injurious behaviours (Wiepkema, 1987). Concepts such as respect and submission can have negative welfare consequences for horses when applied within the context of unwelcome or problematic behaviour. In the minds of some, the terms 'respect' and 'submission' may justify delayed punishment ('He knows what he did wrong!'), as well as poor timing of signals and reinforcement ('He knows what I am asking for!').

Communication between Horses and Humans

Horses communicate with each other via visual, auditory, olfactory and tactile signals. In contrast, communication between humans is primarily based on auditory signals via our well-developed linguistic skills. We may therefore tend to put too much emphasis on auditory signals in our communication with horses, which may be problematic, since differentiating between words and voice tones may be difficult for horses. Horses can learn to respond to certain words or to a tone of voice via the process of classical conditioning, if they have experienced several occasions where that particular word or voice tone predicted an outcome. It is commonly assumed that horses have an inherent understanding of harsh voice cues that would be used as reprimands versus soothing voice cues that would be used as a reward or to calm the horse down. However, recent research shows that soothing vocal cues did not enhance a horse's performance in a novel, potentially frightening task (Heleski *et al.*, 2015).

Thus, we may overestimate the horse's ability to understand voice tones, unless these have been reliably paired with a pleasant or unpleasant outcome.

Horses can also learn to respond to human visual cues, and their ability to use human pointing gestures as a communicative cue (e.g. for indicating the location of food) has received some scientific attention. Maros et al. (2008) tested 20 horses for their ability to recognise different human gestural cues in a choice task, where the horses had to locate a food reward in one of two identical buckets. Four different pointing methods were used:

1) distal momentary pointing (the experimenter pointed briefly, for 1 second, with an finger extended towards the correct bucket, which was at least 80 cm away from the finger, and then lowered the arm so the cue was not present when the horse was making its choice);
2) distal dynamic-sustained (the experimenter's pointing hand was still at least 80 cm from the bucket, but was kept in the pointing position while the horse made its choice);
3) proximal momentary pointing (same procedure as in (1) but the experimenter's pointing hand was only 10 cm from the bucket); and
4) proximal dynamic-sustained pointing with gazing (same procedure as in (2) but only 10 cm from the bucket and the experimenter was now also looking at the correct bucket, whereas in the previous three methods the experimenter was looking at the horse).

The horses performed above the chance level in all methods apart from distal momentary pointing. This corresponds to findings in other animals and it is suggested that distal momentary pointing may be more cognitively demanding than other pointing styles (Maros et al., 2008).

Similar types of experimental set-ups have been used to assess social cognition of a wide range of species, including cats and dogs, and the relatively good performances in domesticated species has led to the suggestion that

the domestication process could have promoted the ability to rely on human gestures. It has even been suggested that dogs may have some appreciation of the referential nature of human gestures (Soproni et al., 2001). However, it is likely that horses rely on stimulus or local enhancement in human-guided choice tasks, rather than a referential understanding of the actual gestures (Krueger et al., 2011; Proops et al., 2010; Lovrovich et al., 2015).

Proops et al. (2010) confirmed that horses could use distal sustained pointing as a cue to locate food, whereas they appeared less sensitive to gaze alternation and body orientation cues for food location. Horses have previously been shown to use subtle cues, such as gaze and body orientation, when determining the focus of human attention (Proops and McComb, 2010), but were unable to use these cues in the object-choice task presented in Proops et al. (2010). In a follow-up study, Proops et al. (2013) compared the performance of young and adult horses across two object-choice experiments and found that their performance was comparable; the participating horses appeared able to correctly choose a rewarded bucket using marker placement, pointing and touching cues, but could not use body orientation, gaze, elbow pointing or tapping cues. It was further reported that horses seem to develop the skill of attending to subtle human cues as they age and that lifetime experience plays an important role in this development. Taken together, these results do not support the theory that horses are innately skilled at using human cues. Rather, horses' ability to use human visual cues in object-choice tasks reflects a more general learning ability (i.e. pointing predicts food), whereas gazing is not a salient cue.

It is often assumed that the individual level of socialisation with humans will affect an animal's ability to respond to human visual signals (e.g. as shown in wolves) (Miklósi et al., 2003). Similarly, in horses, socialisation and other lifetime factors could contribute to the development of responsiveness towards human-gestures (Krueger et al., 2011; Proops *et al.*, 2013). A small study investigated whether horses with different training backgrounds varied in their ability to use human pointing gestures to locate hidden food (Dorey *et al.*, 2014). The authors compared 10 horses originally trained using 'traditional' training methods with 10 horses originally trained using natural horsemanship, which often uses human visual gestures during training because trainers instruct the horse from the ground, whereas traditional riding tends to rely more on tactile cues.

To assess the effects of these different training histories on gestural responsiveness, the authors used a momentary distal point to indicate the rewarded bucket in a pair of two identical buckets. It was reported that neither of the two groups performed above chance level in this task, which accords with the results reported by Maros *et al.* (2008). However, when allowed an additional 60 trials, the horses in the natural horsemanship group learned to follow the cue with significantly greater success than those in the traditionally trained group (Dorey *et al.*, 2014). Clearly, the results of this small-scale study should be interpreted with care, and more controlled studies are needed to determine whether past training style or other lifetime factors may influence horses' success in human-guided tasks and other areas of cognitive ability.

An interesting aspect in relation to human–horse communication is that humans also appear to communicate with horses unintentionally through slight changes in body signals or perhaps other cues. One study found that a heart-rate increase in riders or trainers due to expectation of a frightening event was reflected in a similar heart-rate increase in their horses (Keeling *et al.*, 2009) (Figure 3.5). Interestingly, it was not possible to identify the potential changes in human body posture that led to this perception of human arousal by the horses. Similar results were obtained

Figure 3.5 A nervous handler (a) or rider (b) may cause the horse to become more fearful. In this study, the handlers (n = 20) and riders (n = 17) were asked to lead/ride their horses around a riding arena four times. They were told that during the fourth round an umbrella would suddenly appear from behind the barrier, which would probably frighten the horse. However, the umbrella was never presented, so the increase in the handlers' and riders' heart rates on the fourth round likely reflects their anticipation of their horse's fear response. It is interesting to note the similar increase in the horses' heart rates. The pathway for transmission of arousal from humans to horses remains to be identified. (Reproduced from Keeling *et al.*, 2009).

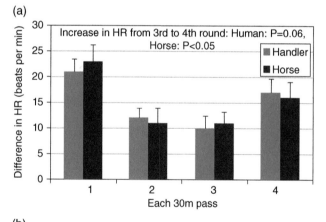

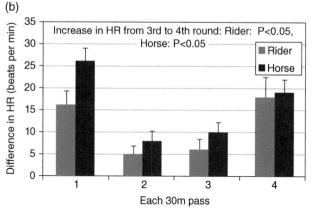

by von Borstel *et al.* (2007) and Merkies *et al.* (2014), whereas von Lewinski *et al.* (2013) reported that a heart-rate increase in riders during a show with spectators did not result in a similar heart-rate increase in the horses. However, the latter study was conducted on a limited number (n = 6) of highly experienced show horses, which may have habituated to the riders' reactions to the show performance. For prey species, it is likely adaptive to respond to arousal cues in other species, because such cues could signal danger. Further research is needed to identify whether slight changes in body posture are the pathway to this inter-species transfer of arousal, as well as whether the ability to perceive human arousal signals is a learned rather than an innate response.

A recent paper explored the potential use of symbols as a means of communication between horses and humans (Mejdell *et al.*, 2016). The authors report that the participating horses appeared able to use symbols to communicate their preferences for blanketing (i.e. the choice of symbol was not random but dependent on weather): the horses chose to stay without a blanket in mild weather, and to have a blanket on when the weather was wet, windy and cold. This was suggested to indicate that the participating horses understood the consequence of their choice on their own thermal comfort, and that they had

successfully learned to communicate their preferences by using the symbols. However, to validate this method for testing horses' preferences, further studies that control for both human unintentional cues and the effect of using food as a primary reinforcer for making a choice are needed.

The Human–Horse Relationship

A relationship may be defined as a series of interactions that occur over time between two or more individuals: these individuals will have expectations of the next interaction on the basis of the previous ones (Hinde, 1987; Hausberger *et al.*, 2008). Understanding that a relationship is built on a succession of interactions is important, as it suggests that attention must be paid to the positive and negative valence of each interaction as a step for the next (Hausberger *et al.*, 2008). Research suggests that horses can recognise and remember individual trainers and riders and whether past interactions with those individuals were pleasant or unpleasant. Sankey *et al.* (2010c) reported that horses trained with food as a reward for correct responses (positive reinforcement) spent more time close to the experimenter compared to horses trained without food. The horses appeared to generalise between the familiar and an unknown experimenter (Figure 3.6).

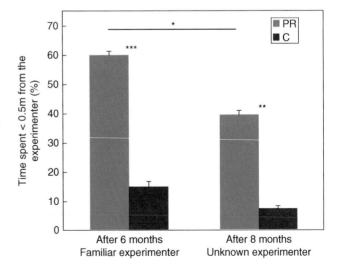

Figure 3.6 Horses appear to have long-lasting memories of their interactions with humans. Horses that had been trained using food as a reward for correct responses (positive reinforcement, PR) spent more time close to both a familiar and an unknown person than horses trained without food (control, C). (Reproduced from Sankey *et al.*, 2010c).

It was also suggested that using food as a reward may be more beneficial than grooming just three strokes at the withers in terms of both facilitation of learning a task (in this case, to remain immobile in response to a verbal command) and human attachment (Sankey *et al.*, 2010a). Nevertheless, Normando *et al.* (2003) reported that horses' heart rates can be lowered by stroking on the neck and, at least during riding, this may be a more feasible reward than feeding them.

Horses appear to use multisensory information, including visual, auditory and olfactory cues, to distinguish between humans, and can distinguish human faces and voices and match familiar voices to familiar faces (Proops and McComb, 2012). A study by Lampe and Andre (2012) found that when cues were incongruent (e.g. when a familiar person came into the visual field of the horse while an audio recording from another person was played), the horses spent more time looking towards the person, compared to when the cues were congruent. In another study, it was reported that horses looked for longer at an unfamiliar person, compared to a known person, when they were giving the same familiar verbal cue ('stay'), which was interpreted by the authors as indicating that the horses were surprised to hear the familiar cue given by an unknown voice (Sankey *et al.*, 2011).

In addition, it has been suggested that horses are able to discriminate between happy and angry human facial expressions in photographs; Smith *et al.* (2016) reported that horses showed a left-gaze bias (a lateralisation associated with stimuli perceived as negative) towards photographs of angry faces and had a quicker increase in heart rate towards angry faces. However, the latter result should be treated with caution because there was no difference in mean or maximum heart rates, and latencies to maximum heart rates have not previously been validated as a measure of negative emotions in horses.

Perception of Human Attention
Another area that has received some scientific interest is the ability of horses to determine the focus of human attention. Proops and McComb (2010) tested the ability of 36 horses to discriminate between an attentive and inattentive person in determining whom to approach for food. The cues provided were body orientation, head orientation or whether the experimenters' eyes were open or closed. It was reported that the horses chose the attentive person significantly more often, suggesting that they can distinguish between attentive and inattentive humans with access to food rewards, preferring to approach humans who are facing and looking at them to those who are not (Proops and McComb, 2010). It has also been shown that the level of attention from an unfamiliar human trainer (looking at the horse versus looking away, or back turned towards the horse) affected the duration of a trained response (standing still in response to a verbal command), whereas the attentional state of a familiar person did not affect response duration (Sankey *et al.*, 2011). In a related study, it was reported that a horse's attentional state is important to its ability to learn the verbal command and that a horse's attention can be manipulated by the type of reward (food versus grooming) offered during training (Rochais *et al.*, 2014).

Other Factors that may Affect the Human–Horse Relationship
Other factors may affect the way horses react towards humans. For example, horses that are singly stabled and thus deprived of social contact are more likely to bite and kick human trainers during training than group-housed horses that have had plenty of opportunity for social interactions with other horses outside the training situation (Søndergaard and Ladewig, 2004) (Figure 3.7). This probably reflects re-directed motivation for social contact in singly housed horses and confirms that horses have a strong need for social contact with other horses (Søndergaard and Ladewig, 2004; Hartmann *et al.*, 2012). It has also been reported that horses with back pain are more likely to show aggressive behaviour towards humans than horses without back pain (Fureix *et al.*, 2010).

(a)

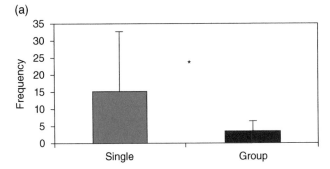

(b)

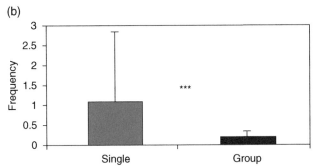

Figure 3.7 Singly stabled stallions are more likely to bite (a) and kick (b) humans during training compared to group-housed horses. This probably reflects their strong motivation for social contact. (Reproduced from Søndergaard and Ladewig, 2004).

It is important to be mindful that whatever we do to horses will affect our future relationships with them. Through the process of classical conditioning, horses readily learn to associate humans with both positive and negative events. If a horse has a series of pleasant experiences with a person, then, via the process of classical conditioning, this person is likely to evoke positive emotional responses in the horse. On the other hand, a person can also become associated with unpleasant events (e.g. a veterinarian who previously conducted a painful procedure, or a trainer who exposed the horse to harsh training procedures, punishment or unrelenting pressure). The formation of such negative conditioned emotional responses during training should be avoided, as it is both unethical and hampers further training (Chapter 6, Associative Learning (Aversive stimuli)).

Horsemanship and Horse-Sense

Is it possible to define good horsemanship? Generally, the word implies practices and skills without regard to learning theory. Its traditional focus has been on training and husbandry that encompassed knowledge of nutrition, conformation, reproduction, farriery and veterinary skills. However, the paramount importance of the deployment of learning processes in training the horse has been overlooked. Because of their love of traditional horselore, horse-trainers have been predictably slow in adopting new approaches (Warren-Smith and McGreevy, 2008a), in contrast to dog-trainers in this regard (Figure 3.8). There is an unfortunate expression: 'You can always tell a horseman; but you can't tell a horseman anything.' This implies that horsepeople are immune to new information but, in fairness, they could not expect to find the same trove of applicable psychology-based training principles that dog-trainers have access to. As previously discussed, horse-training cannot easily be food-based, especially during riding, and the study of training by negative reinforcement is still in its infancy.

Horsemanship tends to reflect detailed knowledge of functional patterns of behaviour typical to the species (Rees, 1997), and is more or less aligned with the correct application of learning theory, even if practitioners do not appreciate the significance of the science in their art. It covers a multitude of skills, including stable-management, horse-keeping and horse-training, but has recently been re-packaged

Figure 3.8 Results of a survey of Australian equestrian coaches (professional, *n* = 830) and dog-trainers (amateur and professional, *n* = 430), showing the distribution of correct, partially correct and incorrect explanations of key terms in learning theory. **Note**: The poor performance of equestrian coaches shown in this chart does not necessarily mean that they were less effective as coaches than dog-trainers, but it does imply that they bring less scholarship to learning theory and developments in training protocols.

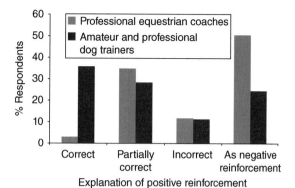

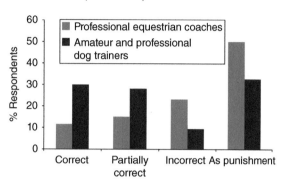

by proponents of so-called horse whispering and Natural Horsemanship. All are underpinned by that highly valuable commodity: horse-sense. Horse-sense is poorly defined but generally refers to the inherent way of being that some people have around horses. Their timing, sensitivity and resolve to pursue a training opportunity allow them to get the best out of their horses.

Horses also train us or, at least, the training process trains humans to modify their training behaviour (e.g. offering the correct response results in the trainer releasing the pressure or using a lighter cue next time). Sensitivity to such cues from horses is a critical element in good horsemanship. Excellent horse-trainers often struggle to describe what it is they do that makes horses respond well to them. From first principles, this must involve timing and consistency. That said, even with the best timing and consistency, some people fail to achieve calmness in horses and, given that calmness is a precursor to optimal training, these practitioners can never excel in training. It has been shown that horses can perceive a lack of relaxation

in their trainers (Figure 3.5), and this may manifest as decreased compliance (Chamove *et al.*, 2002). It is worth noting that there is a persistent belief that a special connection exists between women and horses (Midkiff, 2001) and that this allows them to train with less force than men use. Technological advances (such as those that measure rein tensions and leg pressures) should help to establish the validity of such claims.

Natural Horsemanship

The emergence of horse-whispering ideology represents a range of so-called Natural Horsemanship training techniques and an appealing message. Few horse-owners deny that harmony of horse and human is desirable, but many admit that it can be elusive. The appeal of direct communication between horses and humans is beguiling (Figure 3.9). Clever labelling of human–horse interactions may be designed primarily for educational purposes, but it can also make the interpretations of horse whisperers sound irrefutably plausible and humane. Unfortunately, such

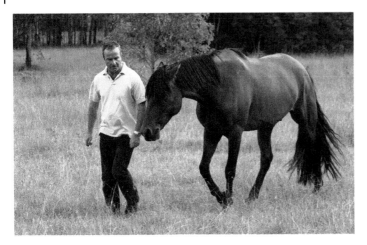

Figure 3.9 Many training methodologies feature the horse seeking to follow a human. This behaviour is a result of the innate tendency of a social animal to follow conspecifics. However, training horses to follow does not train them to be led and subsequent confusion can contribute to conflict behaviours.

labels can be misleading, contradictory and constitute potential barriers to effective training. They can also lead to misunderstanding, conflict and reduced welfare for human and equine participants. For example, some practitioners insist that horses in round-pens signal to their human trainers as they would to high-ranking herd-mates, and that they are motivated to be with those humans simply because they 'respect' them. In contrast, it is possible that horses in round-pens are showing distance-reducing affiliative signals that are being misinterpreted (Goodwin, 1999). However, recent empirical studies suggest that the responses of horses to humans in confined areas, such as round-pens, are context-specific (Krueger, 2007) and may rely more on negative reinforcement than on innate equine social strategies (Warren-Smith and McGreevy, 2008b; Henshall and McGreevy, 2014). These findings prompt us to question the interpretations of a horse's responses to round-pen interventions commonly offered by practitioners and to offer more scientific, measurable interpretations in horse-handling and training.

Dominance and Leadership

The application of dominance theory in the human-horse context implies that unwelcome responses can be explained by the horse trying to dominate the human and achieve higher social status. According to this doctrine, the human should strive for achieving superior high rank and take a putative leadership role to prevent and correct problem behaviour and achieve compliance (Hartmann *et al.*, 2017). Thus, some horsepeople believe that they must be the dominant part of the relationship and the horse the submissive one. Even if horses had a concept such as "top position" in a hierarchy, or that they were aware of the rankings of all members of the group, it is questionable whether that hierarchy would include humans (McGreevy *et al.*, 2009a). Given the complex social organisation of horses and the many factors determining social status within a group, the relevance of dominance theory is likely to be low. Within the group, horses may compete for resources but show no motivation for wanting to dominate others *per se*. Instead, they try to avoid conflict. In established social groups, individual members have learned which horses they can displace and which horses they should avoid during competitive encounters. This knowledge is likely to be based on a series of bilateral relationships, not according to some rank order of all group members. Thus, horses' social status usually only become evident during competition for resources, which is normally absent in a training context. The significant morphological differences between horses and humans also decrease the likelihood that horses would innately respond to human attempts to mimic horse behaviour, as discussed by Henshall and McGreevy (2014). Moreover, as recent results have shown, roles of leaders in groups of horses vary and those individuals acting as leaders may not necessarily occupy the highest rank in disputes over food. Horses, like other species, learn as a result of the reinforcement that follows a behaviour and not because they sense the social rank of the human nor her/his strong leadership skills (Figure 3.10). Therefore, becoming the quasi dominant leader of a horse may have little ethological relevance from the horse's perspective (Hartmann *et al.*, 2017). Anthropomorphism and the embedded appeal of fixed human hierarchies in the form of school, military and ecclesiastical institutions provide fertile ground for such dominance beliefs (McLean, 2013). Fundamentally, behavioural outcomes provided by learning theory furnish the most salient explanation of horse-human interactions.

A relationship based on trust, mutuality and cooperation are what many horse owners are hoping for (Birke and Hockenhull, 2015). Yet, during most work and handling from the ground, horses have negligible autonomy as humans assert control simply because of safety reasons. Attempts to dominate the horse to achieve control often encourage and justify the application of harsh training methods and punishment. Apart from the possible negative effect on the horse's welfare, the working relationship may also suffer. The natural response of a horse to an aggressive opponent is usually to avoid the individual by moving away. If the horse experiences the trainer as aggressive, its predominant motivation will be to avoid the trainer. Therefore, it is of paramount importance that trainers, riders and handlers do not appear aggressive, because this may trigger fear and avoidance responses in the horse.

Similar to horse training, traditional dog training relied on dominance theory for many decades, as it was assumed that dogs misbehave primarily because they are striving for high rank (McGreevy, 2009). This approach has been largely replaced by explaining undesirable behaviour from scientifically sound learning principles and emerged after leading canine ethologists re-evaluated studies on captive and free-ranging wolves and dogs, showing that individuals were not always fighting to gain high rank (Bradshaw *et al.*, 2009).

Similarly, given the complexity and various definitions of leadership in social sciences, using the term 'leader', if not clearly defined, can become blurred in a training context (Hartmann *et al.*, 2017). If horses could decide themselves whether to participate in training, perhaps the presence of peers would be more important than human company. Unless horses have been hand-reared or excessively

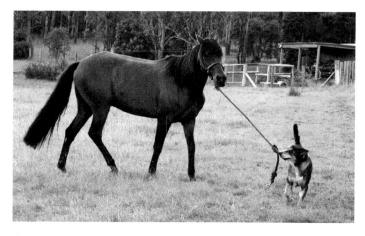

Figure 3.10 Conditioning rather than leadership qualities provides a more plausible explanation of leading behaviours. A horse will lead forward from pressure, even from a well-trained dog.

handled, they typically find conspecifics more salient than humans, which is mirrored in the separation anxiety related responses that are seen in horses when removed from herd-mates and their strong motivation to return to the herd (Jørgensen *et al.*, 2011; Hartmann *et al.*, 2011). This implies that they are not following humans to aversive places away from conspecifics just because they have bonded with the human and regard the human as a trustful leader. Instead, they are responding to operant cues, and in the absence of such cues (e.g. when a rider falls off) they most often return to the herd rather than remaining with the human. Furthermore, if leadership concepts from social sciences are applied at the human-horse interface, then there is the risk of over-estimating horses' cognitive abilities. Since leadership among humans reflects shared expectations and implies that the leader is acting intentionally, then the question arises whether horses are capable of understanding human intentions? Accepting this notion, then blaming horses for knowing what they have done wrong, or that they misbehave deliberately, adds an anthropomorphic label and runs the risk of abuse (McLean and McGreevy, 2010b).

Conclusion

The human–horse relationship is central to the safety of both humans and horses (Hawson *et al.*, 2010a; Thompson *et al.*, 2015). This relationship appears to be dependent on a variety of factors, including the horse's past experiences with humans, the emotional state of the human, and the level of attachment humans feel towards their horses (DeAraugo *et al.*, 2014). In addition, the human–horse relationship is likely to affect learning outcomes if the animal's attentional mechanisms are directed more towards one person than another. Since horses are sensitive to interpersonal contexts that have led to pleasant or unpleasant outcomes in the past, they appear to be good candidates for additional research in relation to attentional states and attachment theory (Brubaker and Udell, 2016).

It is unlikely that horse–horse social status translates to analogues of human-horse interactions, and the concepts of dominance and leadership as advocated in many training manuals proves to be unreliable in the horse as evidenced by several studies. Thus, horses' responses to training are more likely to be a result of reinforcement during which correct responses were clearly and consistently rewarded rather than a result of humans attaining high social rank and a leadership role. Knowledge of horses' natural behaviour and learning capacities are more reliable in explaining training outcomes than anthropomorphic explanations and the application of dominance and leadership concepts that can jeopardize horse welfare and human safety.

Take-Home Messages

- When applied to descriptions of horse behaviour, anthropomorphism is unhelpful and unreliable at best, and at worst, may promote poor welfare.
- There is no evidence that horses comply with human requests because of a 'willingness to please' or a desire to complete a shared goal.
- Horses do not appear to have an innate understanding of human auditory and visual cues.
- Horses can recognise individual riders and trainers and whether past interactions with those individuals were pleasant or unpleasant.
- The human–horse relationship is shaped by all past interactions and influenced by several factors, including human emotional states.
- Horses' responses to training are a result of reinforcement rather than a result of humans attaining high social rank and a leadership role.
- Knowledge of horses' natural behaviour and learning capacities are more reliable in explaining training outcomes than the application of dominance and leadership concepts.

4

Non-associative Learning

Introduction

In Chapter 2, we explored horse ethology and cognition. In this chapter, we will consider the general phenomenon of learning and focus on non-associative learning, which is generally referred to as the simplest form of learning. Non-associative learning comprises habituation and sensitisation. It is about reducing or intensifying a behaviour that is already present in the animal. As we will see, these forms of learning are more important in horse-training than we may imagine and they interact with learning and training at all stages. In addition, habituation of horses to various fear-eliciting stimuli is fundamentally important to both human and horse safety and welfare, and a number of desensitisation techniques are presented in this chapter.

Learning

One definition of learning is 'a process of adaptive changes in individual behaviour as a result of experience' (Thorpe, 1963). As a process, learning is not directly measurable; what *can* be measured is what has been *remembered* as a result of learning. In this way, learning is interlinked with cognitive processes, which refer to the mechanisms by which animals acquire, process, store and act on information from the environment. Cognition includes traits such as perception, learning, memory and decision-making

(Shettleworth, 2001). In scientific studies, an animal's ability to learn a specific task has often been used as a measure of cognitive processes (Figure 4.1). Humans generally make better subjects for learning studies than non-human animals because language facilitates communication. Human learning can be tested by recall, where the subject might recite what has been learned; or by recognition, where the subject recognises the correct answer from an array. Recognition is an easier task because the situation provides stimuli that trigger the memory to the correct answer. When we test an animal in a maze (Figure 4.1), we must rely on observing its behaviour as it traverses the maze. If the horse fails in the maze, we have no way of knowing whether its failure was a failing of learning or of recall, or a lack of motivation for the end-goal in the maze, so there *are* limitations in measuring learning.

Until the 1970s, animal-learning studies were dominated by the contributions of experimental psychologists. Behaviourism, founded by J.B. Watson, firmly established the laboratory rat and the pigeon as the standard species for learning studies. From this foundation sprang new schools of learning dominated by psychologists C.L. Hull, E.C. Tolman and B.F. Skinner, which focused on constructing a system of 'behavioural laws'. These laws were intended to predict conditions under which learning will occur. Following the work of these behaviourists, particularly Skinner, animals were trained,

Equitation Science, Second Edition. Paul McGreevy, Janne Winther Christensen, Uta König von Borstel and Andrew McLean.
© 2018 John Wiley & Sons Ltd. Published 2018 by John Wiley & Sons Ltd.
Companion website: www.wiley.com/go/mcgreevy/equitation

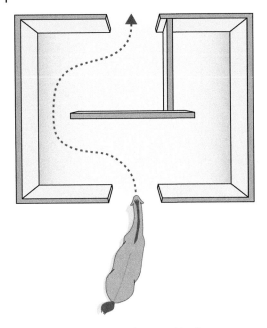

Figure 4.1 An example of a maze. Simple experiments, such as maze learning, allow us to study cognitive processes (e.g. recall). (Reproduced from *Equine Behavior*, copyright Elsevier, 2004.)

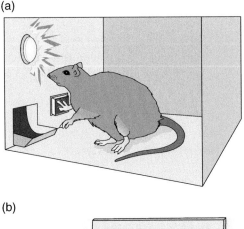

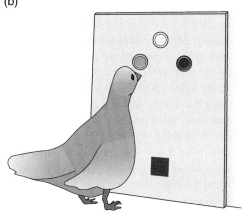

Figure 4.2 An illustration of a rat and a pigeon in so-called 'Skinner boxes', where animals work to obtain rewards such as food or freedom. Skinnerian principles have emerged largely from studies of just these two operant models: rats pressing levers (a) and pigeons pecking keys (b) to obtain rewards. (Redrawn with permission from Sandro Centini.)

not only in laboratories but also in zoos, aquaria and circuses, using these theories and exhibited performing routines featuring increasingly complex trained behaviours.

Early animal-learning studies focused almost entirely on two species, the rat and the pigeon (Figure 4.2). Despite this, when we consider how dissimilar phylogenetically these two species are, any evidence of parallels in learning infers that such abilities could also be expected in other mammals and birds.

After the 1970s, behaviourism fell out of favour for a couple of decades as a result of its purported rigidity as well as sociocultural factors of the era (Skinner, 1971; McLean, 2013). The behaviour of animals was seen to be more complex than the behaviourist models implied. The predominance of behaviourist theory was replaced with cognitive psychology. Behaviour was no longer seen simply as a product of reinforcement or punishment, but as a result of more complex agents. Rejecting behaviourism had both positive and negative implications for our understanding of learning. On the one hand, the rejection of simplistic approaches was an important step forward, but on the other, it resulted in studies of associative learning coming to a virtual standstill for some time. More recently, cognitive ethology has emerged, which is a multidisciplinary blend of behaviourism, cognitive psychology, neurophysiology, cognition and ethology. Shettleworth (2001) pointed out that a multidisciplinary approach is essential for real progress to be made in understanding the animal mind.

Some schools of thought in psychology share a central theme that learning follows some general laws that apply unequivocally in all situations. However, reviews by Seligman (1970) and Manning (1972) suggest that this assumption was too simplistic. Nevertheless, it is helpful to distinguish various categories of learning while keeping in mind that those categories may be arbitrary and seamless. The chief merit of such categories lies in their capacity to illuminate our understanding of learning processes. To this end, it is helpful to distinguish between two basic categories: non-associative learning and associative learning.

Non-associative Learning

Whereas associative learning describes the formation of an association between stimuli, non-associative learning, by contrast, occurs when exposure to a single stimulus results in either habituation or sensitisation. Both are fundamental to effective horse-training and are interconnected at almost every stage of training. Despite this, there has been little published research on the non-associative learning abilities in the horse (Nicol, 2002) until the recent work of Christensen (2007; 2013; 2016), Christensen *et al.*, (2006; 2008b; 2011c) and Leiner and Fendt (2011).

The Evolution of Habituation and Sensitisation

Central to evolutionary theory is the necessity for animals to exploit their environments optimally and their energy efficiency is of crucial importance. In short, it is a waste of precious energy to react to stimuli that prove innocuous and, on the other hand, it is critical to become sensitised to stimuli that predict predation, pain or injury. Thus, habituation and sensitisation are both adaptive processes that enable organisms to function effectively in their environments. Habituation is a form of learning in which an individual ceases to respond to a stimulus after repeated presentations. Animals are constantly bombarded with stimuli from the environment, and habituation is about learning which stimuli can safely be ignored; thus habituation is one of the most fundamental learning processes that allow animals to adapt to dynamic environments (Figure 4.3). For example, animals may habituate to repeated loud noises when they learn that these have no consequences. It should be remembered, however, that aside from learning, behavioural responses to a stimulus can also change because of motivational factors, physiological variables, sensory adaptation or fatigue, and these factors must be ruled out when the interest is in habituation as a learning process. Within equitation, horses habituate to diverse and dynamic aspects of the physical and social environment, and to the equipment used in training, as well as to having humans on their backs.

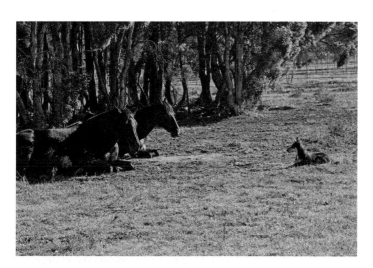

Figure 4.3 Horses can habituate to potential predators.

Sensitisation is the opposite process of habituation, whereby an individual enhances its response intensity. If an individual experiences an arousing stimulus, sensitisation describes the likelihood that it will respond more quickly or with more intensity to this or another stimulus that is presented soon after. Sensitisation is often characterised by an increase in response to a whole class of stimuli in addition to the original one. For example, pigeons that are exposed to painful stimuli (small electric shocks) become more responsive to loud noises (Siqueira *et al.*, 2005). It is worth considering that similar associations may arise in horse training, where horses exposed to painful or frightening stimuli show increased responses to both the original and other arousing stimuli.

Dishabituation, on the other hand, is the recovery of a habituated response. It describes the situation where the presentation of a stimulus, which differs from the one the animal has habituated to, results in an increase in the decremented response to the original stimulus (Rankin *et al.*, 2009). There is some discussion as to whether dishabituation is caused by sensitisation or by a disruption of the habituation process (Steiner and Barry, 2014; Schmid *et al.*, 2015). In horse training, dishabituation can explain the return of a previously decremented response.

Habituation and Desensitisation Techniques

Habituation is regarded as a prerequisite for all other types of learning, because it allows animals to filter out innocuous stimuli and focus selectively on important stimuli (Rankin *et al.*, 2009; Schmid *et al.*, 2015). For example, horses that live beside railway lines or airports can initially show a strong reaction, but this reaction may fade and trains or planes no longer elicit any response. This type of habituation happens without human interference, but there are also situations where habituation does not happen naturally – for example, because the horse is only occasionally presented with the stimulus or situation, such as during training.

Desensitisation techniques refer to the methods applied by humans to achieve habituation. Given the importance and implications of horses' fear reactions for human safety, surprisingly few studies have explored habituation to novel stimuli and the effects of different desensitisation techniques on horses. In one experiment, horses were negatively reinforced (through halter and rope pressure and gentle whip-tapping on the shoulder) to approach novel objects placed on the ground. These horses subsequently showed a shorter latency to approach the same objects, compared to control horses that had been free to explore, or avoid, the objects (Christensen, 2013). This suggests that motivating horses to come close to novel objects speeds up the habituation process, but the study also showed that this approach led to increased stress reactions in the horses (Christensen, 2013). It is therefore important to pay attention to behavioural signs of stress in the horse and decrease the intensity of the fear-eliciting stimulus and/or apply an appropriate desensitisation technique as described below, if the horse appears to become increasingly stressed during the procedure.

Horses are innately neophobic (fearful of the unfamiliar) and their behavioural responses are characterised by avoidance, ranging from a slight increase in distance from the frightening object to a rapid and powerful flight response. Avoidance is usually followed by alertness towards the stimulus and, finally, by investigative behaviours. The intensity and duration of the response varies from seconds to minutes and depends on the stimulus characteristics as well as individual differences in fearfulness, curiosity and prior experience (Lansade *et al.*, 2008; Christensen *et al.*, 2011c; Marsbøll and Christensen, 2015). This tendency of a horse to explore novel objects can also be exploited during desensitisation training; if the horse is allowed to keep a distance from the object of its fear, it may eventually show a natural motivation to approach (see the description of a desensitisation technique *Approach conditioning* below).

One important point to remember during training is that a fear response may be associated causally or coincidentally with the removal of the fear-provoking stimulus. Consequently, the response will be reinforced and thus it is likely to be repeated at future exposures. Also, if an arousing stimulus is removed *before* habituation occurs, the opposite process, sensitisation, may result. For example, if a horse avoids a novel object on the ground and thereby increases its distance from the object, the horse learns through negative reinforcement that avoidance is an appropriate response. The horse may therefore intensify the avoidance response and become more likely to show this behaviour the next time it discovers this or another novel object on the ground. Such responses may be difficult to eliminate if the horse is not given the opportunity to explore the stimulus and learn to tolerate it. If the horse's reaction is inconsistent with the threat posed by the stimulus, several desensitisation techniques can be employed to change such undesired responses. Four main techniques can be derived from the applied animal behaviour literature (McLean, 2008; Mills *et al.*, 2010).

Systematic Desensitisation

Systematic desensitisation is a commonly used behaviour-modification technique for the alleviation of behaviour problems caused by inappropriate arousal. The process in animals is an adaptation of a psychotherapy technique for humans (Wolpe and Lazarus, 1969). In a controlled situation, the animal is exposed to low levels of the arousing stimulus according to an increasing gradient, and rewarded when it remains relaxed or shows an appropriate response. An increase in the level of the stimulus is not made until the animal reliably fails to react to the previous level. In this way the technique aims to raise the threshold for a response. For example, police horses are often systematically desensitised to noise, smoke, flags, rapidly advancing people and objects (Figure 4.4).

Counter-Conditioning (Response Substitution)

Counter-conditioning (response substitution) refers to conditioning of an incompatible response to the undesired one, so that only the desired reaction occurs. The term literally means training an animal to show a behaviour that is counter to the one the trainer wishes to eliminate. The technique is widely used in combination with systematic desensitisation. By ensuring that the preferred behaviour is more rewarding, the animal

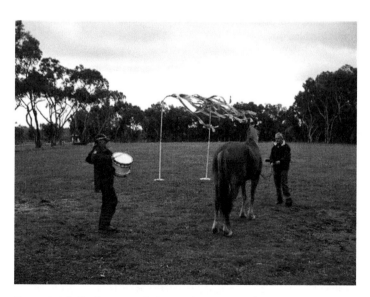

Figure 4.4 Police horses are habituated to a range of stimuli and situations that would normally elicit fear through systematic desensitisation.

learns to perform the new behaviour when exposed to the problem stimulus. In practice, the animal is presented with the problem stimulus simultaneously with another stimulus (e.g. food) that inherently arouses an alternative response (eating), which is counter to the underlying problem behaviour (fear reaction). Eventually the animal should learn that the problem stimulus is now a predictor of a pleasant (rather than aversive) event (Taylor, 2010).

Overshadowing

Overshadowing originally refers to the effect of two signals of different intensity being applied simultaneously, such that only the most intense/relevant will result in a learned response. For example, a trainer may wish to train an animal to respond to a verbal command but unintentionally uses a visual cue concurrently with the command; the animal may initially appear to have learned to respond to the command, but in fact it has not because the command was overshadowed by the visual cue. The term overshadowing has also been used to denote a desensitisation technique where habituation to a stimulus is facilitated by the simultaneous presentation of two stimuli that elicit an avoidance response (such as lead-rein cues and clippers

or a needle (McLean, 2008). As a desensitisation technique, the term describes the phenomenon whereby habituation to the least salient stimulus takes place when two or more stimuli that are competing for the same response are presented concurrently (McLean, 2008). Overshadowing is considered to differ from systematic desensitisation and counter-conditioning, principally because of the use of mobility responses (Figure 4.5).

Flooding (Response Prevention)

Flooding (response prevention) was originally developed to treat human phobias and was claimed to be more effective and less time-consuming than systematic desensitisation (Baum, 1970; Hussain, 1971). The aim of the procedure is to enable the individual to either habituate or learn an alternative appropriate response to the stimulus through the removal of reinforcement for the fear response (Hussain, 1971). The method consists of restraining the animal to remain in the situation it fears, until its apparent resistance ceases. In the original flooding procedure, there is no gradual habituation to the aversive stimulus. Instead, the animal is forced to endure the aversive stimulus at full intensity, usually for a protracted period. For elimination of the response to occur it is necessary

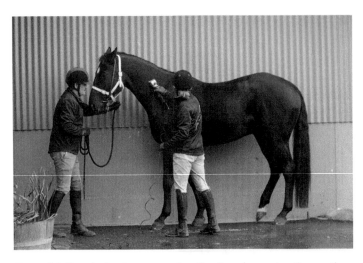

Figure 4.5 Overshadowing an aversive stimuli, such as noisy clippers, through the use of lead-rein pressure can be used as a desensitisation technique. The method should preferably be used in combination with systematic desensitisation.

that the stimulus is not withdrawn before cessation of the response occurs; if the animal remains in a state of heightened arousal and the stimulus is withdrawn, the response may be negatively reinforced and consequently strengthened. Such incorrect implementation of flooding is one of the significant risks of the procedure. Another cause for concern is that, if an animal is being restrained and exposed to uncontrollable aversion, learned helplessness may result. In this case, the animal will be apathetic and may superficially appear to tolerate the aversive stimulus, but its welfare is significantly compromised.

In practice, various desensitisation techniques often overlap and variations of elements from the above techniques can form the basis for other desensitisation techniques based on learning theory and equine ethology, which can be relevant in horse-training. Some examples of such additional techniques are described below and practical examples are given in Table 4.1.

Approach Conditioning

Approach conditioning exploits the natural tendency of horses to explore and approach unknown objects. The horse is stimulated by the trainer to approach the object of its fear while another trainer moves the object back as the horse approaches. In this way, the approach behaviour is negatively reinforced through the retreat of the object. In addition, the horse is less likely to perceive an object as threatening if it is slowly retreating. The horse is stopped before it closes in on the object so that the object retreats further, which will typically motivate the horse to approach again. The method has been successfully applied to horses that are afraid of tractors, diggers and motorbikes.

Stimulus Blending

Stimulus blending uses a stimulus to which the horse has already habituated to systematically desensitise the horse to the original fear-inducing stimulus. The fear-inducing stimulus is applied gradually and concurrently at the lowest threshold of fear together with the known stimulus, and then systematically increased in intensity. For example, a horse may be afraid of aerosol sprays but unafraid of being hosed (Figure 4.6). The aural and tactile characteristics of the problem stimulus (aerosol) are gradually mixed with the habituated one (the hose) making identification of the formerly aversive stimulus difficult and perceptually different. The old benign stimulus can then be diminished and finally terminated, after which the horse will show habituation also to the new stimulus.

As also noted above, the techniques can be highly overlapping and can be used concurrently (e.g. it is almost always beneficial to apply systematic desensitisation in combination with the other techniques). It is always important to consider the stress imposed on the horse; while one desensitisation technique may work appropriately with one horse in one situation, it may not be appropriate for another horse in the same situation, or for the same horse in another situation. Good trainers always evaluate the horse's responses and adjust their training method accordingly. For example, it may be necessary to decrease the intensity of the stimulus to achieve an appropriate response that can be rewarded.

The speed and likelihood of habituation depend on the nature of the stimulus, the rate of stimulus presentation and the regularity with which it is presented (Rankin *et al.*, 2009). It is important to continue presenting the stimulus to the animal regularly, well past the point of initial habituation. Ceasing the stimulus early can cause the fearful behaviour to return suddenly, in a process called spontaneous recovery (Marks, 1977). Even when the habituation is reliable, a prolonged absence of the stimulus can eventually cause the original response to return.

Habituation is easily confused with extinction. Habituation usually refers to a reduction in innate behaviour, rather than behaviour developed during conditioning, in which the process is termed 'extinction'. There are other behaviour-modification techniques, originating from human psychology that can also be relevant in horse-training. For example,

Table 4.1 Examples of desensitisation techniques (adapted from McLean and Christensen, 2017).

Technique	Example	Technique	Comments
Systematic desensitisation	The horse is fearful of aerosols and jumps away when the trainer attempts to apply the spray.	A solution in terms of systematic desensitisation is to initially stroke the horse on the body with the bottle without spraying. This is to habituate the horse to the visual characteristics of the aversive stimulus. When the horse shows no avoidance responses, a next step is to stand some metres from the horse and spray in the opposite direction, preferably with water (i.e. a fluid with no smell). This is to gradually habituate the horse to the aural characteristics of the aversive stimulus. The trainer gradually steps closer to the horse, and when the horse shows no response to the trainer standing next to it and spraying in the other direction, the trainer can gradually spray closer to the horse. Before spraying directly on its body, the trainer should stroke the horse with a hand and spray gently on the hand.	At all stages, it is important to ensure that the horse is only rewarded for appropriate responses (i.e. the aerosol should be briefly removed or spraying terminated when the horse stands still). Positive reinforcement (e.g. food, wither-scratching) can be used as an additional reinforcer for appropriate behaviour.
Counter-conditioning	The horse is fearful of objects on the ground. When the horse discovers, for example, a piece of plastic on the ground, it shows a strong avoidance response.	A solution in terms of counter-conditioning is to place some highly appreciated food on or next to the plastic, i.e. a stimulus that elicits desired responses – approach and eating that are counter to the undesired avoidance response. The horse should be free to explore the object and discover the food.	If the horse is frequently presented with objects on the ground, which all contain food, the horse is likely to learn that the original problem stimuli are now a predictor of a pleasant event. Instead of showing avoidance towards novel objects on the ground, the horse will be likely to expect a pleasant outcome and show approach behaviour.
Overshadowing	The horse is afraid of electric clippers. When the horse sees the person approaching with the clippers, it becomes hyper-reactive and pulls against the trainer's lead-rein tension to escape.	A solution in terms of overshadowing involves the horse being trained to step back and forward from lead-rein cues so that the horse's reaction is elicited from the lightest of lead-rein cues. Next, the person with the clippers approaches the horse and as soon as the horse displays even the smallest of fear responses, the person stops, so that the distance between the horse and the clippers stays constant. The horse is then signalled to step back one step and perhaps then forward a step. Initially the horse delays and does not react to light pressure because its attentional mechanisms are overshadowed by the clippers, so the trainer then increases the motivational pressure of the lead-rein so that in a few repetitions the horse is now responding to light signals of lead-rein. The horse's fear reaction to the clippers has, at this distance, decreased. The clippers are now brought closer to the horse and as soon as the horse shows the slightest fear reaction, the process is repeated. This process continues until the horse's response to the clippers has diminished.	Positive reinforcement enhances acquisition of the lowered arousal. The lead-rein signals and their associated mobility responses are likely to achieve control of the horse's locomotion and thus overtake the clippers for salience. The procedure is most successful if the process is begun at the lowest levels of arousal (McLean, 2008).

Method	Problem	Solution	
Approach conditioning	The horse is fearful of tractors, motor bikes or trams and attempts to escape to lower its fear.	A solution in terms of approach conditioning is to reverse the process whereby the horse approaches the retreating machine; this will usually lower the horse's fear because the machine itself escapes. In best practice, when the horse closes in on the machine the horse is stopped, thus allowing the machine to increase its distance from the horse. The horse is then stimulated to approach again and each time it draws closer to the machine before being stopped. Stopping the horse apparently increases its motivation to approach. This is continued until the horse actually makes contact with and investigates the machine.	Adding positive reinforcement for making contact with the machine will motivate the horse to show further exploratory behaviour.
Stimulus blending	The horse is fearful of aerosols and jumps away when the trainer attempts to apply the spray.	One solution is to blend a stimulus to which the horse has already habituated with the problem stimulus. If the horse is used to hosing on its body, the aerosol is introduced during hosing and on the hosed patches of skin. The sound and feeling of the usual water on the horse's body will blend with the novel sound and tactile feeling of the aerosol, making it less distinct. Eventually, hosing can be terminated while the spraying continues.	Spraying should start at a very low intensity and only gradually be increased when the horse reliably fails to react to the previous level.

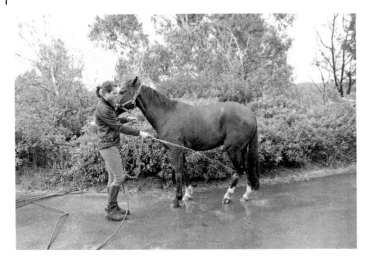

Figure 4.6 If a horse has habituated to hosing, this situation can be used to desensitise the horse to other stimuli, such as aerosols, through *stimulus blending*. The aural and tactile characteristics of the aerosol can be gradually mixed with the hosing making identification of the aerosol difficult, and the hose can gradually be turned off.

differential reinforcement describes the use of positive and negative reinforcement in a structured manner so that only the desired behaviour is reinforced, whereas extinction (i.e. discontinuing reinforcement of previously reinforced behaviour), is applied to other responses.

Desensitising Hypersensitive Body Regions

A biological characteristic of all species is that all traits show some variation, which is central to natural selection. The variation in sensitivity and subsequent learned reactivity of various parts of animals may have selective advantages in survival, because protection of vital body parts may result from subsequently learned reactivity. Hypersensitivity to tactile stimuli may be generalised across the whole body. We see that, alongside head-shyness, horses may show hypersensitivity around the thorax, flanks and legs. When contact with specific body sites elicits hyper-reactive withdrawal responses, there is usually an epicentre of heightened reactivity surrounded by a less reactive area (Figure 4.7). Reactivity positively correlates with proximity to that epicenter (e.g. in most cases of head-shyness, the horse's ears represent the epicentre of reactivity).

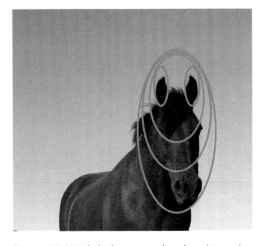

Figure 4.7 Head-shy horses tend to show increasing sensitivity towards an epicentre of the ears or a single ear.

Many trainers, particularly those skilled in behaviour modification, recognise the importance of maintaining the stimulus until some habituation has occurred. Let us consider the example of head-shyness further. Head-shyness is a reaction with a significant learned component (the reaction can become stronger), even though it is likely that there is also a genetic predisposition for such behaviour. The development of this reactivity is easy to imagine. The human unwittingly touches the young horse on or near the ear, which is immediately and rapidly withdrawn. This withdrawal response becomes faster and is reinforced by the removal of the human's hands (negative reinforcement), so the response becomes amplified and the withdrawal response becomes increasingly violent. The human hand touching even a formerly neutral site on the animal's head now elicits a violent withdrawal response. The horse is now sensitised to the tactile stimulus of being touched on the ear. If the trainer had not removed his or her hand in the first place, then habituation might have occurred. The sensitisation of the horse to the human hand occurs after the immediate removal of the hand. It is easy to see how neatly sensitisation processes dovetail with negative reinforcement. Resolution of head-shyness is discussed in Chapter 7, Applying Learning Theory.

Social Transmission of Habituation

Although horses do not appear to show social learning of complex tasks (e.g. Lindberg *et al.*, 1999; Ahrendt *et al.*, 2012; Rørvang *et al.*, 2015b), some studies have shown that in frightening situations there appears to be at least some transmission of information between individuals. Christensen *et al.* (2008a) found that naïve horses paired with a habituated companion horse showed reduced fear reactions towards a suddenly moving object, compared to naïve horses paired with an unhabituated companion horse (Figures 4.8a,b). The reduction in fear response remained three days later when the horses were exposed to the stimulus alone without their companion (Figures 4.8c,d). Similarly, Rørvang *et al.* (2015a) found that observation of a habituated demonstrator horse crossing a linen surface reduced heart rates of naïve observer horses when they subsequently had to cross the novel surface themselves. Studies have also been conducted at group level where only one horse was habituated in groups of four (i.e. one habituated demonstrator and three naïve group members). It appeared that if the habituated demonstrator was young (2 years

old), the naïve group members sometimes caused the previously habituated demonstrator horse to become dishabituated, whereas if the habituated demonstrator horse was old (7+) and the naïve group members were young (1–2 years old), the demonstrator reduced fear reactions in the naïve group members, compared to control groups with unhabituated demonstrators (Christensen, unpublished data). This suggests that the ratio of habituated to naïve horses as well as the age of the horses influence the likelihood of social transmission of habituation among individuals.

Recent research investigated the effect of habituating pregnant mares to various stimuli and allowing the mare to demonstrate her habituation to the foal in the first eight weeks of the foal's life during brief weekly demonstrations. This procedure led to the foals showing significantly reduced fearfulness towards a range of stimuli, including entirely new objects that were not present during the demonstrations with the mare, compared to control foals (Christensen, 2016) (Figure 4.9). This result accords with results from Henry *et al.* (2005), who demonstrated reduced fear of handling in foals after observation of their mother being handled during days 1–5 after birth. The same authors found that the effect was less pronounced if the mare-handling procedure was carried out 6 months after birth, indicating that maternal influence may be more pronounced at an early age (Henry *et al.*, 2007). In these experiments, the effect of maternal transmission was interlinked with the opportunity for individual learning in the foals during the demonstrations. In practice, it is not feasible to separate the effect of these two factors, and it is highly likely that a calm mare acts to facilitate individual learning because the foal will be more prone to approach the potentially frightening stimuli, whereas a nervous mare is likely to transmit her nervousness to the foal, which in turn will be less likely to approach and explore the stimuli (Christensen, 2016). These findings provide a promising potential for reduction of fearfulness in foals through maternal transmission of information at an early age.

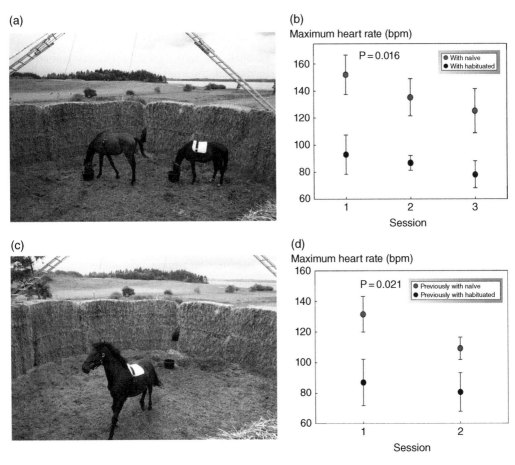

Figure 4.8 Young horses reacted less to a suddenly moving object (a plastic bag pulled up from the ground) when paired with a habituated companion horse, compared to when paired with a naïve companion horse (a). The graph (b) shows the maximum heart rate (beats per minute; mean and standard error) of the horses in the two groups during three subsequent stimulus presentations (session 1–3). This pattern remained when the horses were presented with the same moving object again three days later without companion horses (c,d). (Reproduced from Christensen *et al.*, 2008a).

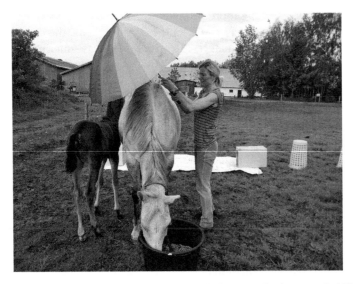

Figure 4.9 The dam is an important source of information for the young foal. The habituated mare can help decrease fearfulness in the foal if they are exposed to usually fear-eliciting situations together and the mare remains calm.

Habituation and Stimulus Generalisation/Discrimination

One phenomenon related to habituation is stimulus generalisation, i.e. when habituation occurs in response to other stimuli that share some similarities with the original stimulus. The opposing process, stimulus discrimination, describes the situation where habituation to other stimuli does not occur, i.e. only the reaction towards the original stimulus is affected. A few studies have investigated whether habituation to some objects is likely to result in reduced fear reactions towards other objects (i.e. whether habituation is generalised to other objects). Leiner and Fendt (2011) found that habituation to an umbrella did not affect horses' reactions to a plastic tarp. In another study, Christensen *et al.* (2008b) habituated horses to six differently shaped and coloured objects in a balanced order: the horses were presented with (and then habituated to) a novel object placed next to a familiar feed container in a known environment every day for six days. The horses showed no signs of stimulus generalisation and reacted with a similar intensity to object number six as to the first object (Figures 4.10a,b). In a second

(a)

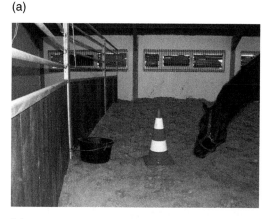

(b)

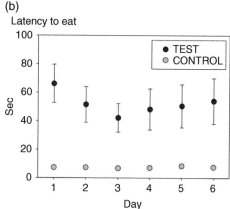

(c)

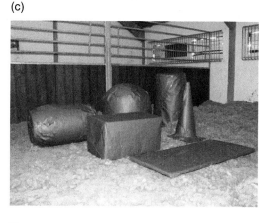

(d)

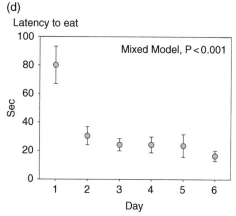

Figure 4.10 Horses do not appear to generalise between objects if these vary in both shape and colour (a, b). The graph (b) shows the latency (mean and standard error) for the test horses to eat from the familiar feed container on days 1–6; every day a novel object was presented in front of the container. Control horses also entered the test arena (without objects) and their latency times reflect the time taken to walk from the entrance of the test arena to the feed container. Test and control horses differed significantly within days, but there was no reduction in the latency time across days (i.e. test horses reacted with the same intensity to object number six as to object number 1). However, when the same objects were wrapped (i.e. all the same colour), the horses did show stimulus generalisation (i.e. their reaction towards new blue objects decreased significantly once habituated to one blue object (c,d)) (Reproduced from Christensen *et al.*, 2008b).

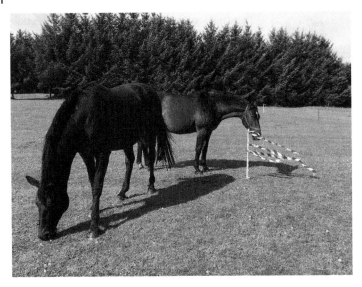

Figure 4.11 It may be possible to reduce general fearfulness in horses if they are routinely exposed in their paddock to various objects that usually elicit fear. The natural tendency of horses to explore objects in their home environment will eventually make them overcome their fear and they will habituate to the objects. It is usually possible to speed up the habituation process if food items, such as small pieces of carrot, are distributed around the objects.

part of the study, the authors wrapped the six objects in the same wrapping paper and found that horses showed stimulus generalisation already with the second presentation of a similarly coloured object. These results suggest that horses show stimulus generalisation only if there are sufficient shared characteristics between the objects (Figures 4.10c,d). This is an important aspect of habituation, which is very relevant in horse training (i.e. horse trainers should change only one variable at a time to provide the best opportunities for stimulus generalisation).

In a follow-up study (Christensen *et al.*, 2011c), horses were habituated to a range of objects simultaneously instead of one by one as in the previous study. It was found that this procedure led to stimulus generalisation as the habituated horses reacted significantly less towards a novel, differently shaped and coloured object compared to control horses. The result may relate to the level of stimulation that a horse experiences in its environment; once habituated to an environment with several objects, the horse may become less disturbed by the presentation of yet another object (Christensen *et al.*, 2011c).

Thus, it may be beneficial to stimulate horses in their home environment (e.g. by routinely placing novel objects, such as balls, secured tarpaulins, poles with flapping plastic tape and other non-harmful items) on the horses' pasture (Figure 4.11). The effect of such procedures on the general fearfulness of horses requires further study.

Habituation to Aversive Stimuli/Discomfort

The young horse must habituate to various equestrian paraphernalia, including the bit in its mouth (Figure 4.12). Restraint, and therefore low-intensity flooding, is frequently used when it comes to habituation to the bridle, saddle, saddle blankets, numnahs, covers, rugs and girth pressure. The girth constricting the thorax can represent a challenge to habituation in horse-training (see also Chapter 8, Training). Some horses respond with persistent hyper-reactivity when first girthed, and this reaction may reflect variations in thoracic sensitivity (McLean, 2003) (Figure 4.13). Horses exhibiting such behaviours are known as girth-shy. There are also claims that girth hypersensitivity is due to birth trauma, but there are no evidence-based data (double-blind trials and age-matched controls) to support this interesting possibility.

The horse must also habituate to the presence of a human on its back. During foundation training, the horse may be habituated to having a person above him (e.g. on a fence beside the horse), and instead of completely mounting the horse, the trainer may break this down into small stages, gradually getting higher and higher onto the horse's back. The trainer may stretch the desensitisation procedure out further and progress to lying along the horse, placing each leg on the horse's sides and then sitting up very gradually (Wright, 1973) (Figure 4.14). A typical desensitisation procedure would entail the rider repeatedly

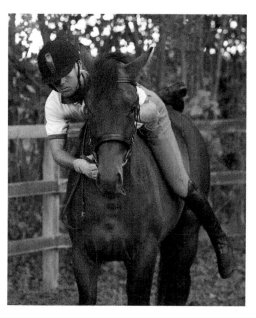

Figure 4.14 Mounting the horse bareback during foundation training is employed by some trainers. This has a number of advantages in habituating the horse to human body contact and separates it from the sometimes troubling girth/saddle experience with a human astride.

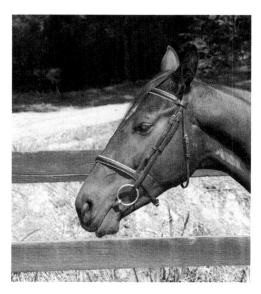

Figure 4.12 During foundation training, horses are expected to habituate to the bridle and the bit.

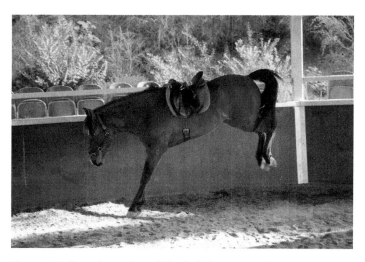

Figure 4.13 Some horses have difficulty habituating to the constant pressure of the girth. (Photo courtesy of Christine Hauschildt.)

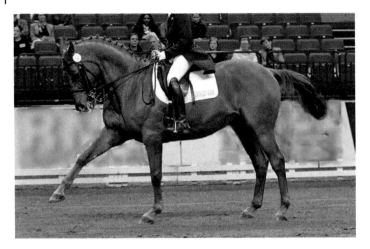

Figure 4.15 Horses are expected to habituate to a certain level of rein tension (called 'contact'). However, when exposed to strong inescapable tension, horses are likely to develop conflict behaviours and, in the worst-case scenario, learned helplessness (Photo courtesy of Minna Tallberg).

putting weight on one stirrup, then when the horse shows adequate habituation, quietly standing on that stirrup and holding the pommel (top front) of the saddle. Next, the rider swings his or her leg to the other side of the horse and when the horse has habituated to this activity, the rider may place his or her right foot in the stirrup and gradually begin sitting upright. At each of these stages, habituation has occurred when the horse no longer attempts to escape the primarily aversive stimuli and shows relaxation (McGreevy and McLean, 2007).

In most forms of equitation, the horse learns to respond to signals provided by the bit in its mouth and signals from the rider's legs (McLean, 2003). This is learned through the operant process of negative reinforcement (Chapter 6, Associative Learning (Aversive stimuli)), in which the removal of the aversive stimulus is reinforcing. Hence, in most equestrian codes, the bit and the rider's legs are not neutral signals. In other words, the horse must not habituate to these signals; if it does, conflict behaviours and stress may ensue. The terms *hard mouthed* or *dead sided* are used to describe horses that have, to some extent, habituated to the bit and rider's legs and possibly spurs. Habituation is a more plausible explanation than 'laziness' for sluggish or inadequate responses to the

rider's acceleration signals (McGreevy, 2004). Clinical experience suggests that habituation of the mouth results in more expressions of conflict (such as rearing, shying and hyper-reactivity) than habituation of the sides (McLean and McLean, 2008) (Figure 4.15). Because the problem is a result of human intervention rather than noncompliance of the horse, it has been suggested that the term habituation should be used in such cases (McGreevy and McLean, 2005). This is an example of the way in which the language of learning theory can make training more logical and accessible.

Repeated habituation to painful stimuli increases the likelihood of learned helplessness. For example, when riders resort to using ever-more-severe bits on horses that fail to slow appropriately, a process of progressive habituation may set in as the horse stops responding to lower/lighter pressures. While habituation to relatively innocuous tactile stimuli may not affect the animal's wellbeing, there is a point on the pain continuum where habituation may escalate into learned helplessness. This term, which describes an animal's apparent habituation to painful stimuli, is discussed further in Chapter 6, Associative Learning (Aversive stimuli). Similarly, when riders resort to using spurs because the horse fails to respond to the lighter leg signals, habituation and the possibility of a degree of learned helplessness may ensue. When a rider applies two or more signals at one time, such as the opposing signals of go and stop (legs and reins), habituation of one or both may occur. Again, learned helplessness may result from such a situation.

Contact

While optimal training requires that reins and leg signals should not become neutral, one exception to that rule occurs in the sport of dressage (including its offshoots, eventing and show-jumping). Here, some amount of bit and leg pressure *is* neutral. This, together with the seat, is known as *contact* (Decarpentry, 1949; German National Equestrian Federation, 1997; Hinnemann and van Baalen, 2003). Rider skill is critical here since the benefits of continuous contact, which relate to delivering subtle signals, may be outweighed by excessive, relentless tension and random hand movements. Current dressage practice requires that for all locomotion, including intra-gait and inter-gait transitions, the reins must be straight and the rider's legs must be in direct contact with the horse's thorax (German National Equestrian Federation, 1997). Recent research investigated the average rein tension applied by eight professional riders, riding three different horses each, in routine dressage training. The authors reported mean tensions at walk (short rein): 14–15 Newtons (N); sitting trot: 20–23 N, and sitting canter: 25–28 N (Eiser48 *et al.*, 2015). Christensen *et al.* (2015) reported mean tensions of 23–31 N applied by 10 professional riders, riding 10 horses each, in a 10-minute standard dressage competition programme containing medium-level exercises. Interestingly, König von Borstel and Glißman (2014) found that mean rein tension during performance testing differed significantly between test stations (9–22 N), suggesting that the training style of the head coach may influence the amount of force applied during riding. Newton (N) is the international unit measuring force. One Newton is about 0.22 pounds of force (lbf) or about 0.10 kilogram of force (kgf). Using kitchen-bench science, 20 N corresponds to the weight of a 2 kg bag of sugar. These reported mean tensions exceed the level of tension accepted by young, inexperienced horses in a voluntary test design (Christensen *et al.*, 2011b). Since horses can be trained to respond to very subtle cues, this highlights the need for further research to be conducted on the pressures applied to horses and, importantly, the subsequent education of riders and trainers so that horses are not subjected to unnecessarily strong pressures.

Sensitisation

The opposite process to habituation is sensitisation (i.e. an increase in the elicited behaviour from repeated presentation of a stimulus). Although it is generally regarded as a non-associative learning process, there are some examples of sensitisation described later that involve associated stimuli. This again shows the seamless and interactive nature of natural phenomena, and how they resist discrete labelling.

Unlike habituation, sensitisation evolved to ensure that animals paid attention to a variety of stimuli because of potentially dangerous consequences (Kandel, 2006). Some of these consequences reflect innate predispositions while others emerge from direct aversive experience, such as injury. Sensitisation may last from just a few minutes to the longer term, depending on the characteristics of the sensitising stimuli. Established learned responses can subsequently be enhanced by sensitisation or inhibited by habituation. Sensitisation plays a significant role in the ontogeny of behaviour problems (e.g. escape learning). A sudden aversive event can sensitise a horse to a previously innocuous stimulus (e.g. electric fences sensitise a horse to ordinary wire) (Figure 4.16). The faster the horse can escape the now-aversive stimuli, the more likely the escape reaction becomes. If a horse is hurt or

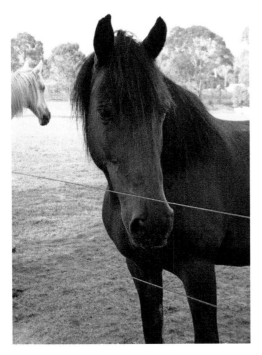

Figure 4.16 If a stimulus, such as an electric shock, is highly aversive, the horse may become sensitised to previously innocuous stimuli, such as an ordinary wire.

frightened inside a trailer, it learns to rush out of the trailer very fast. While shying frequently involves aversive classical conditioning (Chapter 6, Associative Learning (Aversive stimuli)), it can also arise when a previously innocuous stimulus becomes sensitised. A rabbit that suddenly scuttles from the bushes beside a letterbox can, if the horse's reaction is strong enough, sensitise the horse to the letterbox. Similarly, in Hong Kong, a sound is emitted from the apparatus of the starting gates just before they open. The racehorses sprint out and that escape sensitises them to the preceding sound.

Prior to foundation training, horses may offer no response to the rider's light signals from the reins and legs, so training involves the sensitisation of the horse to these signals. If the rider's timing is suboptimal, some horses may become dull to the signals as training proceeds. It is generally seen that it is more sensitive horses, those prone to

hyper-reactivity, that become dull to the stop response of the bit, and it is less sensitive horses that are prone to become dull to the rider's go signals. In both cases, the response must be retrained: generally, sensitive horses require sensitisation of the stop signal, while less sensitive ones are more likely to require sensitisation of the go signal. Here, it becomes clear that isolating sensitisation from negative reinforcement is impossible.

Imprinting and Early Handling

Imprinting is a form of learning in neonate animals at a highly sensitive time in their development, when they are receiving their very first stimulation from the outside world. It is considered a separate category of learning. The first to make systematic observations of this phenomenon was Spalding (1873), who reported that shortly after hatching, young chicks followed any moving object. However, it was Lorenz (1937) who made the topic popular among behavioural scientists. He described imprinting as a unique process in precocial birds characterised by a sensitive period outside of which the process was less likely to occur. During the sensitive period, 2- to 3-day-old hatchlings would imprint on a 'mother figure'. Typically, of course, this would be their actual mother, but Lorenz recognised that they would follow almost *any* moving object during their growth period. The tendency to follow any moving object made imprinting a popular practical ethology topic in universities throughout the world. Ethology students imprinted chicks onto all sorts of moving inanimate objects such as themselves or moving balloons. Lorenz described imprinting as a rigid phenomenon that was irreversible and determined future mating partners. Indeed, birds hatched by other species have been shown to court and attempt to mate with the foster species.

With horses and other mammals, it is questionable whether imprinting occurs. Miller (1991) suggested that the sensitive period for foals is within the first 48 hours of life when the 'following response' is developed.

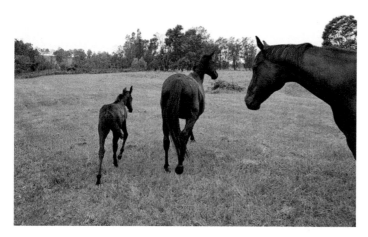

Figure 4.17 Dr Robert Miller's contention that a young foal can imprint onto humans is based on his interpretation of its neonatal tendency to follow its mother.

The foal apparently learns to follow its mother, which is usually the nearest large moving creature in its world (Figure 4.17). Miller not only described imprinting as a process in foals but also introduced the prospect of *Imprint Training*, in which the foal is handled intensively shortly after birth, in the belief that this procedure should reduce the prevalence of aversive reactions as well as sensitise the foal for pressure release (Miller, 1991; 2001). However, most scientific evidence suggests that Imprint Training does not correspond to any natural analogue and that the foals frequently resist strongly and endure high levels of stress while undergoing Imprint Training (Diehl *et al.*, 2002; Sigurjonsdottir and Gunnarsson, 2002). In addition, Henry *et al.* (2009) found that foals handled according to the Imprint Training procedure for one hour after birth showed patterns of insecure attachment to their mothers (strong dependence on their mothers and less play behaviour) and impaired social competences (increased social withdrawal and aggression) at all ages. It is unlikely that the early stress imposed by the Imprint Training procedure, and the associated short- and long-term consequences on social behaviour, can be justified in terms of later benefits (Hausberger *et al.*, 2007b). For example, Williams *et al.* (2002, 2003) reported that when foals were handled at birth and/or

12, 24 and 48 hours after birth, there was no beneficial effect on their later behaviour when tested at 1, 2 and 3 months of age (Williams *et al.*, 2002) or at 6 months of age (Williams *et al.*, 2003).

Distinguishing among the benefits of habituation, any equine analogue of filial imprinting (as described in birds) and the more radical elements recommended by Miller (1991; 2001) is far from simple. So, it is not surprising that some studies have shown some positive effects of Imprint Training. For example, foals handled early tend to approach familiar humans (Simpson, 2002) and accept having their feet lifted (Spier *et al.*, 2004) more readily than unhandled ones. That said, acceptance of aversive stimuli was not facilitated by Imprint Training. Fitting halters or clipping was just as traumatic for handled foals as for unhandled foals at 3 or 4 months of age (Simpson, 2002; Williams *et al.*, 2002; Spier *et al.*, 2004). Significantly, imprinted foals without regular handling were as difficult to approach as controls (Sigurjonsdottir and Gunnarsson, 2002). Some of the studies on Imprint Training have been summarised by Houpt (2007), as shown in Table 4.2.

Research on the effects of handling after the putative sensitive period also suggests only transient benefits (Lansade *et al.*, 2005). While Mal *et al.* (1994) showed no beneficial effects

Table 4.2 Results of imprint training.

Imprint age	Repetitions	Test	Age of	References
14 days	Until 24 weeks	Hoof[a], lead[a], approach[a]	6, 12, 18, 24 months	Jezierski *et al.* (1999)
24 hours	Daily for 42 days	Halter, lead[a]	85 days	Mal and McCall (1996)
6 hours	Daily for 14 days	Halter[a], hoof, lead[b]	16 days, 3 months, 6 months, 1 year	Lansade *et al.* (2005)
10 minutes	24 hours	Restrain, halter, worm, vaccinate, hoof[a]	90 days	Spier *et al.* (2004)
Birth	Daily for 7 days	Approach responses to stimuli	120 days	Mal *et al.* (1994)
2–8 hours	Daily for 5 days	Approach stimuli[a]	4 months	Simpson (2002)
45 minutes	12, 24, 28 hours	Approach stimuli	1–3 months	Williams *et al.* (2002)

Source: Adapted from Houpt (2007), with permission from Elsevier.
a Significantly better than non-handled.
b Three-month results.

when foals were handled during the first 7 days, later research showed that when handled in the same way (stroking, haltering, picking up feet) at 14 days of age, the foals at 3 months were more tractable than non-handled foals. However, when tested at 6 months of age, there were fewer differences between handled and unhandled foals, and by 1 year of age there were no differences at all (Lansade *et al.*, 2004).

Heird *et al.* (1986a) and Lansade *et al.* (2004) reported higher trainability and easier handling, respectively, of foals handled regularly from weaning. Similarly, Hausberger *et al.* (2007b) suggested that the beneficial effects of early handling rely on regular repetitions of handling. Handling foals 5 days per week (tasks included catching, leading, picking up feet, grooming and being approached by an unfamiliar human) until they are 2 years of age results in improved manageability at 12, 18 and 24 months compared with unhandled foals (Jezierski *et al.*, 1999). However, the optimal time for handling seems to be at weaning and this should be followed up with regular handling. This would reduce the chance of interfering with the mare–foal bond, which presents a significant risk in Imprint Training (Henry *et al.*, 2009).

Hausberger *et al.* (2007b) concluded that there is no clear evidence in foals for the existence of a sensitive period in development, which may facilitate the establishment of a foal–human bond. It is appropriate to reflect on the direct benefits for the foals themselves of being near humans. What's in it for them? Especially prior to weaning, they seem to find being scratched highly reinforcing, but Søndergaard and Halekoh (2003) proposed that unhandled 2-year-olds become as familiar as handled animals, probably because humans bring food. As Hausberger *et al.* (2007b) point out, the affiliative qualities of human–horse interactions may be more important than *when* the interactions occur. The reactions of the mare during handling also have an impact on the foal's behaviour. Sigurjonsdottir and Gunnarsson (2002) found a positive correlation between the mare's nervousness and the imprinted foal's resistance to capture, haltering and leading at the age of 4 months. In short, they showed that the calmer the mare, the easier the foal was to handle. This finding could simply reflect the inheritance of flightiness or social transmission. Henry *et al.* (2005; 2006) showed that forcible handling of foals (e.g. where they have been coercively brought to the mare's teat) tended to result in reluctance to approach humans later. On the contrary, a passive human presence tended to induce less flight response than in controls, although the effects were short-lived. As discussed in a previous section, more direct activities such as brushing and hand-feeding of the mare in the presence of the foal have been shown to have a positive effect that may last for some time (Henry *et al.*, 2005). Foals handled in this way have been shown to be more easily approached in the paddock and stroked by a familiar or unfamiliar human a year later, without any handling in the interim. This contrasted with controls that showed greater resistance to capture and to the presence of humans. Hausberger *et al.* (2007b) concluded that establishing a positive human–dam relationship may therefore be an important key to durably enhance the manageability of foals. Of equal importance is establishing clear and consistent interactions with the foals themselves, and as far as training is concerned, to use techniques that fully align with learning theory and, particularly, to time pressure release accurately (Figures 4.18 and 4.19).

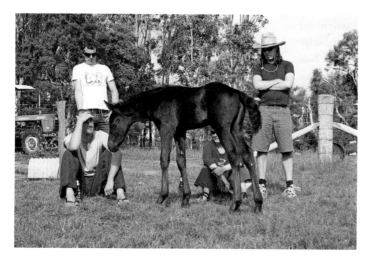

Figure 4.18 It is important to reflect on the effect of the foal's first experiences with humans.

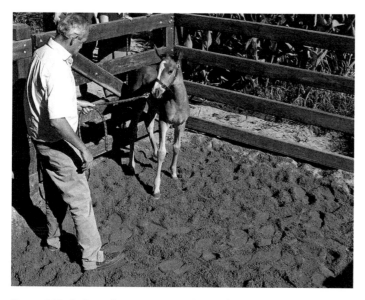

Figure 4.19 Perhaps the greatest contribution from Dr Robert Miller is the assurance that as a precocial neonate, some training, such as lead training, can begin early in the foal's life. This can help ensure safety when veterinary attention is required.

Take-Home Messages

- Non-associative learning occurs when exposure to a stimulus results in either habituation or sensitisation. Both are fundamental to effective horse-training and are interconnected at almost every stage of training.
- Appropriate desensitisation techniques can help the horse to overcome innate fear of various stimuli and situations in the training environment.
- Social transmission of habituation may occur in horses, and mares are especially likely to affect the behaviour of their foals.
- Habituation may also explain the undesired process in which horses decrease their reactions to tactile stimuli such as bit and leg pressure after poor application of pressure or timing or both. Habituation, or learned helplessness, is a more plausible explanation than 'laziness' for sluggish or inadequate responses to the acceleration/deceleration cues.
- When a rider applies two or more signals simultaneously, such as the reins and the legs, habituation of one or both may occur. This is undesirable for both rider safety and horse welfare.

Areas for Future Research

A particularly promising area of research is the possibility to modulate foal behaviour through maternal transmission and further research is required in this area. Since fear reactions are a common cause of horse–human accidents, further studies on desensitisation techniques are also required.

There is also a need for further research to be conducted on the pressures applied to horses via bit, legs, seat and spurs and, importantly, the subsequent education of riders and trainers so that horses are not subjected to unnecessary pressures.

5

Associative Learning (Attractive Stimuli)

Introduction

In order to survive, animals learn to tailor their responses to environmental changes. The way they learn about feeding is a fundamental example. From the first minutes of life, a foal learns the cues that help it to find milk. Its performance in acquiring the teat rapidly improves as long as it is rewarded by milk in its mouth. By learning to avoid pain and discomfort, an animal can make its life more pleasant. Even invertebrates, such as flies and slugs, show advanced forms of learning when avoiding unpleasant stimuli. When animals cannot evade pain or aversive stimuli, they become distressed. We manipulate animals' experience to train them, so there is a huge onus on trainers to keep any distress involved to an absolute minimum.

As the term suggests, associative learning involves an animal experiencing events or stimuli in close association in either time or space. There are two types of associative learning (or conditioning): operant (or instrumental) and classical (or Pavlovian). Broadly speaking, in the context of horse-training, links between two or more signals result from classical conditioning, while links between signals or horses' actions and outcomes develop because of operant conditioning.

Operant Conditioning

An operant response is a voluntary activity that brings about a reward or allows an animal to avoid an aversive outcome, such as punishment. In operant conditioning, the animal must operate within its environment to get what it wants. The learned link between the behavioural response and the reward is what learning theorists call a contingency. This sort of learning underpins most horse-training. The horse must offer a particular response to get the reward. To some extent, the horse can choose whether to respond appropriately or not, so operant conditioning increases the horse's control of its environment.

To study the principles of operant conditioning, US scientist, Edward Thorndike (1911), focused on the behavioural responses of cats in so-called puzzle boxes. The cats were left in a box without food and water (Figure 5.1). They wanted to leave but had to undergo trial-and-error learning to escape. Within the box was a lever that, when pulled, released the catch and allowed the cat to get out. Let us break this down into its constituent elements: to solve this problem, the cat had to see the lever (*the cue*) and pull it (*the operant response*) to obtain liberty (*the reward*). Every operant response has these three core elements. They are referred to as

Equitation Science, Second Edition. Paul McGreevy, Janne Winther Christensen,
Uta König von Borstel and Andrew McLean.
© 2018 John Wiley & Sons Ltd. Published 2018 by John Wiley & Sons Ltd.
Companion website: www.wiley.com/go/mcgreevy/equitation

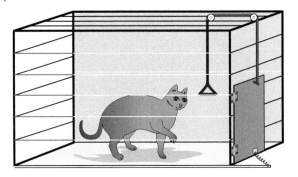

Figure 5.1 A cat in a puzzle box must trial the use of a lever (i.e. *make an instrumental change*) to access its reward (*liberty*). (Redrawn with permission from Sandro Nocentini.)

the operant contingency. Consider a horse that has sensed its rider's leg pressing against its side (*the cue*). The horse moves laterally leg-yielding (*the operant response*) and, if the rider behaves appropriately, is relieved of the irritant pressure on its side (*the reward*). Thorndike referred to this kind of learning as 'trial-and-error learning with accidental success'. At the time, it was widely believed that animals must understand a problem to solve it. Thorndike's investigations blazed the trail for animal learning studies in operant conditioning and provided a model that is of tremendous use when we think about any horse faced with a challenge during training.

Operant or instrumental conditioning consists of presenting or omitting some reward or punishment when the animal makes a specific response (Kratzer *et al.*, 1977). The effect of the reward is to strengthen the likelihood of a correct response being offered again. This strengthening is called reinforcement – the term refers to the process in which a reinforcer follows a particular behaviour so that the frequency (or probability) of that behaviour increases. The relationship between the first event and the second makes an association possible; the links between the two are called stimulus–response–reinforcement chains.

In general, the kind of learning produced by a response–reinforcer relationship, or *contingency*, is now called *instrumental conditioning* since it applies to any procedure in which a response is 'instrumental' in obtaining a reinforcer. In the 1930s, Skinner studied the effects of response–reinforcer relationships on the behaviour of rats and

developed a novel research tool that permitted a major leap forward in the study of instrumental conditioning. His experimental chamber, the now-famous Skinner box, had three main components: something the animal could operate, a *manipulandum* (usually a lever); a means of delivering reinforcers in the form of small food pellets; and a stimulus source, such as a light or loudspeaker, that could be used to signal to the animal a particular response–reinforcer relationship. Using a Skinner box, the experimenter did not have to intervene each time the animal received a reinforcement. Skinner called the response–reinforcer relationships he studied in this chamber *operant conditioning* (Skinner, 1938), since the behaviour 'operates' on, or makes changes to, the animal's environment. So, operant conditioning is a type of instrumental conditioning.

Operant conditioning in the horse has been studied under two sets of experimental circumstances: 'discrete' trials and 'free operant' trials. Discrete trials involve exposing the horse to the learning task, requiring it to make a response and then withdrawing it from the situation. For example, a horse may be led into a simple T-maze and then must choose one of two directions, left or right. In contrast, a free operant involves allowing the horse to operate freely in its environment. For example, it may be led to a paddock and released to do whatever it likes, and then trained by reinforcement of whatever responses it happens to offer. Horses such as those that open their stable doors or dunk their own hay are good examples of free-operant conditioning: they work within their environment to acquire a reward.

It is not difficult to see that learning about the environment and how to make rewards appear will enhance a horse's *umwelt* (Chapter 2 Ethology and Cognition). But, if the contingencies are unreliable and the horse's expectations are not met, we see signs of conflict reminiscent of experimental neurosis. Several studies suggest that lack of control over aversive events can bring about major behavioural and physiological changes (Wiepkema, 1987). For example, after being exposed to uncontrollable electric shocks, rats develop increased gastric ulceration, increased defaecation rates and are more susceptible to certain cancers when compared with individuals that retain control over comparable shocks (Moberg and Mench, 2000). Furthermore, training animals to expect enrichments that are associated with specific cues can increase their anticipation and play (Dudink *et al.*, 2006).

A trained response can tell us a great deal about not just the trainer but also the animal. If all the training is the same and there are differences in the performance of the response from one animal to the next, we can be fairly confident that the motivation of the animal is the chief cause of the difference. This is exciting because we can use this principle to let animals tell us what they want. Operant devices can be used to determine the preference animals have for certain environmental variables. As noted in Chapter 2, Ethology and Cognition, horses can easily be trained to use operant devices in consumer-demand studies. Some have been trained to break photoelectric beams to turn on lighting in their accommodation and, using this device, have demonstrated a preference for an illuminated environment (Houpt and Houpt, 1988). Others have been trained to nuzzle buttons (Figure 5.2) or levers to access resources, such as different levels of social contact (Figure 5.3; Sondergaard *et al.*, 2011).

Training generally means drawing out desirable behaviours and suppressing undesirable innate behaviours. In training horses, we must exploit their need as prey animals to avoid discomfort and, indeed, threats of discomfort. Generally, we apply pressure to

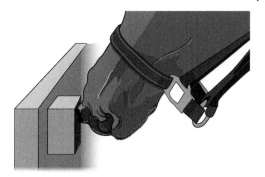

Figure 5.2 A horse nuzzling an operant device to turn on a light.

attain the desired response and remove it when we get the response we want. As we will see, delaying the removal of pressure is appropriate only when we are pushing the horse to try harder; in other words, when we are shaping an improved response (see shaping in Chapter 7, Applying Learning Theory, and Chapter 8, Training).

The aim of training is to install signals that elicit predictable behaviour patterns. For a response to be regarded as being under *stimulus control*, it must satisfy two requirements. First, it must be offered reliably after every presentation of the stimulus (cue) and, second, it must be offered *only* after the cue. At this point, the cue is known as the discriminative stimulus.

There are two main ways to train a discrimination using positive reinforcement: *simultaneous discrimination* and *successive discrimination*. In simultaneous discrimination training, the horse is presented with two or more stimuli at the same time and is rewarded only if it responds to the correct stimulus. In contrast, in successive discrimination training, the differing stimuli are presented to the horse at different times. The trained horse's task includes being able to discriminate not only between general grooming pressures and the trained signals, but also between one trained signal and the next.

A similar approach to discrimination training is called *fading*. This is intended to ensure that few, if any, responses are made to any

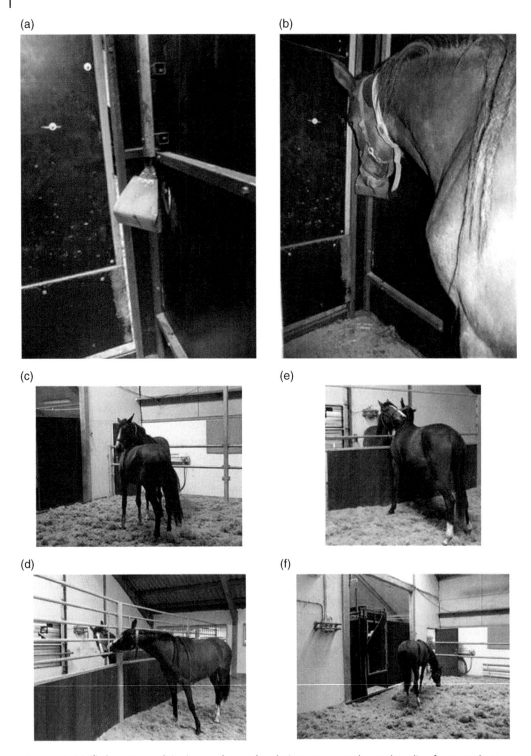

Figure 5.3 (a)-(f). Operant conditioning can be used to design consumer-demand studies, for example, to assess the relative value horses place on different levels of social contact versus social isolation. (a) lever; (b) horse operating the lever; (c) free social interaction possible; (d) social interaction restricted to head-and-neck region; (e) social interaction limited to nasal contact; and (f) social isolation. (Sondergaard *et al.*, 2011).

stimulus other than the discriminative stimulus. If successful, it leads to *errorless learning*. The aim is to reduce the number of errors a horse makes. There are two basic sequential steps in fading: the first step is to train the horse to respond to the discriminative stimulus (critical cues) rather than other stimuli; the second step is to gradually introduce the similar stimulus, or stimuli, that the animal is being trained *not* to respond to. The emphasis here is on gradual introduction. The duration and intensity of similar stimuli must be very gradually faded into the animal's perception. An example occurs in police horse-training, where the horse is trained to attend to the rider's signals, not stimuli coming from people on foot. Once basic distracting stimuli on the ground have been successfully faded, the rider's signals are gradually magnified.

Training horses, whether under-saddle or in-hand, stabled or in the paddock, basic, advanced or remedial, involves operant principles. Before giving a reward, the trainer must wait until the animal produces the desired activity. Rewarding the desired behaviour relates to the law of effect, which states that the behaviour immediately preceding reinforcement will be strengthened. When the association between pressure, response and timely release becomes highly predictable, a habit emerges. If a habit does not develop, the horse may have learned, for example, through incorrect timing of pressure-release, that it cannot offer any response that reliably causes the pressure to be released. Unfortunately, there are many horses in all spheres of ridden and draught work that have developed such apathy and lack of responsiveness. They are often unfairly labelled as dull or stubborn (Chapter 12, Unorthodox Techniques).

The changing role of the horse in developed countries, at least, demands a greater emphasis on humane treatment and more research into horse education. In this context, prevention is better than cure, so correct foundation training of naïve horses is generally preferable to re-training animals with inappropriate experience. There is certainly less detraining

(unlearning) to do and one of the ways in which this manifests is with less frustration. All animals that have learned to expect relief from pressure by adopting a certain unwanted response will eventually stop when the rewards are removed. However, most will show *more* of the response before it disappears completely. For example, a horse that has learned to obtain relief from rein tension by head-tossing may initially try even harder to obtain this relief by the previously successful action of head-tossing; even if subsequently trained by a skilled trainer who maintains a certain degree of rein tension at all times to teach the horse that head tossing is not the desired response to rein tension.

If an animal is exposed several times to a conditioned stimulus before structured conditioning commences (i.e. before reinforcement), its acquisition of a conditioned response to that stimulus will be retarded. An example is a horse that is habituated to sustained pressure on its sides before being trained to produce a locomotory response. The horse has simply learned to ignore the pressure because it has no important consequences.

All therapeutic behaviour-modification programmes identify the motivation, remove the rewarding aspects of the unwelcome behaviour and reinforce a more appropriate alternative. If the strategy does not work, the most common explanations are either that training has been insufficient to establish the new associations or that the reinforcement for the new response is insufficient to overcome gratification from the existing behaviour.

Classical Conditioning

Classical conditioning is the acquisition of a response to a new stimulus by association with an old stimulus. From the outset, it requires a stimulus that evokes an innate or learned physiological or behavioural response. Also labelled Pavlovian conditioning, it has its origins in the studies of gastric physiology conducted by Ivan Pavlov, who spotted his experimental dogs salivating when they heard his technician tinkling a bell as he approached the kennels to feed them (Pavlov, 1927). Determined to establish how accurately dogs could develop these associations, Pavlov replaced the sound of the bell with more easily varied sounds made by a buzzer and then a metronome. To measure the rate of saliva production, Pavlov surgically implanted a tube into the dogs' cheeks and used saliva flow and volume as a measure of the association between the novel cues and the food.

Pavlov linked a novel stimulus (*the buzzer*) to a physiological stimulus (*food in the mouth*) and response (*salivation*) (Figure 5.4). The dogs quickly began to salivate in response to the buzzer, a new stimulus that had previously been irrelevant or neutral. The labels Pavlov created for the elements in this process are still used today. Before the learning experience, only meat powder, the *unconditioned stimulus* (US), produced salivation as an *unconditioned response* (UR). After learning, the buzzer became a *conditioned stimulus* (CS) and the salivation response to the conditioned stimulus became the *conditioned response* (CR, also known as the learned response).

The sound of a buzzer was consistently followed by the delivery of food to the mouth, regardless of what the dog might have done when it heard the buzzer. This is of critical importance in understanding the difference between classical and operant conditioning. Classical conditioning enables the animal to associate events over which it has no control. This increases the *predictability* of an environment. In operant conditioning, the animal operates within its environment to get a reward or avoid punishment and so makes the environment more controllable. The more frequent and consistent the pairing of the neutral stimulus and the unconditioned stimulus is, the more rapidly the association develops. In some cases, usually involving the most critical pain or pleasure, the association is formed with a single experience (Lieberman, 1993).

There are numerous examples of classical conditioning in the horse world. Most stud managers will agree that stallions become aroused when they hear the sound of a particular bridle, if it is the one used to control them in the breeding barn. Racetrack grooms use classical conditioning when they whistle each time they see their charges urinating (Figure 5.5). Once the association between the whistling and urination is made, the horses urinate on cue for post-race urine tests (Chapter 7, Applying Learning Theory).

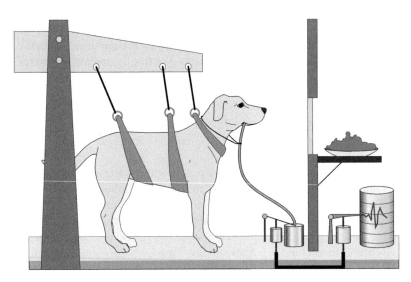

Figure 5.4 Pavlov's apparatus for collecting saliva as a measure of the association between food and various novel stimuli.

(a)

(b)

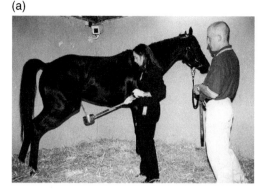
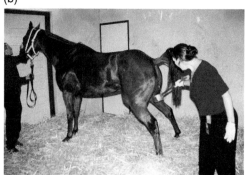

Figure 5.5 Post-race urine samples being taken on cue from a gelding (a) and a mare (b).

Some horse-trainers use it to pair verbal praise (which, of course, means nothing to a naïve horse) with an inherently rewarding outcome, such as food. The strength of associations that are built in this way can be assessed by the extent to which horses will work for these learned rewards. If the associations between primary and secondary rewards are too loose, the quality of the animal's performance will decline, because of a process called extinction. Pavlov found that if a CS, such as the sound of a metronome, was paired with food as a US, it would continue to make the dog salivate just as long as the CS continued to be followed by the arrival of food. If the buzzer was sounded again and again but food no longer arrived, then *extinction* resulted in the disappearance of salivation to the tone. Extinction can apply to all examples of classical conditioning.

Riders use classical conditioning when they replace hand or leg pressure cues with previously neutral signals, such as changes in their position or movement of their seat. Although changes in the rider's position may, to some extent, produce desired responses naturally (as suggested by some riding theories) and without the need for the horse to learn, as the horse, for example, steps to the side to regain balance that was disturbed by the rider's change in position, most riders will agree that it is difficult to train a horse to *stop* from the seat alone. Instead, you must train a *stop* response with an unconditioned stimulus from the rein and then link it with a specific cue from your seat (CS, e.g. bracing against the action). Trail-riding operators sometimes do the same with a whistle (CS) that is linked to bilateral rein signals (US) as a means of stopping horses in an emergency should novice riders lose control. Training responses to a piece of string around a horse's neck is largely the product of a similar approach (Figure 5.6b). The critical skill in training a classical conditioned association is to ensure that the links are made frequently because the associations will not last indefinitely. In a study that used classical conditioning to fear-condition horses for research purposes to a specific tone, three sessions of nine associations between the CS and the US (various moderately frightening stimuli, such as a ball thrown at the horse or a popping balloon) were sufficient to produce elevated heart rates in response to the CS alone for up to eight days after the last training session (von Borstel, 2008). Nevertheless, there are limited scientific data available on minimum requirements for classical conditioning to occur in horses, and it may well be that fewer sessions would have been sufficient, or that the association lasted for more than eight days. In building associations, it is important to present the CS before or at the same time as the US. Presenting the CS after the US leads to no association, simply because this order of events cannot increase the predictability of an environment.

A particularly useful variant of classical conditioning is called *counter-conditioning*, a

(a)　　　　　　　　　　　　　　　　(b)

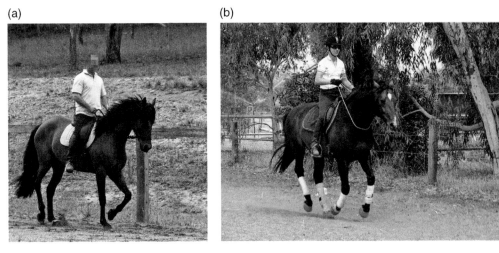

Figure 5.6 Horses being ridden without a bit (a) and without a bridle (b). (Photos courtesy of Pierre Malou and Portland Jones.)

procedure that changes an aversive or noxious stimulus into one that is positive for the animal. The first known example comes from Pavlov's lab: he used a mild electric shock, which initially elicited signs of pain, as a conditioned stimulus. After the shock had been paired repeatedly with food, it began to elicit salivation and there was no sign that it was still painful. Counter-conditioning can be very useful in animal-behaviour therapy and in getting animals to accept painful therapeutic interventions. An example is when clippers (an aversive outcome that elicits fearful responses in many horses) are associated with feeding (an attractive outcome for all horses).

An important feature of classical conditioning is that it is selective and is dependent on the relative closeness of competing stimuli. So as one particular stimulus, such as the noise from a clicker, becomes strongly associated with some important event, such as food, we see a weakening of the associations between other stimuli and food.

An example of this selectiveness and the effect of competing stimuli is *overshadowing*. A trainer may intend that the horse learns to associate a certain word with food or with an appropriate response. However, if the trainer always makes an unintended hand gesture or body movement when uttering that word, the visual cue from the hand or body may become the effective conditioned stimulus instead. In this case, the body language signals have overshadowed the spoken signal or command. Consequently, they need either to become the cue in the trainer's mind or to be watered down by making them more variable. We will see more examples of overshadowing in Chapter 8, Training.

Selective learning is seen in a process called *blocking*. If a stimulus is established as a consistent and reliable signal for a reinforcer, learning about a second stimulus that accompanies the first, is retarded or blocked. So, if a hand signal on its own has already become a strong conditioned stimulus, the later addition of a verbal command, even if issued at the same time as the hand signal, is likely to remain ineffective. If your aim is to train with clarity and consistency, avoid blocking and overshadowing because they impede training programmes. Fundamentally, good trainers are careful to make sure that only the intended stimulus can serve as a signal to the horse.

Another important characteristic of classical conditioning is that associations between two events are more rapidly acquired if the events are *novel*. If a horse is exposed to a conditioned stimulus on several occasions before the conditioning procedure commences (i.e. before it is paired with the US), the conditioned response to that stimulus will be acquired more slowly. It is as if the animal has simply learned to ignore the stimulus because it has no important consequences, and this association must be unlearned first. When pre-exposure to a stimulus produces retardation of learning, it is called *latent inhibition*. An example from a stableyard might be the relative sluggishness with which a stallion would learn to get aroused by a headcollar, if he had been led around by that piece of equipment for years and then it was only used to lead him to the breeding barn. Similarly, a horse that has continually been told he is a 'good boy' with no salient consequences (such as the release of pressure or arrival of food) will take longer than an entirely naïve stablemate to learn this as a secondary reinforcer, when associated with primary reinforcers.

So we can see that poor timing and inconsistent signalling can produce only weak, and sometimes even unwanted, associations. Good trainers have excellent timing and consistency, often without having to think about it.

Like all good scientists, Pavlov kept a notebook and it is from this source that one of his most telling observations emerged. He noted that his dogs would race ahead of their handlers and jump onto the table in the experimental area. Instead of waiting for any stimuli (either unconditioned or conditioned) that made their mouths water, the dogs would actively try to place themselves into situations and perform activities that led to rewards. This resulted from trial-and-error learning and foreshadowed the other important category of associative learning: operant conditioning.

Cue Salience

The relative salience of auditory tactile and visual cues to horses remains unknown. In other species there is some literature on the impact of different types of stimuli as conditioned stimuli (CS). The best-known work,

pioneered by Garcia and Koelling (1966), showed that rats can learn the association between a taste and illness (nausea) very quickly, but learn much less readily about exteroceptive cues (visual and auditory) that predict nausea. Conversely, rats can learn quickly about the relationship between the same exteroceptive cues and pain (a brief shock), but learn very little about taste–shock associations. Therefore, at least some animals have innate predispositions to learn certain CS–unconditioned stimulus (US) associations more readily than other associations. For rats, evolution is likely to have favoured learning a taste–illness association because of the dangers of a diverse foraging lifestyle, where taste would be more relevant in a foraging context than visual or auditory stimuli. Conversely, tastes are unlikely to predict pain and, again, evolution may have selected for the reverse bias in associability. This is an important area for future research in equitation science. It is critical to consider the horse's adaptations as an open grassland forager and social prey animal, in understanding its evolved stimulus preferences.

Reinforcement and Punishment

Reinforcement, whether it is positive or negative, will always make a response more likely in future. Conversely, positive or negative punishment will generally make a response less likely in future (Table 5.1). Both punishment and reinforcement are central to operant conditioning because they can be applied as consequences of behaviour. Many trainers who claim not to use negative reinforcement are simply confused by its unpleasant connotations (Warren-Smith and McGreevy, 2008(a)). In the scientific study of cognition and ethology, negative is used in the arithmetic sense referring to the subtraction or removal of something from the animal's world, while positive refers to an addition. Negative reinforcement differs from positive reinforcement, not least because of the point at which stimulus control is achieved. When using positive reinforcement, trainers may

Table 5.1 Punishment versus reinforcement – effect of the treatment (with examples).

Reinforcement	Punishment
Response becomes more likely in future	*Response becomes less likely in future*
Positive reinforcement (titbit offered directly following a horse's nicker reinforces nickering)	Positive punishment (applying tension on the rein directly after the horse starts bucking increases discomfort in the mouth, and makes bucking less likely)
Negative reinforcement (easing tension on the rein directly after the horse produced a halt, reduces discomfort and reinforces stopping in response to rein tension)	Negative punishment (stopping to scratch a horse when it attempts to respond with allogrooming the person, extinguishes the allogrooming response)

wait until the shaped behaviour is offered before expecting it to come under stimulus control, whereas with negative reinforcement they are obliged to begin each pressure with a light version of the signal to prevent distress arising from the pressure and thus rapidly focus the horse on the light signal.

Using Attractive Stimuli

A reinforcer is any event that increases the frequency of a behaviour that it follows. Whether some event is called a reinforcer is related purely to the effect it has. So the value of a reinforcer can be measured only in terms of the degree to which it makes the behaviour more likely in future. If a trainer's saying 'Good boy' in response to a horse's leg-yielding has no effect on the horse's future behaviour then, according to this definition, reinforcement has not occurred. The trainer's words have had a neutral effect. A scratch on the head may be less reinforcing than a scratch at the withers or other preferred body parts, but a good trainer watches the animal to see how it responds, not just to these comparable interventions but also to whether they genuinely make the preceding behaviour more likely.

Therefore, *many* different contextual features associated with both stimuli and reinforcers can be integrated to maximise differentiation and thus enhance performance (Nicol, 2002). Palatable foods are generally more reinforcing if they are not normally part of the horse's diet. However, this is less likely in naïve horses because of neophobia (literally, fear of the new). Horses that have been exposed to highly valued foods and do not receive them as part of a daily ration may perform with a higher level of consistency for such reinforcers. They recognise these foods as highly palatable and seem more motivated to work for them because they receive them infrequently. Clearly, this has a bearing on the rewards used in training since it explains why some horses appear to become rapidly sated (over-faced) with one type of food reward.

A horse's ability to discriminate between colours improves if the reward outcome differs. For example, in a discrimination task, if the colour of a central panel signals that either a left or a right lever response was correct, horses perform best when different reinforcers (food pellets for one lever, chopped carrot for the other) were linked with each lever, than when reinforcers were randomly assigned or identical (Miyashita *et al.*, 2000). This suggests that the cues for one reward are learned by classical conditioning, so the horses would probably show a preference for one reward over the other and this preference would eventually affect their motivation to choose both panels equally.

Significantly, horses work to avoid aversive stimuli, even when this interferes with their access to positive reinforcement (Nicol, 2002). Acquiring food is generally rewarding but when the mouth that chews it contains a bit, enjoyment may be compromised by discomfort from the metal. If, additionally, tight nosebands are present, there is an added risk of choking as the tight noseband may prevent the horse from properly chewing the food. In practical terms, this adds to the problem of blending negative and positive reinforcement (Warren-Smith and McGreevy, 2007(c)).

A significant problem when trying to use food reinforcers is the difficulty in delivering food immediately after the ridden horse offers a desirable response. Leaning out of the saddle after every good response is likely to train horses to slow down and halt, since this is the response they make immediately before we can easily flex forward from the saddle. So, the use of secondary reinforcement could be a solution, or alternatively, devices that instantly deliver rewards to the mouth allow the time between performance of the desired behaviour and its reinforcement to be minimised, effectively enhancing the speed of learning. In trials with positive reinforcement alone, some horses took longer than control horses to complete a maze; this apparent stalling may reflect the nature of innate foraging strategies in horses. In other species, similar effects called contra-free-loading are observed. The term describes the tendency for animals to continue working for access to food or to continue searching for foods at additional sites, even if there is an abundance of food freely available at a known site. Possibly, the exploratory behaviour *per se* may be rewarding (Forkman, 1996). Also, in the presence of fear, the motivation to feed may be greatly reduced relative to the motivation to avoid aversive stimuli, such as pressures from negative reinforcement. This

is probably due to the inhibiting effects of stress on the digestive system and is adaptive, as food intake is temporarily of secondary importance in a potentially life-threatening situation, while avoiding bodily hindrance or harm remains an important goal to maintain fully functional flight responses. This highlights the importance of reducing fear and other stressors during training to achieve optimal learning performance.

So-called reward devices or sugar-bits, which deliver food rewards (such as molasses or carrot juice) orally, via a remotely controlled hollow bit, have been used successfully in combination with bit pressures in experimental situations (Warren-Smith and McGreevy, 2007(c)) (Figure 5.7).

Reinforcers can be either primary or secondary. Primary reinforcers are any resources that animals have evolved to seek. When the animal needs them, acquiring them is rewarding. In contrast, when the animal has just satisfied its need for them (i.e. it is sated), such resources are no longer rewarding. If the animal's motivation can be correctly predicted, food, water, sex, play, liberty, sanctuary, gentle scratching, and companionship can all be used as primary reinforcers. Secondary reinforcers are stimuli that are not

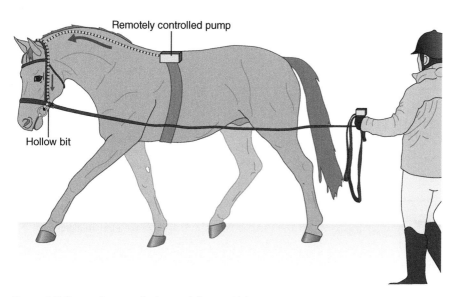

Figure 5.7 Remotely controlled reward devices (delivering positive reinforcement) can be used in combination with bit pressure (negative reinforcement).

intrinsically rewarding but that have become linked (by classical conditioning) with a primary reinforcer of some kind. These associations make great sense in evolutionary terms, since an auditory, olfactory or visual cue that has become reliably linked with a primary reinforcer provides the horse with information on opportunities to enhance its biological fitness (e.g. by obtaining food or a chance to reproduce).

It is worth considering the innate value of things we class as rewards (Figure 5.8). Horses are often praised with tactile stimuli, chiefly with a scratch at the withers or a pat on the neck. Horses have evolved to find grooming one another (allogrooming) rewarding, so a scratch on an appropriate part of the body is a primary reinforcer. By comparison, the far more common practice of patting horses on the neck, if too forceful, can even be aversive or at best neutral to the horse (Thorbergson *et al.*, 2016). Patting is reinforcing only if the owner has coupled the pat with something inherently pleasant (McGreevy, 2004). Horses have not evolved to be motivated to offer certain responses for pats on their necks, so patting, if it is going to

be used at all, must be conditioned as a secondary reinforcer. We have seen already how two stimuli can become linked via classical conditioning. An interesting example is the way in which the bridle used for restraint during mating, the environs of the breeding barn, and the dummy used for semen collection can all become arousing for breeding stallions because they become reliable predictors of sex. The inadvertent emergence of similar links can easily arise during feeding time. Horses have not evolved to eat discrete meals, so the appearance of concentrated food in bulk causes inordinate excitement, especially for horses that do not have foraging opportunities between meals. This means that the sight of feed buckets, the sound of feed buckets and even the arrival of humans who frequently supply feed may all become secondary reinforcers. It is important that personnel who work around horses are aware of this possibility, because they may inadvertently reinforce inappropriate behaviours such as pawing and aggression at the time of feeding. Feeding horses immediately after inappropriate responses is not advisable. Clearly, feeding cannot be achieved without

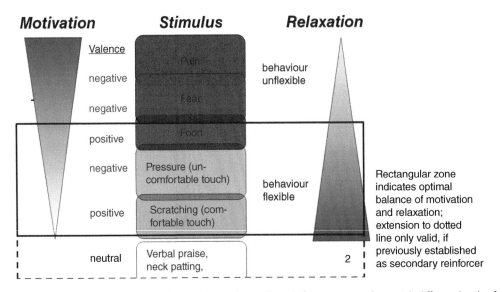

Figure 5.8 Different rewards used in positive and negative reinforcement go along with different levels of relaxation and are of different valence (negative or positive) and value to the horse, depending on its general (e.g. the horse's innate level of tactile sensitivity) and temporal situation (e.g. the horse's current degree of hunger). Choosing an appropriate type and intensity of reward for a given horse to balance motivation and relaxation is crucial to training success.

some noise, so the best advice for owners of horses that get boisterously over-excited at feeding times is to feed plenty of roughage (so that horses are not frustrated by periods without food) and to stagger feeds throughout the day so that noise and the sound of feed buckets (being used to deliver food to *other* horses) become less likely to predict the delivery of food. In this way, any inadvertently rewarded responses will become extinguished. There are many ways in which we inadvertently reinforce our horse's responses. Just because we are not intending to train a response does not mean that the horse will not be learning something. Horses are learning all the time since they make no distinction between associations built through regular handling, regular riding, training and competition.

Given what we know about the horse's ability to discriminate between cues that are linked to a given reward (Miyashita *et al.*, 2000), in the most elegant case, a specific secondary reinforcer tells the animal that it will reliably encounter or receive a certain primary reinforcer. In this way, a trainer can mark excellent responses with a secondary reinforcer that delivers the resource for which the horse is most highly motivated.

Horse-trainers rarely need to question whether a technique is based on classical or instrumental conditioning, but it pays to look at possible interactions between the two types. Declines in performance of trained behaviour can sometimes result from competition between classically and instrumentally conditioned responses. They arise when unwanted responses that would be innate responses towards resources in more natural settings are offered in response to learned cues. A useful example is seen when a horse feeding from a bucket begins pawing at the ground; pawing is thought to be an innate activity horses use to expose edible roots in the soil or forage covered by snow and so is a natural response to slightly frustrating feeding in a domestic context. This reversion to innate responses is known as *instinctive drift* (Breland and Breland, 1962).

Trick-trainers risk instinctive drift when they build a chain of instrumental responses that produces the reinforcer. For example, they may train a horse to pick up a hat, carry the hat and then relinquish it into the correct receptacle (e.g. the trainer's hand) to receive food. As performance improves, an increasingly consistent relationship develops between the stimulus, the hat, and the food; the hat becomes a conditioned stimulus that reliably signals the arrival of food (the unconditioned stimulus). This CS–US relationship produces classical conditioning, and so the hat acquires the properties of a surrogate food item and the horse will tend to hold onto it rather than let it drop. Responding to the hat as a food object, therefore, competes with the operant response of releasing it, so that this trained response is performed more slowly and less reliably.

Ethical Considerations on Positive Reinforcement

Various pleasant stimuli can be used as positive reinforcers (e.g. scratching and stroking, or other forms of social contact), but the most commonly applied stimulus is food. However, some trainers deplore the use of food, because they either consider that food will induce mugging behaviour or that it is ethically inappropriate to treat horses like circus animals and to employ their desire to eat for our entertainment. From the perspective of learning theory, either food or scratching constitutes a positive reinforcer and, depending on a horse's current individual motivation to eat or to be scratched, one or the other reinforcer may work better. However, given the horse's natural feeding behaviour and the relative importance of food over tactile contact to biological fitness, it seems plausible that for most adult, healthy horses, food will serve as one of the most salient reinforcers. However, the strong motivation for the reward is not without risks. In various animal species, repetitious locomotory activity such as pacing behaviour (Staddon and Simmelhag, 1971) and wheel-running (Segal, 1969; 1972; Staddon, 1977), as well as aggression (Looney and Cohen, 1982) have been induced by using food-reward schedules. The discontinuous delivery of food during shaping and variable schedules of reinforcement can, in some individuals, also contribute to raised arousal levels that can induce these unwanted effects. In horses, stereotypies such as weaving and crib-biting have also been shown to be associated with food. While positive reinforcement provides an important and powerful training protocol, it should be remembered that frustration can occur. This outcome may not only be distressing for the horse but can sometimes be dangerous for humans if equine frustration escalates to aggression.

Another problem may occur when a signal reliably precedes an appetitive event and, as a result, the subject's approach responses are conditioned to the signal or the person delivering it, rather than the desired behaviour. This is known as 'sign tracking', where the subject becomes obsessed with the rewarding agent and attempts to remain near it with excessive frequency (Hearst and Jenkins, 1974). It is commonly seen in horses on positive-reinforcement schedules in that they harass the trainer for food, known as 'mugging'. For this reason, many astute trainers initially teach the horse that food is only delivered when the horse looks away.

The use of positive reinforcement has a very important place in training. However, trainers should always be mindful of its pitfalls. Training is essentially an exploitative event and there is no ubiquitous training modality – all have advantages and drawbacks.

Reinforcement Schedules

Until a given response behaviour is under stimulus control, the trainer must be consistent in applying cues and providing rewards. If consistent reinforcement is not provided for correct responses, the horse's behaviour becomes unpredictable. Once a response is consistently elicited as a conditioned response, it can be made more resistant to extinction by means of a variable reward schedule. The desired behaviour can then be rewarded unpredictably. Horses respond to different *fixed-ratio* positive-reinforcement schedules, in which partial reinforcement is delivered on the basis of the number of correct responses made, and *fixed-interval* positive-reinforcement schedules, in which reinforcement becomes available again only after some specified time has elapsed (Myers and Mesker, 1960). This aligns them with other animals that are trained using positive reinforcement. When shaping novel responses, practitioners find that continuous-reinforcement schedules rapidly increase the response rate (McCall and Burgin, 2002). However, once the response has been shaped and is under stimulus control, intermittent reinforcement can be used (with a resultant increase in its resistance to extinction).

Horses cannot be expected to learn well if reinforcement is delayed, because the delay prevents them from relating the reinforcement to the behaviour. Previous work has shown that horses have short-term spatial recall of less than 10 seconds in a delayed-response task (McLean, 2004). It is also necessary to obtain the same results in multiple locations for the behaviour to become generalised and not context-specific (some training systems refer to this quality as 'proof', e.g. McLean and McLean, 2008).

Although the neural pathways involved in negative and positive reinforcement are the same, much of what we know about positive reinforcement cannot automatically be applied to negative reinforcement (i.e. horse-training in the ridden context). With negative reinforcement, trainers cannot choose to reinforce sometimes and not others (as in a variable reward schedule), since maintaining pressure leads to habituation. If, in a negative reinforcement system, riders delay reinforcement (release of pressure), they should do so only when shaping an alternative response. The horse subjected to sustained pressure may try harder to offer a response that solves its current problem but the trainers must know what they are waiting for in terms of an improved response, since failing to reward the improvement will again lead to habituation. It pays to consider why this practical skill is so hard to teach to riders. There is evidence that judges (and so, presumably, coaches) fail to detect lightness in observed riders (de Cartier d'Yves and Ödberg, 2005). This means that they are likely to fail to spot removal of pressure and so are currently poorly placed to comment on the rider's most critical means of reinforcement.

Shaping Behaviour

Shaping is the principle of reinforcing successive improvements that are approximations of the final response. Trainers seeking to reinforce particular responses can either wait for the behaviour to occur spontaneously – it can be readily reinforced if the behaviour occurs frequently – or they can shape the behaviour pattern. Using this technique, trainers can move from a point where it is impossible to reinforce a desired response (because that response never occurs), to one where basic attempts are offered and reinforced, to one where the response is offered with increasing reliability. A common characteristic among good trainers is their ability to recognise an opportunity to reinforce improved 'approximations'. While less-effective trainers complain that their animals fail to understand what is being asked of them and feel that the animals have peaked in their training, superior trainers have the skill and patience to capitalise on each tiny improvement as the only way of moving towards the final response.

Crucially, shaping relies on reserving the reinforcement so that the animal must keep trialling new responses or responses that are developments on those that have previously been reinforced. For example, when training a horse to approach a target (in so-called target training), rewards are given chiefly when the horse travels closer to the target or does so faster than on previous occasions. While shaping a new response or, for that matter, modifying an existing one, it is important to reward target responses immediately. To delay in delivering reinforcement is to allow intervening responses to be linked with the reward.

Clicker Training

If every delivery of a reward depends on the close presence of a human, its effect can quickly become context-specific to human proximity, so that a horse fails to perform the behaviour at any distance from its trainer. The cue of a human is an important contingency for these animals. Clickers that can be used to reinforce at a distance really come into their own here. These devices are currently the most popular example of a secondary reinforcer, and are being used by thousands of trainers worldwide (McCall and Burgin, 2002).

Clickers developed in the field of marine-mammal-training, a context in which restraint of the animals during training is impractical and in which the application of pressure for negative reinforcement or punishment is virtually impossible. By creating a classically conditioned association between the particular sound and the arrival of a primary reinforcer (most commonly a food reward), the trainer can *bridge* the gap between the moment an animal performs a response correctly and it receiving the reward. Essentially, the clicker comes to mean, 'Yes, that's good, a reward is coming'. When a clicker is first used, the correct association is established by making the sound just before giving a highly valued reward. Repetition of the pairing between the two stimuli assures the animal of the signal's reliability.

Some trainers deplore the use of food in training, since they see it as a cause of biting. This may be true in horses and ponies that have been allowed to 'mug' their owners for food. Good clicker trainers never feed unless they have made a clicker noise, so their subjects expect food only on cue. These trainers also feed only at some distance from the receptacle containing the store of food (usually from a pocket or pouch on a belt). This breaks any direct connection between the food and its source and restricts the horse from helping himself. Moreover, consistency in this practice places the feeding response itself under stimulus control and extinguishes begging or nuzzling responses, which are never reinforced (and if they have been previously reinforced by another trainer, they are rapidly extinguished). It is certainly unwise to use food to lure horses during training, since this makes desirable responses contingent on the presence of food ('no food, no deal').

After establishing desirable responses through negative reinforcement, trainers can use clicker training to help maintain the acquisition of the light signal. The benefits of positive reinforcement as applied in clicker training are largely to do with the ephemeral nature of light pressure signals and the likelihood that it may be more humane than traditional negative reinforcement training. With clicker training, 'what you click is what you get', so if your observations and timing are not perfect, you will inadvertently shape some responses you do not want. Subsequent adjustments that remove this reinforcement mean that these inadvertently shaped responses are extinguished. So, while poor timing can make clicker training ineffective, the same trainer error in traditional negative reinforcement training could amount to abuse (Chapter 6, Associative Learning (Aversive stimuli)).

Commercial clicker devices make a sharp and distinctive noise. The brevity and clarity of the click facilitates precise capture (reinforcement) of transient responses, such as the horse bringing forward its ears. Also, being pocket-sized or attachable to keyrings, clickers are very convenient, but they are not an obligatory item for so-called clicker training. An important caveat on the topic of clicker training is that its focus on the clicker sometimes obscures the fundamental message: that any secondary reinforcer, when developed appropriately, can be a powerful training tool. Virtually, any discrete auditory stimulus can be linked to a primary reinforcer to become a secondary reinforcer.

Some horses are fearful of the click *per se* and are, therefore, candidates for such alternative secondary reinforcers. Indeed, as long as they cannot be confused with words that appear in common parlance, any consistent vocalisation by a trainer (so-called clicker-words) will be effective. 'Yes!' or 'Good boy!' are examples, but it is worth emphasising that

the reinforcing value of any noise is a function of the degree to which it is associated with a primary reinforcer. Trainers, who click (or say 'Good boy!') without delivering a primary reinforcer just afterwards, are diluting the impact of the secondary reinforcer. This explains why horses show a rapid decline in interest to respond to the secondary reinforcer only, and the temporal link between the primary and secondary reinforcers is also critical (McCall and Burgin, 2002). Also, when choosing a 'clicker-word', it is advisable to choose words or ways of pronouncing them, that make the auditory stimulus distinct from other words horses may regularly hear during human–human or human–horse conversations. Indeed, when horses are first trained using words as secondary reinforcers, they may initially react to any word, or even any sound, including, for example, the sounds of the horse's own intestinal peristalsis. This reflects the horse's ability to generalise. Only when the secondary reinforcer continues to be one unique word or sound, does the horse learn to distinguish this meaningful sound from irrelevant noise. Thus, the fundamental rules of learning theory apply, and trainers who maintain the horse's motivation for the primary reinforcer and build the firmest association between the primary and secondary reinforcers can most effectively shape desirable responses.

A secondary reinforcer is most effectively established when presented before or up until the presentation of a primary reinforcer. Simultaneous presentation of a reward and a novel secondary stimulus is less effective, because the primary reinforcer will block or overshadow the new stimulus. Presentation of the secondary stimulus after the primary reinforcer is entirely unproductive because, although an association may exist between the two, it will not help the animal to predict the arrival of a reward.

The use of secondary reinforcement seems to increase a horse's interest in performing novel tasks (Myers and Mesker, 1960) and this creativity in the horse's approach to problem-solving accounts for the growing appeal of clicker training in behaviour-modification programmes and some higher movements (such as piaffe, see Figures 5.9b and c), especially where traditional remedial approaches have failed (Chapter 12, Unorthodox Techniques and Chapter 14, Ethical Equitation). Furthermore, the principles of clicker training can be very helpful in shaping and modifying

(a)

(b)

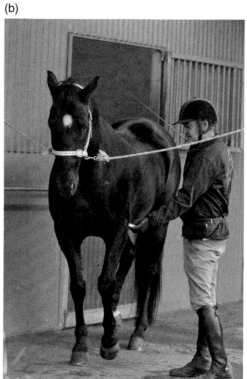

(c)

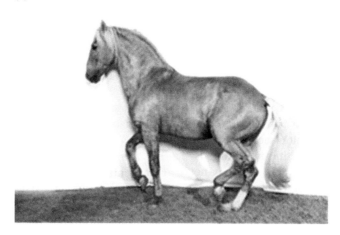

Figure 5.9 (a) A horse stretching (i.e. making an operant response) towards a target, as a part of being trained to traverse a ground-based obstacle. (b) A horse in early training of piaffe being reinforced using positive reinforcement. (c) A horse trained to piaffe at liberty using positive reinforcement. (Photo (c) courtesy of Niels Stappenbeck/Diana Krischke.)

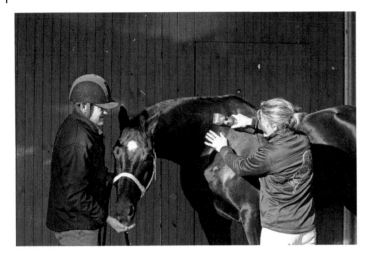

Figure 5.10 Horse being clipped in the presence of food, an example of counter-conditioning.

unwanted responses. By deconstructing a series of undesirable responses that arise in a set context, we can counter-condition fear responses (Figure 5.10). For example, by training a trailer-shy horse to approach a target and then moving the target towards a ground-based aversive stimulus (such as a tarpaulin, see Figure 5.9a), we can shape approaching hazards and then ultimately the trailer without using any pressure.

When selecting primary reinforcers, experienced trainers observe the horse's responses to determine the reinforcing value of a novel reward. Many horses respond well to carrots as the primary reinforcer in a clicker-training protocol, but more so if carrots are not routinely offered in regular meals. The relationship between motivation and the reinforcing value of any food should be considered here. The speed or strength of learning increases with the value of the reinforcer. This explains why horses will learn to run faster to the sound of a rattling bucket (a secondary reinforcer associated with concentrate foods) than they will to the rustling of a hay-net (a secondary reinforcer associated with hay).

In general, the larger the reinforcer, the greater is its effect on behaviour. This may suggest that big is always better, but the effectiveness of a reinforcer may decline when many reinforcers need to be given within a short period. An obvious example of such a satiation effect is the use of a food reward to a hungry animal that will soon lose its appetite when given frequent large rewards. So many trainers use small rewards within a session and then end when the horse completes a 'high note' – that is, performs particularly well – at which point it is given a large reward, a 'jackpot'. Learning theory suggests that jackpots should be used sparingly, since once the horse starts to expect large reinforcers in a set context, small reinforcers may start to lose their effectiveness. Therefore, it is advisable to start training with large rewards and short sessions and progressively move towards smaller rewards given in longer sessions. Sometimes horses get overexcited by large rewards so they should not be allowed to see jackpots before they are given (i.e. conceal rewards in a pouch).

Contiguity

The principle of temporal contiguity states that events that occur closely in time become associated. As we will see in the next chapter, the longer the delay between a warning sound and the arrival of an aversive outcome, the weaker will be the horse's fear response to the sound. Similarly, giving a carrot to a horse two minutes after a pat on its neck will not make the pat reinforcing. The carrot would have to arrive within seconds of the pat if reinforcement is to occur. The interval between stimuli is usually, but not always, the most important criterion for the establishment of an association. Events distanced by time can still become associated if there is a high predictive link between them. The best example of this is food-aversion learning, which helps animals avoid food items that have previously made them ill. Novel flavours are more likely to be associated with later sickness and, therefore, horses may be alert to this possibility when they consume novel foods. Operant conditioning has been used to indicate the behavioural effects of drugs. So, for example, a horse trained to press a lever can be monitored before and after the administration of a pharmaceutical test. Since the reward for pressing is usually food, a decrease in the rate of demand suggests that the drug has either depressant or anorexic effects. Food-aversion learning has also been used by scientists interested in the consequences of proprietary drugs on horse welfare. The aversive effect of drugs can be calibrated by the degree to which a food associated with it is subsequently avoided.

Combining Positive and Negative Reinforcement

Most early research involving positive reinforcement with horses has been conducted on non-equitation-related activities such as mazes (e.g. Haag *et al.*, 1980; McCall *et al.*, 1981; Heird *et al.*, 1986(b); Marinier and Alexander, 1994) and so, while they may yield valuable results, they are not always directly transferable to traditional equitation (Dougherty and Lewis, 1991). Haag *et al.* (1980) found a significant correlation with the learning ability of a group of ponies in both a shock-avoidance trial and a single-choice maze. More recently, several studies directly compared learning outcomes when using negative and positive reinforcement. In general, it appears that both training methods yield comparable results as regards learning speed, although it has been suggested that the

success of the methods may also be task-dependent as well as context-dependent (Döhne *et al.*, 2014). For example, tasks that require the horse to stand still while the trainer is moving away may, at least in the initial stages of training, be achieved faster with negative rather than positive reinforcement, because with the latter, horses are probably more inclined to maintain a short distance from the trainer (who is the source of a valuable resource). However, even though speed of learning appears to be similar for positive and negative reinforcement, most studies noted additional advantages of training regimens based on positive reinforcement, such as an improved horse–trainer relationship, compared to horses trained by negative reinforcement alone (Heleski *et al.*, 2008).

Visser *et al.* (2003) used an avoidance test that involved punishment (puffs of air being given for the wrong choice) and measured learning performance by percentage of correct responses, and in a reward test, measured performance by latency to obtain the reward. Some horses did not respond to the aversive stimulus.

Employing a remotely operated pump that delivered a small food reward into the horse's mouth via a hollow bit (Figure 5.7, above), Warren-Smith and McGreevy (2007(c)) assessed the effectiveness of a blend of both positive and negative reinforcement in shaping responses to a halt stimulus. They found that, although it did not increase the speed of learning, horses subjected to this blend nodded their heads and mouthed the bits less and were more likely to lick their lips than those reinforced with negative reinforcement only. It will be interesting to see how research in this domain develops.

Long-Term Potentiation

As learning proceeds, memories encoded in short-term memory begin to become established as more durable long-term memories, which is known as long-term potentiation. Implicit in this transition is the neurotransmitter serotonin, and experimental studies have shown that five spaced deliveries of serotonin over a period of 1.5 hours have produced long-term changes lasting several days. Studies both in animals and with cells *in vitro* indicate that long-term memory is an extension of short-term memory. As short-term memory develops into long-term memory, they are seen to share many physical similarities, such as broadening of the action potential, an increase in excitability and enhanced release of transmitters of sensory neurons. However, long-term memory is also characterised by synthesis of new protein molecules (Castellucci *et al.*, 1989), as well as further structural changes (Bailey and Chen, 1983). The persistence of structural changes correlates with the behavioural duration of the memory (Bailey and Chen, 1983). This more elaborate memory structure confers stronger resistance to forgetting, which characterises long-term memory (Kandel, 2006). For example, long-term memory is more resistant to various chemicals and traumas than short-term memory.

Take-Home Messages

- Just because a horse can be trained to offer a particular response, we should not assume it enjoys giving that response. After all, dogs can be trained to salivate in response to electric shocks.
- Horses are learning all the time and they make no distinction between associations built through regular handling, regular riding, training and competition.
- Effective trainers are clear and consistent in their signals and the way in which they set up challenges for animals to solve (i.e. the way in which they pose questions).
- Effective training relies on timing and consistency.
- Detraining can take the form of inconsistency and variable timing.

Ethical Considerations

- The reliance on pressure and release in horse-riding distinguishes it from training in most other species. Animal-welfare considerations put the onus on trainers to use minimal pressure and release it immediately.
- Should novice riders (including children) be taught the principles of cause-and-effect with positive reinforcement before being permitted to ride, balance and use negative reinforcement?
- The governing bodies of horse sports should encourage research into the most humane application of pressure and alternative means of communicating with horses and reinforcement during training.
- Ethical investigations into the use of positive and negative reinforcement should compare and contrast the motivations of hunger and pressure removal.

Areas and Anticipated Limitations for Further Research

- There are many questions remaining about positive reinforcement as it can be administered to horses. Results to date are in no way the full story.
- Can we discover practicable ways to deliver 'jackpots' (a primary reward that is substantially bigger than usual and comes as a surprise) to ridden horses?

6

Associative Learning (Aversive Stimuli)

Introduction

While the previous chapter focused on training with attractive stimuli, aversive events are far more critical with the ridden horse. This chapter explores the use in horse-training of aversive stimuli, most of which are tactile. The trainer is well placed to deliver tactile stimuli, because the ridden or led horse is in direct physical contact with her/him. Aversive stimuli underpin the horse's learning of responses evoked by the rider's legs, reins and lead-reins, as well as whips, spurs and possibly seat and weight signals. No matter how much we positively reinforce velocity and directional mobility responses, any tactile signals that elicit them are necessarily aversive, at least initially. Moreover, the acute sensitivity of horses to cutaneous irritations is well known, so the fundamental challenge in the initial training of horses is that they must respond calmly, yet sometimes powerfully, to aversive stimuli.

Equestrian technology has undergone very few quantum leaps. The chief milestones have been the bridle, the curb bit, the stirrups and the (saddle's) tree. Although horse-riding may have benefited from adjustable trees, air-filled panels and spring-loaded stirrups, it is essentially a low-tech activity. Despite the contribution of some innovative technologies, a successful partnership between horse and rider still relies predominantly on the skills of the rider. It is the development of such skills that have enabled humans to manipulate and control the behaviour of the horse. The use of aversive stimuli to control horses has a long history. There is archaeological evidence of restraint artefacts from around the end of the third millennium BC (Levine, 2005). Xenophon, writing more than two millennia ago in his treatise *Hippike*, wrote extensively about the varied uses of aversive stimuli to control horses.

Experimentally, our understanding of aversive learning is comparatively recent. The famous Ivan Pavlov mostly used food in his learning experiments, but a Russian contemporary, Vladimir Bechterev, also experimented on dogs using electricity. He showed, perhaps unsurprisingly, that if a conditioned stimulus (CS) such as a buzzer was repeatedly presented just before a dog's hindpaw was shocked, the dog very quickly learned to lift its leg in response to the buzzer alone. Bechterev's experiments provided the first objective study of aversive learning in animals. Animals generally find an electric shock so aversive that they resist habituation to it, even at mild levels.

Escape and Avoidance Learning

In Bechterev's experiments, the dog's innate response to electric shock was escape. If the escape behaviour successfully terminated the aversive stimulus, this behaviour was negatively reinforced and the dog would be likely

Equitation Science, Second Edition. Paul McGreevy, Janne Winther Christensen,
Uta König von Borstel and Andrew McLean.
© 2018 John Wiley & Sons Ltd. Published 2018 by John Wiley & Sons Ltd.
Companion website: www.wiley.com/go/mcgreevy/equitation

to show the same behaviour with increased intensity upon the next exposure. In similar, nasty, experiments scientists can get a rat to jump off a platform into cold water, which it would normally hesitate to do, by mildly electrifying the platform. As the rat jumps, it escapes the shock; the jump is termed *escape behaviour*. Escape learning transforms to avoidance learning if the animal is given a signal just before the aversive stimulus. Through the process of classical conditioning, the animal will only require a few occurrences before the signal alone produces an *avoidance behaviour*. This type of learning happens very quickly and is highly persistent. For example, if a flashing light precedes the electrifying of the platform, the rat will quickly learn to react to the visual signal and jump into the water without waiting for the electric shock (Figure 6.1). The warning signal gives the rat an opportunity to control the aversive stimulus because it can perform a behaviour that prevents the stimulus. Interestingly, the rat will keep on jumping into the water in response to the flashing light, even if the platform is no longer electrified. This happens because the avoidance response is negatively reinforced through relief. The self-reinforcing properties of avoidance learning were clearly demonstrated by Richard Solomon in his so-called shuttle box experiments on dogs. Solomon placed dogs in large two-chamber cages with a low wall between the two chambers and conditioned the dogs to jump to the other chamber in response to an auditory warning signal to avoid floor electricity. After the shock generator had been turned off, the dogs continued to jump to the other side in response to the sound signal, and the avoidance behaviour never extinguished. This happened because the dogs did not allow themselves to discover that the aversive stimulus was no longer present. It is, of course, possible to change the avoidance behaviour if the animal is forced to discover that the warning signal no longer predicts the threat, and extinction of the avoidance response will occur faster if the warning signal is now paired with a pleasant stimulus, such as food.

The role of avoidance and escape learning in equitation is profound. It is not difficult to interpret the locomotory responses to rein and leg signals in trained horses as examples of avoidance learning. The experiments with rats and dogs also explain why horses learn to respond to the most salient of competing aversive stimuli. For example, to drop off a bank into water to avoid whip, spur or leg pressure. Solomon's experiments also explain the uptake of light or unrelated cues that predict stronger pressures. In the same way, light cues (e.g. seat or postural cues) can predict aversive pressures and thus confer controllability over them. This highlights the equitation imperative of keeping cues light and minimally invasive.

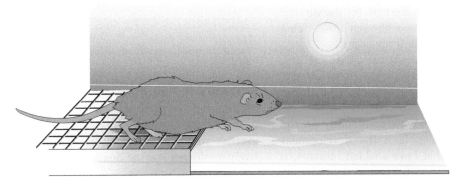

Figure 6.1 Rats show avoidance learning when they respond to a flashing light that heralds an electric shock. Avoidance responses are learned through classical conditioning and are highly persistent.

(a)

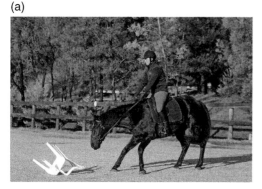

(b)

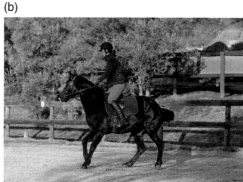

Figure 6.2 Even an up-turned chair (a) can be perceived as a novel object worthy of fear and horses may learn to shy away suddenly (b) from stimuli they perceive as aversive.

In addition to discomfort or pain resulting from tactile stimuli, fear-eliciting events are also aversive for horses. Novel fear-eliciting stimuli may be encountered by the horse during riding (Figure 6.2), and avoidance responses are negatively reinforced through removal of (i.e. increased distance from) the object of its fear. Furthermore, even rider anticipation can cause horses to become aroused and subsequently fearful. For example, when riders were told to expect a fear-eliciting stimulus to appear suddenly, their horses' heart rates rose, indicating that they were mirroring their rider's increased arousal (von Borstel *et al.*, 2005; 2007; Keeling *et al.*, 2009). As with the examples for aversive tactile stimuli above, horses are also naturally motivated to avoid frightening stimuli and avoidance responses are quickly learned and can be difficult to erase.

Negative Reinforcement

You will recall that in positive reinforcement the animal's behaviour is reinforced by a primary reinforcer (e.g. food) and perhaps a secondary reinforcer (e.g. a clicking noise). It is easy to imagine the rewarding effects of providing an animal with something it likes. What, then, could be so reinforcing about aversive events? The answer lies in the animal being able to terminate, escape or avoid the aversive event. Where possible, running away provides the simplest solution for an animal faced with an aversive stimulus. In negative reinforcement (NR), learning occurs because the stimulus is taken away, *subtracted* (Chance, 1993). Good examples are where a horse is motivated to remove itself from pain, discomfort or a predatory threat, but there are also more commonplace responses, such as moving to the shade when the sun becomes too hot. The removal of the aversive stimulus reinforces the behaviour, thereby making it more likely in the future.

Negative reinforcement may occur in many subtle situations, such as when you advance towards a horse and it retreats. There will be a learned response: the horse will retreat (i.e. remove you) when he sees you approach (clearly, this will happen only if the horse is motivated to remove you). Another example is when the farrier touches the horse's hindleg and the horse swings away, removing the farrier's hand. In this case, NR has occurred and the swing away will occur more rapidly next time the farrier touches or even approaches. Therefore, farriers, veterinarians and all personnel must understand that by such removal, habits of escape are rapidly acquired and elements of hyper-reactivity may also become attached to the response (Figure 6.3).

All responses in-hand and under-saddle begin with pressure, but can later come to be elicited by other signals. Thus, the reins, the trainer's legs, whips, spurs, lead-reins and halters are all potential instruments of negative reinforcement.

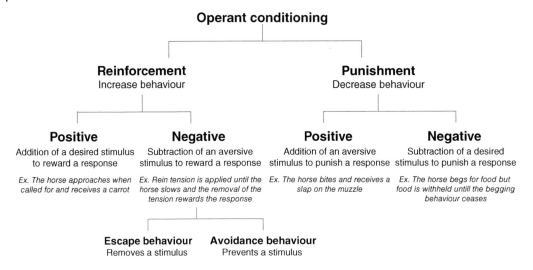

Figure 6.3 Operant conditioning comprises reinforcement and punishment, which can be further subdivided into 'positive' (addition) and 'negative' (subtraction). Escape and avoidance behaviour are negatively reinforced through the removal of an aversive stimulus.

Releasing the Pressure

It is the removal of pressure that initially trains the responses required in equitation, and this can take some time. Horses learn to *stop* to release rein tension, to *turn* to release turn-rein tension, to *go forward* to release pressure from the trainer's two legs, and to *step sideways* to release the trainer's single-leg pressure. Similarly, in-hand, the horse learns to *stop* to remove the posterior lead-rein tension and to *go forward* to release the anterior lead-rein tension. With repetitions, horses learn to perform these manoeuvres from very light pressures, because they perceive the initial increase of tension of the rein or pressure from the leg, and learn to respond to it to avoid the stronger pressures. Thus, in correct training practices, the application of all pressures must begin with very mild pressure. Soon, the horse perceives that stronger pressure can be avoided by reacting to the initial light pressure. Even though light pressure is the same modality as stronger pressure, this step arguably represents the conversion of response initiation from operant to classical conditioning. Similarly, horses can easily learn to react to, for example, a sound to avoid leg or bit pressure,

because the sound cue will act as a classically conditioned signal for the application of pressure (i.e. avoidance learning).

Control and Predictability

In any operant contingency, contiguity (the closeness of events in space or time) is essential (Lindsay, 2000). Horse-trainers refer to this as timing. In negative reinforcement, the behaviour learned by the horse is the one that leads to the release of pressure. The response solved the aversive problem, so it offers the same response more frequently in the future. From the horse's standpoint, offering responses that switch off aversive stimuli gives it *control* (McGreevy, 2004). As the animal increasingly responds to salient elements of the aversive pressure, such as the initial onset of pressure, it acquires a second element essential to its wellbeing: *predictability*. These psychological elements, control and predictability, are well known to influence the impact of stressors on animal welfare (Sapolsky, 2004). The more unpredictable the stressor, and the lower the degree of control the animal has over the aversive stimulus, the stronger the negative impact of that stimulus (Sapolsky, 2004). Similarly, other psychological factors, such as *outlets for frustration* and *social support*, also influence the impact of aversive stimuli on horse welfare. These factors will be further addressed in Chapter 13, Stress and Fear Responses.

Trialling Responses

A key feature of operant conditioning is the tendency to trial a range of responses to solve the current challenge (hence, the alternate term of trial-and-error learning). When faced with an aversive stimulus (e.g. from the rider's leg when learning to *go forward* under-saddle), the horse may trial going backwards, kicking out or biting the rider's leg before it trials going forward, at which point the trainer must immediately release the pressure to reinforce the correct response. However, the trainer can set up the situation so that the horse is more likely to offer the correct response. For example, if the horse has already learned to *step forward* from lead-rein tension, a trainer from the ground can apply this signal just after the rider starts to apply leg pressure. In this way, the horse is more likely to offer a step forward. In addition, learning can be facilitated by the use of a complementary aversive stimulus; for example, if the horse has learned to *step forward* from whip-tapping, this stimulus can be used to complement the rider's leg cues until the horse offers the correct response.

Because of the tendency of animals to trial a raft of responses when presented with an aversive stimulus, it is interesting to investigate the range of responses an animal may offer to various pressures. McLean (2005(a)) conducted trials involving 50 young horses (Thoroughbreds and European Warmbloods undergoing foundation training) that were habituated to the presence of a rider astride but naïve to stimulus control from the rider. Horses offered an array of responses when the rider applied the *go* signal (closing/nudging both legs) on the horses' sides (Table 6.1).

Table 6.1 Distribution of trialled responses that arise from the closing pressure of the legs of the rider.

Response to leg pressure	Percentage of horses
No response within 5 seconds	32
Move neck and head up	18
Move head to side	14
Step forward	12
Step laterally	10
Flight response (hunch back, buck, rear, spin)	8
Step back	6

The large percentage of horses that did not *step forward* from the leg pressure of the rider suggests that stepping forward represents a learned association, trained by negative reinforcement when the trainer releases the pressure of the legs after the horse gives the correct response by going forward. In other words, the trainer maintains the pressure throughout an incorrect response until a near-correct response is offered, whereupon the pressure is released. It is not difficult to understand how incorrect responses can be accidentally reinforced in foundation training, and that in such circumstances the young horse is at the mercy of the horse-trainer's knowledge or skills in the correct use of learning theory. Disturbingly, this highlights the ease with which a young horse can be trained to show undesired behaviour.

How to Use Negative Reinforcement

Stimulus control can be defined as the degree to which a response occurs in the presence of a specific stimulus and does not occur in the absence of this stimulus (McGreevy *et al.*, 2005). In horse training, achieving stimulus control of the basic locomotory responses is essential for safety, especially so that the horse can be stopped or slowed at any time.

The correct use of negative reinforcement can enable this important control; however, from the horse-welfare viewpoint, training must deploy the best-practice use to avoid the many perils of the incorrect use of negative reinforcement. To this end, the following steps have been proposed (McLean, 2005(b)):

1) The response to be trained is 'targeted' by the trainer. It is important that *only* the targeted behaviour results in the removal of pressure/discomfort.

2) The pressure (aversive stimulus) should be maintained or increased during the 'incorrect' behaviour until the targeted response emerges. During this phase, the pressure must not fluctuate or decrease, because this constitutes a lowering of pressure and, thus, could be reinforcing.

3) If intermittent pressures are used (e.g. nudging by the rider's legs or tapping with a dressage whip), there should be no change to the frequency of these pressures, so that the horse does not perceive this transient relief as reinforcing.

4) At the *onset* of the targeted response, the aversive stimulus should immediately be removed. Removal of the aversive stimulus must be contingent upon the onset of the 'correct' behaviour (Figure 6.4).

A Continuum of Reinforcing Possibilities

One of the interesting characteristics of negative reinforcement is the sliding scale of aversiveness (Figure 6.5). If pressure B is greater than pressure A, then it follows that relief from pressure B is more reinforcing than relief from pressure A. For example, consider mouth pressures on a linear scale from 1 to 10, where 1 represents the mildest of aversive stimuli and 10 represents the most painful, fearful and unendurable level of aversiveness, intolerable even for the shortest duration.

In practical horse-training, these mouth and body pressures are real; light cues occur in the lower scale, while the more motivating aversive pressures lie in the higher scale. At some point along the scale lies a threshold, where the tolerable escalates to the intolerable. When horses have unfortunately desensitised to the bit or to the rider's legs through incorrect negative reinforcement, effective trainers can rehabilitate such horses by increasing the motivation of the aversive pressure for a short duration and then releasing the pressure at the onset of the correct response. In other words, the

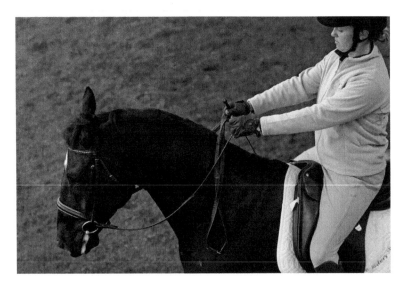

Figure 6.4 Horses learn to *stop/slow* from the release of pressure through trial and error. This highlights the need for trainers to release at the appropriate moment: the onset of the targeted response.

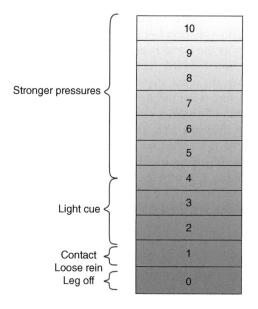

Stronger pressures

Light cue

Contact
Loose rein
Leg off

Figure 6.5 An arbitrary scale showing that the neutral stimulus, the classically conditioned cue (the lightest pressure signal) and the stronger motivating level of pressure can be considered a linear scale of pressure.

operant contingency must be re-established. Re-training responses that were incorrectly trained originally by negative reinforcement unfortunately require deployment of greater motivational aversiveness than would otherwise be the case. This is why it is imperative that learning theory becomes part of every horse-trainer's education, so that it may be applied consistently both at the start and throughout every horse's training.

Because equitation generally relies on a foundation of aversive stimuli, it is important to mention that, as most highly skilled trainers have noted, best practice is embodied in the use of the least aversive stimuli (the lightest cues). To ensure horse welfare during training, the level of aversiveness should always be kept to a minimum and trainers should be very careful to avoid invoking fear reactions during training. Provoking fear in animals is unethical and fearful horses are difficult to handle and can become dangerous. As described previously, escape reactions easily become negatively reinforced when the horse succeeds in increasing the distance between itself and the aversive

stimulus, and the horse will be likely to show the escape behaviour more frequently and with greater intensity. Consequently, fear reactions can be difficult to erase and training systems that routinely induce fear reactions are unethical and should be avoided.

Round-Pen as Negative Reinforcement

Round-pen work, such as has been popularised by the commercial methodology Join-up (Roberts, 2000), has been described as a method based on an element of the social ethogram of the horse in which a dominant member of a group will chase another to become its leader, force its compliance or win its respect. However, round-pen work can be more accurately described as another example of negative reinforcement, where the human in the centre of the round-pen pressures the horse to move around the pen but removes the pressure for various responses, including slowing. The horse's approaches towards the human in the centre of the round-pen are reinforced, and the approach behaviour is shaped through progressive improvements. However, if the horse stops approaching, pressure is applied again to move the horse around the pen until it actively approaches the human again. Join-up can be established because it effectively uses learning theory and, in particular, negative reinforcement.

Negative Reinforcement in Foundation Training

The job of the foundation trainer is to install mobility responses clearly so that the stimulus–response (S–R) associations develop to the point where they are elicited by diminutive versions of the relevant pressure signal. The training programmes of all ridden animals, such as elephants, camelids and bovids, similarly centre on the use of negative reinforcement. Whether the use of negative reinforcement is correct or not always merits consideration (Jones *et al.*, 2015) and, if not, this highlights welfare issues that need to be addressed.

A well-trained young horse may be described as having a perfect temperament, yet so much of the horse's future behaviour depends on the clarity of the early responses learned during foundation training. Indeed, every domestic horse has a 'negative reinforcement profile' that is the sum total of all negative reinforcement interventions beginning with the first time a human touched it as a foal. If the foal ran away and successfully removed the human hand, this may feature as a fundamental lesson. A significant proportion of behavioural dysfunction is a result of incorrect negative reinforcement (McGreevy and McLean, 2005).

Negative Reinforcement in Horse-Training – In-Hand

In-hand, the negative reinforcement process, involves training the horse to *lead forward, turn, stop* and, sometimes, to *step back*. As far as *leading forward* is concerned, the aim is to train the horse to step forward from anterior lead pressure. However, horses are stronger than humans and when faced with the two choices of relenting or not to the forward lead pressure by stepping forward, many choose to tolerate and possibly desensitise to the poll pressure. Most horsepeople, therefore, prefer to pressure the young horse slightly sideways (~45 degrees) because this way, as the horse relents, it can be moved a fraction forward more easily (Figure 6.6). When the horse steps forward, the lead-rein pressure is immediately released. This termination of pressure reinforces the embryonic step forward and the horse increasingly offers this response each time the *lead forward* pressure is presented in a similar context. Typically, the horse offers responses more consistently from anterior pressure and some time later will offer a number of steps and respond to increasingly light signals. As well as training the horse to lead in a straight line, by using negative reinforcement in the form of pressure release the trainer may also reinforce faster or longer steps from subtle differences in the duration of anterior lead signals.

The *stop* and *step-back* responses are trained using negative reinforcement in the same way, except that pressure is delivered by the posterior-facing lead-rein. Here again, the pressure is released as soon as the animal gives the correct response and, again, the signal can be modified to elicit slowing and shortening of the stride responses. Similarly, during lungeing, the trainer negatively reinforces the horse's forward response using the lungeing whip for acceleration and the lunge rein (albeit at an oblique angle) for deceleration.

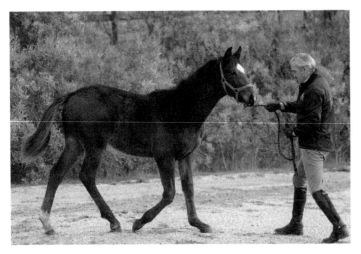

Figure 6.6 Training a naïve horse to *lead forward* involves reinforcing a single step of the forelegs slightly sideways. Sideways facilitates the *step forward* by inhibiting backward resistance.

Negative Reinforcement in Horse-Training – Under-Saddle

Under-saddle, notwithstanding minor differences in equestrian pursuits, the following basic mobility alterations predominate: going forward, stopping, going backwards, changing direction with the forelegs or hindlegs and going sideways to right or left. These variations in mobility are trained via negative reinforcement in that one or both reins or one or both of the rider's legs elicit the appropriate response through pressure and its release. Again, further developments can take place where the strides can be quickened, slowed, shortened or lengthened through the training of variations in pressures from rein or rider's leg (Figure 6.7). These alterations typically involve variations in duration or magnitude of pressure. Horse-riders also use rein or leg pressure to effect alterations in head- and neck-carriage as well as body posture (longitudinal and lateral bend) and also to increase engagement.

Whips and spurs are used by many riders under the very same principles of negative reinforcement to effect control where the rider's legs fail to produce a sufficient response. When whips or spurs are used to trigger certain desirable behaviours, their intermittent pressure is maintained or increased until the desirable behaviour emerges (Table 6.2). Intermittent pressures such as those from whips and spurs have two modes of interaction: their effect is a result of their magnitude and/or the frequency of use, both of which can be varied. The same is true for any intermittent pressure, such as the rider's legs (kick, squeeze, nudge) and the reins (pull, squeeze, vibrate). Similarly, curb bits with lever-action shanks produce a dramatic increase in pressure in the horse's mouth that depends largely on the length of the curb shank. Such technologies have been used for centuries because they can inflict greater discomfort on the animal compared with standard rein and leg pressures. They are effective because they breach well into the pain threshold of practically all horses, regardless of sensitivity, overshadowing all other salient stimuli in the animal's immediate perception. They represent pressures that every horse will want to terminate.

When Negative Reinforcement Goes Wrong

Negative reinforcement is also the responsible mechanism behind what are known as evasions. Head-shy horses manage to stop having their heads touched by learning to throw their heads and remove a person's hand. Girth-shy horses, if they are successful, might manage to buck the saddle and girth off. Clipper-shy horses effectively remove clippers from their vicinity. Leg-shy horses remove human hands from their legs, and

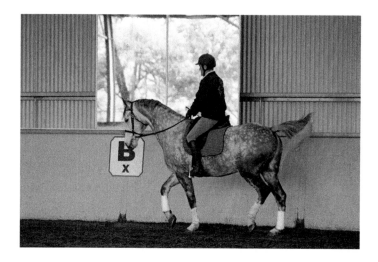

Figure 6.7 Shortening the strides can be trained by variations in the duration and magnitude of rein tension that become associated with seat characteristics.

Table 6.2 Facilitating the learning of locomotory responses: the relationship between applying various aversive stimuli and the negative reinforcement of removing them.

Required response	Aversive stimulus	Negative reinforcement
Acceleration and deceleration in-hand	Lead-rein signals	Removal of lead-rein tension
Acceleration under-saddle	Leg signals	Removal of leg pressure
Acceleration under-saddle	Whip	Removal of whip
Acceleration under-saddle	Spurs	Removal of spurs
Deceleration under-saddle	Bit: via reins	Removal of tension

Table 6.3 Learning various unwelcome behaviours: the relationship between various aversive stimuli and the negative reinforcement provided by their removal.

Behaviour problem	Aversive stimulus	Negative reinforcement
Head-shy	Hands touching head	Removal of hands
Clipper-shy	Clippers	Removal of clippers
Needle-shy	Injections	Removal of injection
Leg-shy	Hands touching legs	Removal of hands
Bucking	Rider's control	Removal of rider
Shying	Rider's control	Removal of rider's control
Rearing	Rein and leg pressures	Removal of rider's control
Head tossing	Rein tension	Removal of rein tension
Jogging	Rider's legs	Removal of rider's legs
Pulling back from tethering	Head restraint	Removal of head pressure

needle-shy horses remove veterinarians with sharp needles from their vicinity. Whip-shy horses are effective at removing any hint of whip use and, sometimes, even the rider. Even if a rearing horse is not lucky enough to remove a rider, it generally does manage to render the rider helpless for a moment so that the reins go slack and the rider's legs slide back away from the sensitive site (Table 6.3).

Fear associated with an experience results in associations being formed from single experiences, and also results in recurring fearful reactions in subsequent similar situations. Horses are capable of one-trial learning (McGreevy, 2004) and discover in just a single attempt that bucking is effective, even if the rider is not removed. Bucking is additionally reinforced by the removal of the rider's control during the event. Similarly, during shying, the rider is dislodged and, thus, her/his control is temporarily removed. Because of the context-specific way in which the horse learns, it is likely that an identical reaction will occur at the same site in the future. When horses swerve at jumping obstacles, the reaction is rapidly acquired because of the reinforcement provided by the escape.

Ethical Considerations when Using Negative Reinforcement

In negative reinforcement, the removal of pressure is reinforcing and the timing of removal is fundamentally important. There are at least two problems inherent in the use of negative reinforcement in equitation: first, the reinforcing attributes of negative reinforcement (the pressure reduction) may not be fully understood by riders, trainers and coaches (Warren-Smith and McGreevy, 2006). Riders of all skill levels are often unaware of the way in which they unintentionally negatively reinforce fear or hyperreactive responses, such as rearing and shying, where the horse is accidentally rewarded for the undesirable behaviour. The use of aversive stimuli in horse training, within the context of negative reinforcement, can be sustainable only when the aversive pressure is preceded by a classically conditioned cue (e.g. a neutral cue such as light pressure) and ceases when the correct response is offered. Second, the removal of rein tension requires considerable skill when riding the moving horse in the various gaits. Egenvall *et al.* (2012) showed that the release of rein pressure should be at the onset of the desired behaviour, which may be difficult to recognise or predict. If the release of pressure is late, behaviours indicative of conflict or stress increase. This highlights a cognitive difference between horses and dogs: Mills (1998) posited that it is possible to be later in reinforcing a dog for a behaviour than it is for a horse. Furthermore, the movement of the horse makes it difficult to deliver precise signals. One of the important features of horse-riding pedagogy surrounds the maintenance of a stable connection from the rider's hands to the horse's mouth and the maintenance of a stable leg and seat position (the latter moving with the kinematics of the horse's back in each gait, speed and direction).

Errors in negative reinforcement account for major behaviour problems when subtracted pressures are poorly timed and serve to strengthen incorrect responses, leading to conflict behaviours and prolonged stress (McLean, 2005b). It is therefore essential that riders are trained in the optimal use of negative reinforcement and, clearly, that the correct use of learning theory should be established as a 'first principle' in equestrian coaching.

Negative Reinforcement Versus Positive Reinforcement

Many animal-trainers focus only on training via positive reinforcement, because their subjects are required to perform at a distance, so negative reinforcement (typically, by applying pressure) is irrelevant in these circumstances. Animals such as dolphins, seals, bears, zoo elephants and dogs are, to a large extent, trained via positive reinforcement. In positive reinforcement, the trainer ignores errors made by the animal. If an animal takes fright during training for whatever reason, the trainer waits until the animal chooses to return to the training station. This presents no problem when the subject is at liberty, but when an animal flees with a rider astride, the situation is critically dangerous. Horse, camel and working elephant trainers almost universally use negative reinforcement because they can virtually 'force' the animal to *turn*, *slow* or *go* in adverse circumstances. Herein lies a fundamental difference between positive and negative reinforcement: in negative reinforcement, the trainer does not have to wait for the animal to offer the response – he or she can *contrive* it.

It is appropriate here to reiterate the use of positive and negative in terms of reinforcement and punishment (Figure 6.8). Remember these terms were coined from their mathematical, as in *add* or *subtract*, rather than ethical associations. Yet it is common to hear, even from professional trainers and scientists, positive reinforcement referred to as 'positive training', implying that negative reinforcement is 'negative training'.

Prima facie, the distinction between positive and negative reinforcement is simple: one is concerned with attractive stimuli and the other relates to aversive stimuli. However, if we accept that both positive reinforcement and negative reinforcement are concerned with goal-directed behaviours (acquiring resources or avoiding aversiveness), and therefore associated with drive reduction, we begin to see that there are elements of aversiveness embedded in positive reinforcement. For example, unless an

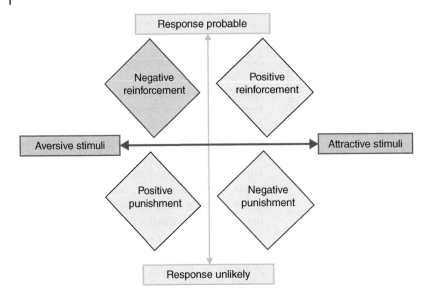

Figure 6.8 The likelihood of a horse in training offering a particular response is a result of the level of the attractiveness or aversiveness of the reinforcer/punisher. Within this structure lie all forms of reinforcement.

animal is completely satiated, it is subject to varying degrees of hunger, which is an aversive state. Authors, such as Perone (2003), have questioned whether the rat presses the lever because such behaviour produces food (the behaviour is positively reinforced) or because it reduces hunger (the behaviour is negatively reinforced). Such opposing, yet identical, propositions remind us that compartmentalising processes assists our understanding of nature on the one hand but, on the other, also narrows our perception. The learning processes of animals are more seamless than our arbitrary labels would suggest (see also Baron and Galizio (2006), Iwata (2006) and Sidman (2006) for an interesting discussion on the distinction between positive and negative reinforcement).

Combined Reinforcement

Positive and negative reinforcement can be used in conjunction, putatively to enhance the reinforcing effects of each other. Whether negative reinforcement training of horses is augmented by primary or secondary positive reinforcement, the actual mechanism of learning is termed combined reinforcement.

Combined reinforcement has been shown to be useful in many training situations, such as with rhesus monkey husbandry and dolphin management (Stacey *et al.*, 1999; Wergard *et al.*, 2015). For example, captive dolphins are positively reinforced for accepting veterinary interactions, but at the same time they are restrained by a net that negatively reinforces immobility. Research has shown that when combined reinforcement is used, the aversive effects of negative reinforcement may be reduced (McKinley, 2004; Warren-Smith and McGreevy, 2007(c)). In addition, combined reinforcement may also be used to increase the probability that the naïve horse shows the desired behaviour, which can then be rewarded through both negative and positive reinforcement (Figure 6.9).

Punishment

Punishment refers to the presentation of a stimulus that suppresses a behaviour (Figure 6.3). It can be divided into two categories: positive punishment and negative punishment, depending on whether the punitive situation arises because of the addition or omission of an event. Smacking,

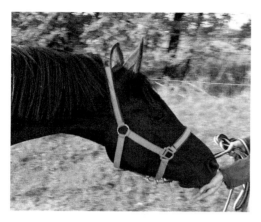

Figure 6.9 Negative reinforcement training (release of pressure) can be augmented by primary (e.g. food or wither scratching) or secondary (e.g. voice) positive reinforcement and this combined reinforcement may enhance the reinforcing effects.

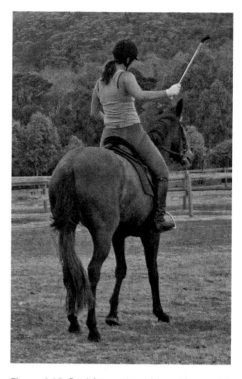

Figure 6.10 Punishment is replete with associated problems that range from a disinclination to trial new learned responses to the development of fearful associations with humans.

slapping, whipping, punching and kicking are typical examples of positive punishment (Figure 6.10). However, the term also embraces even minor amounts of discomfort that suppress any behaviour. Withholding something attractive, such as food, is an example of punishment by omission. Negative punishment is usually not deliberately employed in horse-training, but it does occur occasionally and sometimes inadvertently. For example, if a horse is pawing while tethered, the trainer can walk away, which may negatively punish pawing.

Punishment terminates the behaviour that it follows, whereas reinforcement increases a behaviour. Both learning mechanisms can sometimes be identified to occur in the same situation. Take the example of trailer loading. In some countries, horsepeople have been known to use a long whip on the animal's hindquarters when it refuses to go any farther. However, each time the whip is used, the horse runs backwards faster, the opposite effect to what was intended. What began as a futile exercise in punishment has now turned into a (more futile) process of negative reinforcement, where the use of the whip has trained the horse to run backwards. Unfortunately, the amount of violence

characterised by punishment is often out of all proportion to the behaviour that it is intended to change.

Punishment is associated with certain emotional states, such as fear and frustration (Lindsay, 2000) and is cautioned because of its well-documented side-effects, such as:

a) Lowered motivation to trial new behaviours (Haag *et al.*, 1980);
b) Habituating the animal to punishing stimuli leading to learned helplessness (McGreevy and McLean, 2009a);
c) Deleterious emotional changes;
d) Negative associations with the punisher (Mills, 1998);
e) Learning deficits (Parker *et al.*, 2008); and
f) The possibility of post-traumatic stress disorder emerging, resulting in latent aggression (Bradshaw, 2009).

The formation of a conditioned emotional response (CER) is said to have occurred when an animal makes a reflexive association with a trigger. A CER can be either positive (+CER, i.e. if a signal reliably predicts a pleasant stimulus it is likely to induce a pleasant emotional response in the animal) or negative (−CER, i.e. the signal predicts an aversive outcome and induces a negative emotional response, such as fear). The formation of a −CER during training should be avoided, as it is both unethical and hampers further training.

However, it should be remembered that horse management frequently relies upon punishment. Consider an electric fence, for example. The electric fence is not only a positive punisher but also a highly aversive punisher; it may register as such a serious punitive event that an animal will scarcely venture to touch it a second time. As a punishing stimulus, an electric fence at least offers some controllability in the sense that the horse can actively choose to move away and release itself from the aversive stimulus. Compare this with an electric shock collar, where the controls are in human hands. Here, the animal has diminished control and is at the mercy of the skill of the human. For this reason, many countries have outlawed the use of electric shock collars.

Punishment is commonly used when a horse bites or kicks a human, lunges towards a human, or threatens to do so. McLean (2005(b)) has shown that biting and kicking may correlate with specific dysfunctions of the *go* and *stop* signals in-hand and under-saddle; therefore, it follows that punishing the horse for biting and kicking may be inappropriate, compared with the therapy offered by re-training the dysfunctional signals. Furthermore, punishment may not prevent future biting and kicking, because it does not address the cause. This important caution must apply to all situations where punishment occurs. Punishment, therefore, may provide the wrong answer to a problem and may be too simplistic as a solution.

Non-Contingent Punishment

When horses behave dangerously, such as bucking, rearing, shying or bolting, trainers often feel justified in attempting punishment. Sometimes this may be effective, although it is difficult to conceive any practical way to punish bolting. There are two common issues in the use of punishment. Both relate to the belief, in some circles, that the horse's behaviour was deliberate and that it is aware of its misdemeanours. The first problem is the potential for excessive physical punishment (to 'teach the horse a lesson'), which has no place in a modern training programme, and the second is the use of non-contingent punishment. For punishment to be effective it must be contingent – it must literally be connected to the offending behaviour. For example, when punishing a horse for kicking, the punishment must occur while the horse is kicking or at the precise moment the kick ends. The use of non-contingent punishment is confusing and frustrating for the animals concerned and, as it does with dogs (Lindsay, 2000), will most certainly have deleterious consequences. Because of such problems, punishment is best avoided.

When a jumping horse refuses an obstacle, it is not uncommon for trainers to use the whip as the horse stands motionless in front of the obstacle after its refusal. Punishment at that point is non-contingent and, therefore, devoid of any useful training effect. In some cases, the refusing horse is punished and then turned away for another presentation. When horses do attempt an obstacle after a random act of punishment, it is likely that increased anxiety levels make the horse run and, if the obstacle is in its path, it may well jump over it. At best, this is a haphazard training exercise, destined to have low, if any, efficiency. At worst, it simply trains the horse to default to a flight response in the presence of jumps.

Non-contingent punishment is ineffective. For example, a show-jumping horse that is pulling rails cannot be reformed by punishing it after it lands. In contrast, the importance of contingency has prompted some jumping trainers to resort to another technique: rapping. Rapping is an illegal practice (outlawed by the Fédération Equestre Internationale, FEI, rules) that involves an assistant hitting a horse's forelegs or hindlegs as he clears a jumping obstacle. When this is done repeatedly, there is a temporary alteration in the horse's perception of the jumping effort required for a given height, so the horse makes a short-term increase in jumping effort. Because of the damaging effects of incorrect use, punishment should be used *only* when other avenues have been exhausted. In addition, it is best used in conjunction with an antecedent secondary punisher (such as the word 'No!') so that the primary punisher itself can be eliminated at some stage. The need for caution regarding punishment underscores the importance of teaching horse-riding coaches the fundamentals of learning theory.

Experimental Neurosis

Gaining control over aversive stimuli (e.g. escape or avoidance) is vitally important to animals. When escape is thwarted, control is lost, the animal's wellbeing is threatened and experimental neurosis may develop. Hence, extra care must be taken when using aversive stimuli to train animals, because animals find it imperative to achieve control over such stimuli. Solomon (1964) showed that maladaptive behaviour arises when an aversive stimulus embodies these four conditions:

1) there are sustained raised levels of arousal;
2) the aversive stimulus is unpredictable;
3) the aversive stimulus is uncontrollable; and
4) the aversive stimulus is inescapable.

Numerous studies attest to the problems that emerge when these conditions arise. Pavlov's (1941) experiments with dogs provided one of the earliest accounts of experimental neurosis, based on discrimination training (Chapter 5, Associative Learning (Attractive stimuli)). In one experiment, he rewarded dogs for associating a leg movement with a circular patch of light, but punished them with an electric shock when they responded to an elliptical one. When the dogs had learned these associations, he began some alterations to the experiment: the elliptical patch was made more circular. At some point, the dogs were unable to distinguish between a rewarded shape and a punished one. Some of the dogs became very aggressive, while others tried to escape or gave up responding and fell asleep. Masserman (1950) performed a similar experiment on cats (Figure 6.11). He trained cats to open a box for a food reward when signalled by a light. Later, when the cats opened the food box they sometimes received a blast of air. Again, some of the cats became excitable and hyper-reactive, while others became dull and refused to move. These responses are examples of experimental neuroses.

Because of their reliance on stimuli based on aversiveness, horse-trainers should be very careful to ensure that the cues and pressures they use result in consistent, and

Figure 6.11 Masserman induced experimental neurosis in cats by punishing them with a blast of air after they had learned to open a box for a food reward.

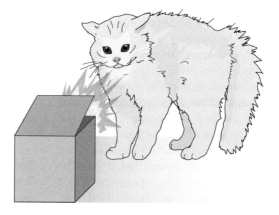

preferably improved, learned responses. The prevalence of hyper-reactivity and dullness among trained horses suggests that the importance of maintaining operant contingencies is not currently well understood among horsepeople. Self-carriage of speed, line and head-and-neck-posture should be maintained as a priority for the ridden, driven and led horse throughout the animal's working life.

Learned Helplessness

When animals are repeatedly exposed to pain as a result of sustained highly aversive stimuli, conditions such as experimental neurosis may escalate so that the animal loses all active control. When the highly aversive stimulus is totally inescapable, learned helplessness may set in. The important distinction here is that the animal no longer tries to cope – it simply gives up and becomes dull.

Learned helplessness was first identified by Seligman and Maier (1967); Maier *et al.*, (1969) following their experiments with dogs (Figure 6.12). After repeated exposure to inescapable aversive stimuli, the animals showed a deterioration of cognitive, emotional and motivational attributes. During the experiments, some dogs were trained to switch off an electric shock, administered to their feet, by moving their head sideways to contact a switch. Other dogs were similarly shocked, but were unable to switch the electricity off. The next day, these two groups of dogs plus another unexposed group were subjected to electric shocks in a shuttle box apparatus, where the dogs could terminate the shocks by jumping a small hurdle. All dogs rapidly learned to jump the hurdle, except some of the group that were unable to avoid the shock during the experiment the previous day. Those dogs were helpless and instead of trialling a response to avoid the shocks, they showed intense hyper-reactivity and then became passive. Weinraub and Schulman (1980) proposed that it was the uncontrollability of the experience rather than the experience of shock itself that interfered with subsequent avoidance learning. It was noted that with sufficient exposures, diminished aggression and loss of appetite occurred and apathy persisted in these dogs long after the experiment.

Investigating the effects of previous exposure and controllable shock with rats, Seligman (1975) showed that past experience in dealing with escapable shock *immunised* subjects from the effects of learned helplessness when exposed to inescapable shock later on. On the other hand, naïve rats that had never been exposed to escapable shock became helpless after exposure to inescapable shock. Furthermore, Hannum *et al.* (1976) showed that rats with previous experience in escaping shock early in their lives performed better in escape-learning tasks than did non-shocked controls. In dogs, it has been shown that individuals repeatedly exposed to excessive punishment, where they have learned to tolerate pain gradually become unmoved by increasing pain (Lindsay, 2000). Similarly, previous exposure to correct pressure/release can partially immunise horses against subsequent bad riding, but bad foundation training can leave a lifetime legacy.

The symptoms of learned helplessness in rats and dogs include anhedonia (loss of pleasure-seeking behaviour), depression and motivational, emotional and cognitive deficits (Seligman *et al.*, 1980; Pratt, 1980). Worse still, in the experiments carried out by Weiss *et al.* (1975), as well as by Seligman and Maier (1967), several rats and dogs died as a direct result of the experimental treatments. These events confirm the importance to animals of predictability and controllability, particularly when they are dealing with aversive stimuli. It is not surprising that learned helplessness has been used as an animal model of human depression and post-traumatic stress disorder (Hall *et al.*, 2007). The neural tissues responsible for generating experimental neurosis and learned helplessness are similar to human equivalents linked to depression (Cabib, 2006); their mechanisms seem to share a profound inhibition of dopamine release in the nucleus accumbens. A novel approach is to test affective states using cognitive bias tasks, which aim to test the choices made by animals (along the lines

(a)

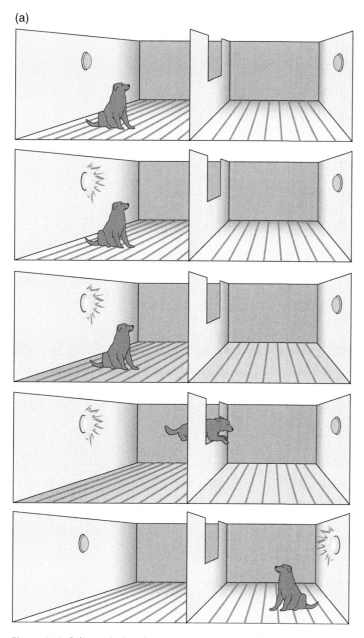

Figure 6.12 Seligman's dogs became apathetic when the warning light inconsistently predicted pain (illustrations (a) and (b)) and avoidance became impossible.

(Continued)

of: is the glass half empty or half full?). For example, individuals in a negative affective state are more likely to interpret an ambiguous event negatively, and to anticipate negative rather than positive events (Paul *et al.*, 2005). In horses, this approach was used by Freymond *et al.* (2014), who reported that horses trained with negative reinforcement were more optimistic, compared to horses trained with positive reinforcement, despite the former showing more negative emotions during training.

Recent experiments with horses have aimed to investigate depression-like symptoms such as reduced attention and anhedonia (Rochais *et al.*, 2016; Fureix *et al.*, 2015).

(b)

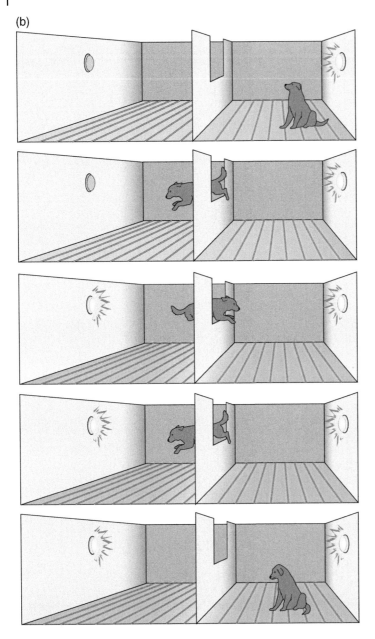

Figure 6.12 (Cont'd)

The authors suggest that a 'withdrawn' state in horses resembles the reduced environmental engagement that is characteristic of depressed humans. 'Withdrawn' horses were defined as displaying the 'withdrawn state' at least once out of approximately 907 behavioural scans (Rochais *et al.*, 2016), which appears to be a very low occurrence. Nevertheless, the occurrence of this state in horses was related to reduced sucrose intake (i.e. anhedonia; Fureix *et al.*, 2015) and lowered attention to novel stimuli (Rochais *et al.*, 2016). The authors suggest that the depression-like symptoms relate to inappropriate living conditions. Similarly, previous researchers have identified the possibility

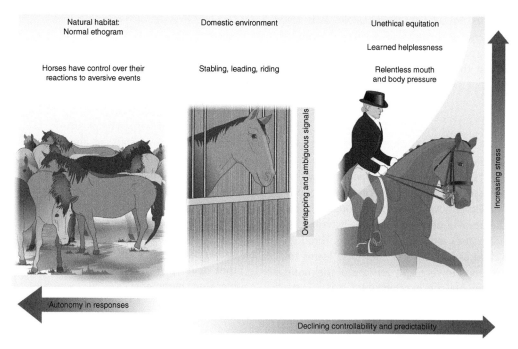

Figure 6.13 From the domestic horse's viewpoint, increasing amounts of losses of control followed by inescapable pain arising from poor equitation can lead to learned helplessness. This amounts to a major loss of controllability.

that learned helplessness in horses can occur (Ödberg, 1987; Lieberman, 1993; Ödberg and Bouissou, 1999). In a review of learned helplessness, Hall *et al.* (2007) indicated that some behavioural responses exhibited by the domestic horse are probably examples of learned helplessness. McLean and McGreevy (2004) pointed out that although many horsepeople assume that the loss of sensitivity in horses with 'hard (desensitised) mouths' and 'dead sides' is the result of accumulated scar tissue, it is more likely to reflect learned dullness. Just where this dullness emerges on the continuum that terminates in learned helplessness is not clear. However, the practice of using contradictory acceleration (leg/whip) and deceleration signals (bit via reins) simultaneously and indeed delivering these signals via amplifiers, such as the (lever-action) curb-bit and rowelled spurs, make the horse a likely candidate for learned helplessness (Figure 6.13). Learned helplessness would show up only after the failure of active coping mechanisms, such as bucking and hyper-reactivity. Established learned

helplessness may compromise horse welfare since an animal in this state has suffered a critical loss of control of its environment (Webster, 1994).

Conclusion

No matter how subtle it is, horse-training is largely based on the use of negative reinforcement. First principles in horse-training, therefore, are that pressure motivates the horse to respond, and its removal trains the response. Horses learn to *stop, go* and *turn* because these responses bring about the release of pressure associated with the rein or rider's leg, both in-hand and under-saddle. The anticipatory processes of classical conditioning result in the horse learning to respond to very light pressure or other cues.

Because the stimuli used in horse-training are based on aversiveness and because many disciplines of equitation may involve the use of severe bits and sometimes spurs, extra care should be taken to ensure that the cues and pressures are as light as possible. It is also important for the animal's welfare that use of pressure results in consistent learned responses and that these operant contingencies remain consistent over the animal's lifetime.

Take-Home Messages

- First principles in horse-training are that the pressure motivates the horse to respond, and its removal trains the response. It is the removal of pressure that initially trains the responses required in equitation. Through classical conditioning, the horse learns to respond to very light versions of the motivating pressure or other cues.
- Reinforcement is very effective and works irrespective of the trainer's intentions.
- Negative reinforcement training can be augmented by primary or secondary positive reinforcement and this combined reinforcement may enhance the reinforcing effects.
- Fear responses should be avoided at all costs because of their rapid acquisition and their resistance to erasure. It is also important to prevent fearful reactions recurring in subsequent similar contexts, so trainers must be very cautious about invoking fear responses during training.
- A significant proportion of behavioural dysfunction in the ridden horse is a result of incorrect negative reinforcement.
- Training is essentially an exploitative event and there is no ubiquitous training method; all have advantages and pitfalls.

Areas for Future Research

- Learned helplessness is an interesting area for future research in horses. Inability to control aversive stimuli (e.g. from relentless and strong rein tension) may lead to certain levels of learned helplessness.
- The interaction of classical and operant conditioning is particularly relevant in equitation. Riders may apply a seat cue that precedes rein tension to classically condition a deceleration response or they may apply the two cues concurrently. It would be of interest to explore the relative strengths of association of these cues, their development, competition and their blocking characteristics.

7

Applying Learning Theory

Introduction

Successful equitation relies upon non-associative and associative learning processes in the horse. This chapter is dedicated to identifying how learning theory is correctly applied to training the ridden horse. Other elements of equitation, including rider position and balance, are described in Chapter 8, Training. The process of correctly applying learning theory can be understood systematically by means of a set of training principles that consider the nature and welfare of the horse and predict the success or failure of training, as well as its optimal efficiency. These training principles are also recommended by the International Society for Equitation Science (ISES, 2017):

1) Train according to your horse's ethology and cognition;
2) Use learning theory appropriately;
3) Train easy-to-discriminate signals;
4) Shape responses and movements;
5) Elicit responses one-at-a-time;
6) Train only one response per signal;
7) Form consistent habits;
8) Train persistence of elicited responses (known as 'self-carriage');
9) Avoid and dissociate flight responses; and
10) Demonstrate minimum levels of arousal sufficient for training.

Horse trainers across all disciplines of equitation should maintain these principles and consider the applications described in this chapter. In doing so, the horse's abilities as a work, sport or leisure animal will be maximised and learning rates accelerated. Furthermore, it is important that equestrian teaching manuals and institutions emphasise these as 'first principles', in order to lower behavioural wastage rates and increase safety for both riders and horses.

Achieving Stimulus Control

The fundamental locomotory capabilities of the horse (to accelerate, decelerate, turn the forelegs and turn the hindlegs) provide the basis for all the movements in all equestrian sports and disciplines and so may be called the four basic responses. These reactions are provided by the biomechanical characteristics of the quadrupedal limbs, such as retraction, protraction, abduction and adduction in either the swing or stance phase and prescribed by the particular gait (as described in Chapter 11, Biomechanics). Cognitive constraints on biomechanics suggest that the most salient moment to apply signals and cues is at the onset of the swing phase of the relevant limb(s) and that this 'window' diminishes as the limb begins to engage in the stance phase, which is preoccupied with proprioception (Maes and Abourachid, 2013).

The basic locomotory responses are the concrete foundations on which are built shoulder-in, half-pass, pirouette, travers, renvers, piaffe, passage, rein-back, side-pass,

Equitation Science, Second Edition. Paul McGreevy, Janne Winther Christensen, Uta König von Borstel and Andrew McLean.
© 2018 John Wiley & Sons Ltd. Published 2018 by John Wiley & Sons Ltd.
Companion website: www.wiley.com/go/mcgreevy/equitation

roll-back and jumping. Many of these involve more than one of the above four basic responses and so are *composite sequences* of the basic locomotory building blocks. Therefore, the aim of trainers, both in-hand and under-saddle, is to place these responses under the *stimulus control* of signals provided by the rider or trainer.

When horses shy, leap or stall in response to environmental events, they are under control of those events more than under control of the rider or trainer. Training and re-training, therefore, are focused on removing environmental influences as much as possible and replacing them with signals issued by humans through correct use of desensitisation techniques and operant conditioning.

Because the currently known mental characteristics of the horse place certain limitations on its information-processing abilities, the precautionary principle should be adopted and the horse should not be expected to extrapolate or understand exceptions to rules or to infer responses when signals are unclear. The horse trainer's task is not to make the horse submissive so that it does what is required (as many people believe), but to *train* it to do what is required by reinforcement and repetition so that it forms desirable habits. Trainers should be very particular about the way they go about training signals, because the task the horse faces is far from simple. Wiepkema (1987) described the importance to animals of consistent outcomes from stimuli so that they gain efficient control of their environment and resources. Thus, the ontogeny of consistent and uniform stimulus–response entities makes for predictability and controllability of an animal's environment.

Application of Learning Theory

Training animals utilises various pre-existing motivations and locomotory abilities. Therefore the effective use of non-associative and associative learning processes accounts for the most effective training. Previously, we have established that most forms of equitation principally involve the use of negative reinforcement, where the rider's legs and the reins or the lead-rein establish stimulus control over the horse's locomotion (McLean and McGreevy, 2004). The effect of negative reinforcement lies in the release of the aversive pressure, so it follows that in training, the timely removal of pressures from rein, leg and lead-rein is vital to ensure a training effect (Figure 7.1). Similarly, with the use of

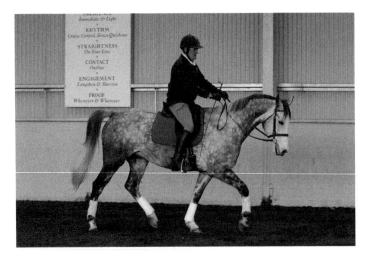

Figure 7.1 As illustrated in the previous chapter, contact is a neutral stimulus and thus obliges the rider to release the reins briefly yet regularly during locomotion to check that the rein contact pressure is not confusing. The horse should maintain his speed, direction and outline if contact training is correct.

positive reinforcement to further establish locomotory stimulus control, timely rewards are essential. Thus, precise timing is fundamental to correct training.

When pressures exerted on the horse by reins, legs, spurs and whip are not released at the correct moment, unwanted behaviours are inadvertently reinforced. If variable behaviours precede the release of pressure, confusion arises from loss of predictability and/or controllability, and conflict behaviours may set in. The horse may become hyper-reactive and tense, or the horse's responses may diminish and it becomes dull to the signals. Finally, inescapable uncontrollable pressure that creates significant pain may lead to learned helplessness. Euthanising horses due to behavioural problems may be the final solution to what begins as ignorance of training processes.

Another important and frequently misunderstood component is the nature of the pressure itself. To be effective, pressure must be sufficiently motivating for the horse to offer a response. Sometimes, however, the animal is reluctant to offer a response if that response is outcompeted by a more salient stimulus. For example, the horse is signalled to go forward into a creek or puddle but perceives the water as highly aversive. It now faces a dilemma: which is the more aversive, the leg/whip combination or the water? Trainers may attempt to overcome this dilemma by increasing the pressure of the leg/whip stimuli until the horse goes forward through the water. While this may be effective with some horses in some situations, this method may lead to escalation of arousal and negative associations in other horses. If so, the rider should either exploit the natural social tendency of horses to follow other horses and allow the horse to follow another habituated horse into the creek, or use an appropriate desensitisation technique. Sometimes simply waiting for 20 seconds or so for arousal levels to lower may stimulate the horse to investigate and enter the creek. It is essential that stress levels are kept low so that only the correct response is learned.

For the same reason, punishment should never be used in this situation.

In training and re-training, the use of a single aversive pressure (positive punishment) instead of the maintenance or an escalation of pressure followed by release (negative reinforcement) is ill-advised. The use of positive punishment in training is cautioned against because of its well-documented side-effects:

1) Punishment only tells the horse what it should not do, and not what it should do, and regular use of punishment reduces motivation to trial new behaviours (Haag *et al.*, 1980).
2) The trainer may unknowingly use far too much pressure, causing an overly fearful reaction. This fear reaction may then be the learned outcome. Furthermore, this incorrect response may be learned in just one trial, particularly if the sudden pressure is interpreted by the horse as highly aversive (see one-trial learning in Chapter 6, Associative Learning (Aversive stimuli)).
3) Fearful reactions may unexpectedly reappear in other challenging circumstances.
4) The horse may form negative associations with the punisher (Mills, 1998). If the rider's legs or whip is used as a punisher, it may lead to deleterious emotional changes (i.e. a negative conditioned emotional response (CER) to the legs and whip, and learning deficits may result when the same stimuli are intended to be used as light cues for desired responses.
5) Punishment may result in the development of learned helplessness (McGreevy and McLean, 2009(a)).

It makes more sense and is more in alignment with learning theory to start with a mild pressure and either maintain it, or if no response occurs, progressively escalate the aversive pressure until the precise moment of the correct response and then release. In this way, the horse has a chance to learn which responses the trainer wants, and not just what the trainer does not want.

Although simply escalating pressure may work for skilled trainers, it may not be a good solution if the horse is fearful. Obviously, training should initially take place in a safe environment as stress induced by environmental stimuli increases the level of pressure required to achieve a response (because environmental stimuli may overshadow signals from the rider or trainer). In subsequent repetitions, the trainer should be mindful of the amount of pressure that resulted in the correct response and aim to reach that level of pressure more quickly than before. Avoiding habituation to pressure is an important caveat in the use of escalating pressure, but it must be reconciled with the necessity of using a uniform scalar increase in pressure. When using the whip, for example, the trainer should escalate the whip-tap sequence. Temporal gaps between whip-taps may constitute reinforcement (by their removal), and although the duration of the time space has not been researched at this point, it is scientifically appropriate to suggest that the temporal gaps should be as short as possible and that the rhythm of the taps should be consistent. Beginning with the lightest of taps is important, because the light tap soon heralds the onset of stronger aversive pressure and thus becomes a discriminative stimulus itself.

So the horse soon learns to respond to light leg signals or light whip-taps.

Another important aspect of the use of aversive pressure lies in the quality of response that is offered. It is important to apply the principles of shaping and progressively build a response to the desired quality. If the basic responses (*go*, *stop* and *turn*) are well consolidated, these will be cued from light signals and will form the foundation for composite movements. Trainers should have a clear picture of their expectations and should also become skilled in breaking these down to the most irreducible blocks of single learned responses.

While the notion that the release of pressure reinforces the preceding response seems simple, trainers do not always understand what actually constitutes pressure. For example, when initially making contact with any part the horse's body, this may be perceived as aversive by the horse and the trainer should remember that if the horse offers any reaction resulting in the person's hand being removed, this removal is reinforcing (Figure 7.2). Thus, horses become increasingly head-shy and leg-shy when their reactions result in the removal of the human contact. This neatly illustrates the importance of the knowledge of learning theory – the remedy is self-evident when it becomes known that removal of

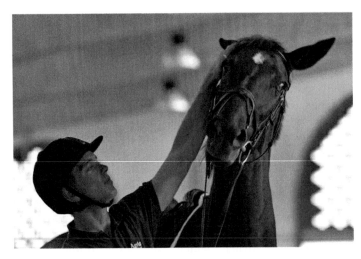

Figure 7.2 Removing your hand at the wrong time from the head of a head-shy horse reinforces head-shyness. (Photo courtesy of Elke Hartmann.)

aversive stimuli is reinforcing. So, to habituate the horse to the human touch, the answer lies in *not* removing the stimulus until the horse is still or calm. In a sensible training programme, it is important not to flood the horse with an aversive stimulus, but to progressively habituate at the lowest thresholds of aversive pressure. It is also important to habituate well past the point of initial habituation (McGreevy, 2004), because there are likely to be unseen physiological stress responses, such as an elevated heart rate, that take longer to return to baseline.

Classical Conditioning

The cognitive processes of classical conditioning provide the neural architecture for acquiring signals. Pavlov showed that efficient acquisition occurs when the new signal is contiguous (joined) with the older already known response in several ways. The new signal can occur just before, overlapping or during the already known response, but no acquisition takes place if the signal occurs after the already known response. The close temporal connection of the preceding signal to the response is important in establishing learning efficiency. The response soon

becomes contingent (dependent) upon the signal so that, from the horse's viewpoint, the signal consistently predicts the response. Therefore, voice commands, postural signals (seat, position) and light diminutive versions of the pressures installed by negative reinforcement should initially be paired each time with the pressures themselves (Figure 7.3).

Signals can also be effectively learned during a response. For example, consider classically conditioned urination (as described in Chapter 5, Associative Learning (Attractive stimuli)): the most effective way to get a whistle to initiate urination is to whistle at the very first sign of urination (each time the horse positions its legs for urination). In other words, the whistle should precede and overlap the behaviour.

Installing Signals

Horses often wear headcollars, halters or bridles for in-hand training. Attached to these are reins or a rope, so trainers can achieve speed and line control. Anterior facing lead-reins exert pressure mostly at the top of the horse's head, which usually provides the motivating pressure for negatively reinforcing the forward response. The lead-rein signal

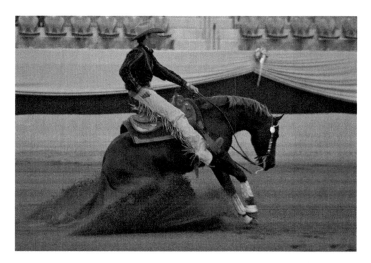

Figure 7.3 In some disciplines such as reining, the rider leans back when using the reins to stop the horse and, by classical conditioning, the horse soon learns to stop from the leaning back of the rider without the reins being used. (Photo courtesy of Julie Wilson.)

may be fortified by rhythmically tapping the horse's sides with a whip until it steps forward. Similarly, the motivating level of pressure for *forward* may arise from the use of a Dually™ halter, which presses on the nasal bones and mandible. In some methods, horses are encouraged to learn to move in response to the trainer's body/feet moving. However, this can be problematic for horses, because there will inevitably be exceptions to this rule and such exceptions are cognitively challenging for horses. For example, when a horse is tethered or loaded into a trailer, the horse perceives the conditioned stimulus to move (the trainer's body/feet moving), but he cannot move. This confusion may lead to increased stress. It is therefore sensible to choose signals that are unique to the desired response.

Posterior facing leads exert pressure on the horse's nasal bones, which negatively reinforce *stopping*, *slowing* and *stepping backwards*. Because of the effects of classical conditioning processes, the horse soon learns that escalating pressure is preceded by a discriminative stimulus, the light lead signal, and so it soon learns to react to that signal (Chapter 6, Associative Learning (Aversive stimuli)). Similarly, the horse also learns to respond to voice commands and visual signals.

The use of negative reinforcement provides an efficient mechanism for rapidly achieving control of the horse's locomotory responses, because it motivates the animal to trial a response. The use of negative reinforcement is termed *Phase 1* in the training process in-hand and under-saddle (McGreevy and McLean, 2007), as shown in Table 7.1.

In correct equitation, the pressures provided by the reins and the rider's legs begin with the lightest pressures and smoothly but rapidly increase to a threshold that prompts a desired response. So, the initial light pressure acts as a discriminative stimulus heralding the onset of stronger pressures that approach this threshold. The subsequent release of pressure reinforces the correct response and

Table 7.1 Examples of the training phases of negatively reinforced locomotory responses during training and riding. In phase 1, the stimulus–response relationship is established through negative reinforcement. In phase 2, the light signal (the discriminative stimulus) becomes the trigger that elicits the response (i.e. avoidance learning). The response to the light signal is acquired through classical conditioning. In phase 3, other neutral stimuli become associated with the response through classical conditioning.

Phase 1	Phase 2	Phase 3	
Original stimulus	Discriminative stimulus (light versions of the original stimulus)	Other discriminative stimuli (examples)	Locomotory response of the horse
Under-saddle			
Both reins via the bit or 'bitless' bridle	Light rein signal	Voice command or seat signal	Inter-gait and intra-gait downward transitions
Single rein	Light rein signal	Seat signal	Turn
Rider's two legs/spurs	Light leg signal	Voice command	Inter-gait and intra-gait upward transitions
Rider's single leg/spur	Light leg signal	Seat signal	Sideways
In-hand			
Anterior direction pressure of the rope/ lead-rein	Light signal in the rope/ lead-rein	Voice command or visual signal	Inter-gait and intra-gait upward transitions
Posterior direction pressure of the rope/ lead-rein	Light signal in the rope/ lead-rein	Voice command or visual signal	Inter-gait and intra-gait downward transitions

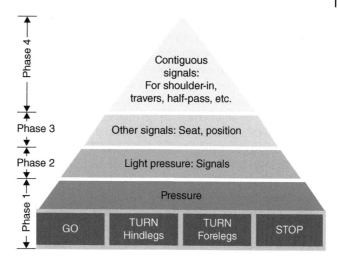

Figure 7.4 Diagram showing that the correct order of training begins with stronger pressure used to motivate *stop*, *go* and *turn* responses. Pressures should rapidly shrink to light versions, and from here other signals can be introduced. Finally, after consolidation of these basic responses, movements that consist of composites of these basic elements can be trained.

then, through classical conditioning, the discriminative stimulus (the light cue) becomes the trigger that alters the horse's locomotion. This transformation is termed *Phase 2* of training (Table 7.1). Ultimately, stimulus control of all locomotory responses, both in-hand and under-saddle, should be achieved via these light signals: the diminutive version of the original rein or leg pressures.

Finally, further discriminative stimuli, such as the seat, posture and voice, can achieve stimulus control. Again, these signals are acquired through the process of classical conditioning. Because the stimuli in this case are not directly related to the diminutive versions of the original pressures, their emergence as discriminative stimuli is termed *Phase 3* of training (Table 7.1).

When the first three phases are consolidated, the horse can be trained to do certain *movements* where the earlier trained single responses are contiguously elicited. This is termed *Phase 4* of training. These movements include, for example, *side pass*, *shoulder-in*, *travers*, *renvers*, *pirouette* and *roll-back*.

It is important to recognise the characteristics of the four phases of training and the different mechanisms of learning (negative reinforcement and classical conditioning) they employ. While desirable responses can be classically conditioned, many undesirable responses can also emerge if the basics are not established unequivocally at *Phase 1*.

The four phases of training can be summarised as follows (Figure 7.4):

- *Phase 1* – Trial-and-error (operant) learning where the horse learns the correct response to the pressure stimulus.
- *Phase 2* – Shrinking the pressures used in pressure/release training so that they become light versions of the same stimuli. Responses are now under stimulus control.
- *Phase 3* – Classical conditioning of light signals to other unrelated cues. This is the phase where new cues achieve stimulus control.
- *Phase 4* – Contiguous responses such as *turn* and *go* are elicited to produce movements. These are then repeated to form habits.

Similarly, for horses trained using visual or verbal cues and positive reinforcement, the original signal, which perhaps was a distinct movement from the trainer, can shrink to a very subtle visual signal, or be associated with other signals.

Combined Reinforcement

As positive reinforcement has become more popular in training riding horses, it is important to accurately recognise the negative reinforcement components of all under-saddle interactions and therefore to be cautious in attributing results solely to positive reinforcement. Since horses did not evolve to be ridden or led, and since they are motivated to remove even the light touch of an insect, then any discomfort exerted by humans is likely to be significantly inconvenient. Whether negative reinforcement training of horses is augmented by primary or secondary reinforcement, the actual mechanism of learning should be termed combined reinforcement, which has been shown to be useful in many training situations, such as with rhesus monkey husbandry and even dolphin management (Stacey *et al.*, 1999). For example, captive dolphins are positively reinforced for accepting veterinary interactions but, at the same time, they are restrained by a net, which negatively reinforces immobility. Combined reinforcement more accurately accounts for much of what many modern-day clicker trainers claim as training done solely by positive reinforcement. Any behaviour elicited by the removal of tactile somatic tension, no matter how light, constitutes negative reinforcement.

While operant conditioning provides a 'toolbox' for trainers, there are other factors that influence the outcome of learning and therefore the learning modality that the trainer might choose. It is critical to remember that animal training is largely dependent on motivation. In the natural world there may be a number of conflicting motivations and the most salient one will be responded to. This is an important concern for safety. While food as a primary reinforcer can achieve a high degree of salience, and may out-compete the motivation for avoidance of aversive stimuli to some extent, it is unlikely to out-compete the motivation for a flight response in strongly frightening situations (McGreevy *et al.*, 2014(a)). In this light, we might see that negative reinforcement and positive punishment could out-compete positive reinforcement and negative punishment for salience. However, this does not account for the insecurity of the particular animal, which may also have an influence on the outcome. For example, a well-trained horse trained through positive reinforcement may be less likely to be fearful than one poorly trained through negative reinforcement in challenging circumstances. Given the high death and serious injury rates of humans in horse–human interactions, the relative salience of positive, negative and combined reinforcement protocols in challenging situations needs to be explored further.

As details of operant and classical conditioning paradigms that explain horse-training have been identified, other more esoteric aspects of training have now come under the research spotlight. Recent work has highlighted the importance of various factors that influence learning outcomes, such as arousal, affective states (Starling *et al.*, 2013) and attachment (McLean *et al.*, 2013). Highly aroused horses may be differently motivated for food or the removal of aversive stimuli and, furthermore, highly aroused states may inhibit learning. High levels of arousal are common with punishment strategies and can sometimes occur with negative reinforcement if pain thresholds are raised. On the other hand, the generally lowered arousal states of positive reinforcement schedules can stimulate a broader attentional focus and therefore increase the tendency to trial new responses. Positive and negative affective states may also influence learning. These states are fundamentally about optimistic and pessimistic outlooks, where animals may tend to trial new responses or become risk-averse. One study suggested that although negatively reinforced horses showed more negative emotions during training compared to positively reinforced horses, the former were more optimistic in a judgement bias test (Freymond *et al.*, 2014). This may be explained by the difference in reinforcement contingencies: in optimal negative reinforcement, the reinforcement is continuous, whereas in positive reinforcement, the reinforcement often switches from a continuous schedule to a variable schedule. Furthermore, during shaping, the animal may offer many unrewarded responses before it chances upon the correct response. Thus combined reinforcement may provide the most expedient and welfare-friendly mode of horse training, given the strengths and limitations of operant conditioning strategies. In addition, the bond between horses and humans may be explained by attachment theory and this in turn is likely to affect learning outcomes if the animal's attentional mechanisms are directed more toward one person than another (Fureix *et al.*, 2009; Sankey *et al.*, 2010(c); DeAraugo *et al.*, 2014; Payne *et al.*, 2015). While it is now widely accepted that the dog–human relationship can be explained by attachment theory, the horse–human relationship has not been thoroughly explored. Because the horse is a social animal, there is a strong possibility that attachment theory underpins the horse–human relationship also.

Perseveration

In traditional equestrian training based on negative reinforcement, the horse is required to maintain a behaviour, 'keep going' (i.e. if signalled to trot, it must keep trotting until signalled to do something else). It is possible that there is an element of the unreinforced process of perseveration in maintaining certain responses in horse-training. Perseveration is the term used to describe the behaviours of animals that continue to offer a trained response, even when it no longer yields rewards. It is recognised as a feature of stereotypic birds and rodents (Garner and Mason, 2002), but more recently has been reported in horses (Hemmings *et al.*, 2007; Roberts *et al.*, 2015). Interestingly, the studies have found that crib-biting horses displayed a bias towards habitual response patterns, even in the context of minimal training. Roberts *et al.* (2015) reported that stereotypic horses (both crib-biters and weavers) acquired an initial response faster than non-stereotypic control horses, whereas Hemmings *et al.* (2007) did not find a significant difference between crib-biters and non-stereotypic controls in response acquisition. However, both studies concluded that crib-biters required significantly more unreinforced trials before the previously learned response was extinguished. This resistance to extinction may

potentially be beneficial in traditional horse-training based on negative reinforcement, and trainers rarely dislike stereotypic horses for reasons other than management problems. That said, it should be noted that the equine studies in this domain have positively reinforced subjects for pressing levers, so there is a need for caution when applying these findings to the ridden horse that is trained almost exclusively with negative reinforcement.

The basal ganglia are implicated not only in stress but also in stereotypic behaviours and alterations in learning. Inside the basal ganglia, the striatum filters and relays information to and from cortical structures and is integral in motivation, action and learning. Chronic stress has been shown to alter dopaminergic modulation of the striatum. For example, crib-biting horses have been reported with significantly higher receptor subtypes in regions of the basal ganglia associated with reward (the nucleus accumbens) and significantly lower numbers of receptors in the basal ganglia region known as the caudatus, the tissue involved in determining action and outcome (McBride and Hemmings, 2005). In rats, inactivation of the dorsomedial striatum impairs both reversal learning and strategy switching and is, thus, implicated in the perseverance of behaviours, including stereotypies (Ragozzino, 2007). In horses, there appears to be a difference relating to the type of stereotypy displayed: horses with an oral stereotypy (crib-biting) acquired habitual response patterns (i.e. they performed significantly more operant responses during an extinction phase, where the response was unrewarded) compared to horses with a locomotor stereotypy, such as weaving, and non-stereotypic controls (Roberts *et al.*, 2015).

Contact

In some sports, such as reining, the rider maintains his or her legs away from the horse, only making contact to initiate movements. Similarly, the reins are loose until the rider wishes to effect a *slowing* or *turn* response. In these sports also, turns of both forequarters

(a)

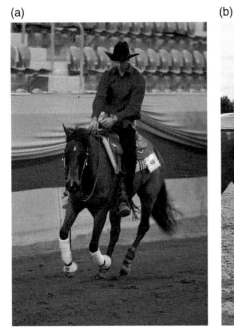

(b)

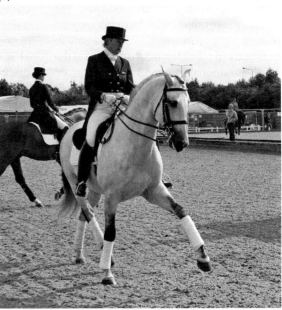

Figure 7.5 The presence or not of constant rein contact is one of the chief differences between reining (a) and dressage (b) training. (Photos courtesy of (a) Julie Wilson and (b) Kyra Kyrklund.)

and hindquarters are sometimes trained from the turn signals of the rein(s). In the Olympic sports of dressage, jumping, eventing and allied sports, such as showing, the rider maintains contact of the legs (calves) and reins at all times (Figure 7.5). Thus, low-level pressures of rein and leg contact become neutral. Turns of the forelegs are elicited only by the rein(s). Turns of the hindlegs are trained and elicited by a single leg moved back along the thorax by approximately 10 cm. The turn of the hindlegs is negatively reinforced by the rider's single leg, and the horse learns the discriminative stimulus of the light pressure. During forward motion, the horse is generally not required to pivot around the forelegs but to go sideways. So, here the turn of the hindlegs around the forelegs develops into a sideways movement.

Using the Whip

The use of the whip warrants some discussion (the debate around its use in certain sports is discussed in Chapter 14, Ethical Equitation).

Whips are often seen as tools for punishment and their use as such is common in horse-training. When used as a tool of punishment, the force of the whip does not tend to diminish, whereas in negative reinforcement it *should* and *does* diminish, because the strength of the horse's reaction will dictate it. In punishment, the whip is used for non-compliance to the rider or trainer's demands. So, here the whip is used to punish the horse for *not* responding in the hope that the horse will reconsider the signal. This represents a very complex task and, coupled with poor timing and an inconsistent tapping rhythm, can lead to anxiety, confusion and conflict behaviours. It is even more contradictory if the whip is used to punish the horse for not responding to the reins for slowing.

It is far more effective if trainers and riders think of the whip as simply another signal (an extension of the fingers). They should, therefore, train the horse to respond correctly to the whip by using it in a light rhythmical tapping that increases in frequency, but not necessarily in intensity, and that targets a specific site on the horse's body for a specific

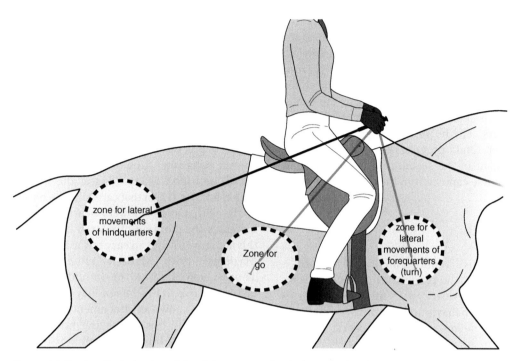

Figure 7.6 Precise discrimination of signals is necessary for the horse both in-hand and under-saddle. It makes sense to use the same regions on the horse's body to train the horse to respond from tapping with the whip for both in-hand and under-saddle training. The zones should be used consistently, but may differ between different training systems in relation to which area is used to elicit which response.

activity (Figure 7.6). For example, both in-hand and under-saddle, the whip can be successfully used on:

- the mid-thoracic region to motivate forward;
- the hindquarters to motivate turning the hindquarters and leg-yielding; and
- the (horse's) shoulder to motivate the turn of the forelegs.

As with all signals that manifest as negative reinforcement, it is crucial that the motivational pressure is maintained or, if no response is elicited, increased and then released as soon as an improved or correct response appears. Therefore, even with intermittent whip-taps, the tapping should not reduce in frequency or intensity until the desired response emerges. It is optimal to increase the frequency rather than the intensity and only increase the intensity as a very last resort. Furthermore, as training proceeds, the whip-taps naturally reduce as the horse learns the beginning taps as discriminative stimuli.

This reduction can develop into training the horse to respond appropriately to either quicken the steps or lengthen the steps. For example, two taps can be trained to signal quickening the steps, while one tap can signal lengthening the steps if negative reinforcement is used correctly.

Clucking

Horse-trainers commonly use a clucking noise made by the tongue in an *ad hoc* way rather than beginning and ending at a specific part of training a response. It may be perceived as an aversive stimulus and, therefore, it should be used in the format of negative reinforcement. Rather like a mild whip-tap, it can be used when the horse fails to respond to a signal. So, optimally, it occurs when the signal is given and continues without any alteration in rhythm or intensity except for an increase in intensity but not a decrease (as this can be reinforcing for some horses) and is ceased at the precise moment the horse offers a correct response. To illustrate, consider when a canter signal fails to elicit the canter and instead the horse simply runs faster at the trot. In this instance, the clucking should occur at the moment the canter signal is applied and continue until the horse canters. The horse will progressively canter earlier and progressively closer to the moment of the signal. In a few repetitions, the horse canters from the signal alone.

Rewards

In negative reinforcement, the reward is intrinsic – the removal of pressure is reinforcing. However, when the horse performs random behavioural responses that the trainer deems worthy of reward, primary reinforcers, such as food, or tactile rewards (caressing) can be administered, or else secondary reinforcers, including voice or patting, can be trained. The training clicker or whistle are also sometimes used as secondary reinforcers. Because of the risk of competing stimuli, it is prudent to use positive reinforcement when the motivating pressures of negative reinforcement have been diminished to light cues (McLean and McLean, 2008).

Secondary reinforcers should be carefully trained if they are to become effective as rewards (Figure 7.7) (also Chapter 5, Associative Learning (Attractive stimuli)). For example, verbal praise should be trained using the same approach as clicker training, where a precise vocal stimulus marks the correct behaviour (this must be accurately timed) and food or caressing at the wither region follows. Given that caressing the horse at the wither region lowers heart rate and increases the duration of relaxed behaviour, this activity provides an easy reward (Feh and Mazières, 1993; McBride *et al.*, 2004; Thorbergson *et al.*, 2016). In addition, the tactile rewards in this region may be aligned with what is known as 'attachment theory', in that the tactile rewards to the horse may consolidate the bond between horse and rider. The effects of tactile soothing rewards on human–human relationships and human–companion animal are well-documented (Fraley *et al.*, 2011; Odendaal and Meintjes, 2003). However, they are yet to be fully explored in horse–human interactions and represent a promising field of research.

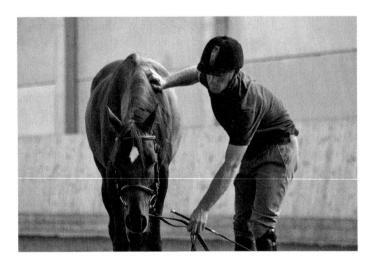

Figure 7.7 Judicious use of the term 'good boy' followed by wither caressing provides a convenient means of secondary reinforcement in training. Here a horse is trained to lower his head. (Photo courtesy of Elke Hartmann.)

Shaping

All equestrian disciplines involve progressive improvements in responses considered by trainers and judges to be correct. These improvements result from *shaping*. In most disciplines, horse-trainers attempt to control all the movement directions (forward, backwards and sideways). For each of these responses, however, there are several alternative reactions of its locomotion and posture that the horse can offer (e.g. not responding at all, delaying its reaction, only responding to strong signals, quickening, slowing, swerving and altering its head posture). Because it is the horse's locomotory abilities rather than its posture that present the greatest potential to thwart success and, furthermore, because locomotion is the most essential feature of the equid as a vehicle, trainers have long recognised that controlling locomotion is of primary importance. With sports, such as horse-racing, polo, hunting, camp-drafting and some Western disciplines, posture of the head and neck is clearly secondary to correct locomotory responses.

In some sports, particularly dressage, the postural requirement is highly significant to the extent that many trainers and riders today prioritise head-and-neck posture above locomotory responses. This has not always been the case, and classical dressage theorists believe that the body tonus, relaxation, and head-and-neck posture are consequences of consistent training of the horse's locomotion (Henriquet, 2004). Focusing on the head-and-neck posture at the expense of locomotory responses is implicated in conflict behaviours because the horse learns to prioritise, for example, shortening the neck before slowing its legs from the rein signals (McLean, 2003; McGreevy and McLean, 2005; McLean and McLean, 2008) (Figure 7.8).

So, training locomotory responses in terms of speed and direction is fundamental to all forms of horse-training. The shaping stages are also similar, regardless of what the horse is used for (Figure 7.9). From the standpoint of learning theory, it is essential

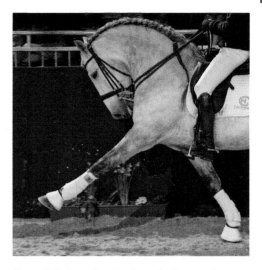

Figure 7.8 A modern tendency in dressage has been to achieve neck flexion from rein tension. Altering the horse's outline with the reins can confuse the *stop/slow* response and result in hyper-reactive behaviours and further deleterious effects. (Photo courtesy of Minna Tallberg.)

to recognise that the first locomotory aspects to be reinforced for any of the basic responses are the offering of a near-correct attempt in the chosen direction. Sometimes this is referred to as offering a good try (Parelli, 1995). Responding to pressure is the hallmark of *Phase 1* (Figure 7.4). Next, it follows that the horse should initiate its response without delay. This immediate responding ensures that the horse is moving beyond the trial-and-error stage of learning and the response to the signal is now more akin to being rote learned. During this phase of learning to respond immediately, the negative reinforcement (release of pressure) is swift and the horse learns that light pressure predicts stronger pressure. Through classical conditioning processes, the horse now learns to respond to light signals (*Phase 2*). The pressures have shrunk to much lighter versions of the original pressures for the particular response, so stimulus control is now achieved, even though speed and direction have not yet been shaped. At any point now, other signals (e.g. voice and seat) may be acquired, so stimulus control is further elaborated. When the horse is offering

(a)

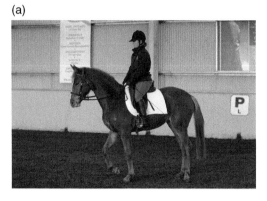

(b)

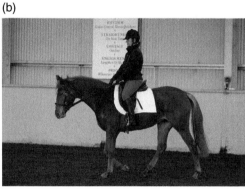

(c)

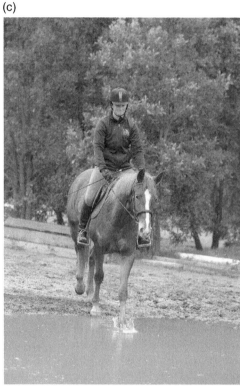

Figure 7.9 The '*go*' response requires several shaping stages, beginning with training a single step (a), then a stride followed by multiple strides (b) and ultimately training in new environments (c).

responses to light signals, there is a most significant opportunity to begin to positively reinforce, typically in the form of secondary reinforcement (e.g. 'good boy'). Earlier, when pressures were higher, they would be likely to outcompete any secondary positive reinforcement, because their removal would be generally seen as more salient (Warren-Smith and McGreevy, 2007(c)).

While the horse may be offering near-correct responses from light signals, it may still be exhibiting speed and line anomalies. Directional line refers to the response where the horse follows the precise track dictated by the rider or trainer. Because speed offers more danger (such as bolting) and because it is the greatest manifestation of fear responses compared with direction and line issues, it seems logical to shape speed control before line. Moreover, biomechanical studies on laterality suggest that losses of straightness may occur due to the different propulsive

characteristics (different power and speed) of the two diagonal couplets (Chateau *et al.*, 2004); Murphy *et al.*, 2005; Clayton *et al.*, 2007(a),(b); Colborne *et al.*, 2009). The horse is trained to maintain a particular speed through negative reinforcement via the reins or rider's legs. For example, if the horse quickens, the rider slows it; if it slows, the rider quickens it, but does nothing when the horse maintains its speed. In some equestrian disciplines, such as dressage, speed control may be shaped further so that the horse shortens and lengthens its strides from the rider's signals.

The final aspect of locomotory control is training the horse to maintain its direction and cease drifting to one side or the other. This is achieved through tension in the reins or pressure from rider's legs. In many horse-training methodologies, shaping also involves gradually refining the head, neck and body posture in addition to shaping locomotory responses that culminate in a 'rounded' outline, where the neck is to some extent arched and the nasal plane is slightly in front of the vertical plane.

The term 'straightness' is frequently used to describe a horse that is not flexed laterally in its vertebral column and its hindfeet track into its foretrack. The antithesis of straightness is crookedness. A horse that is crooked is not only asymmetrical in its gait but also drifting sideways to a greater or lesser extent or attempting to drift (McLean, 2003; McGreevy *et al.*, 2005; McLean and McLean, 2008). This attempting to drift lies at the heart of the problem of straightness. Equestrian texts pay scant attention to the loss of direction or attempts at losing direction that manifest as losses of straightness, yet are contained by uneven signal pressures of the rider. For this reason, we include directional line and straightness as synonymous.

In some sectors of contemporary equitation, the horse is not trained to maintain its own speed and direction but instead speed control is achieved by containing the horse between constant rein tension and pressure from the rider's legs, and directional control is achieved by containment between the rider's legs. The difference here is that if the rider relinquishes rein tension, such a horse may quicken, or if the rider removes leg contact, the horse may drift. Thus, in these situations the horse is not trained to maintain its speed and direction but trained to habituate to rein tension and leg pressures where the removal of them negatively reinforces the opposite response. Such training, where the removal elicits an opposing response and the horse is forced to habituate to certain pressures, is an inadvertent recipe for conflict behaviour. Nevertheless, to achieve some amount of speed and line control, training necessarily involves the progressive shaping of the same qualities of responses as described earlier for all equitation codes. The following qualities are, therefore, common to most methodologies of horse-training:

1) The correct locomotory responses emerge through trial-and-error learning (negative reinforcement).

2) The locomotory responses come under the stimulus control of the discriminative stimuli of the appropriate light signals of the rein(s), lead or rider's leg(s).

3) The correct locomotory responses occur within a distinct time-frame and locomotory structure.

4) Persistence without additional cueing of rhythm and tempo of locomotory responses.

5) Persistence without additional cueing of line and directional locomotory responses.

6) Persistence without additional cueing of the horse's head, neck and body postures.

7) All the above in different environments, ensuring that the horse is consistently under stimulus control in the face of other aversive and potentially competing stimuli.

We propose this as a basic training scale (and therefore to inform a dressage judging scale) for every learned response and movement. We stress that achieving stimulus control of locomotion is most important, and therefore, the ultimate outcome. Any training scale should be subject to peer review and refinement. It may be that training scales will eventually be informed by training profiles such as those conceptualised in the SMART models (McGreevy *et al.*, 2009(b)) (also Chapter 16, The Future of Equitation Science). Here, stimulus control is represented as responses with the greatest likelihood of being produced in response to the rider's stimuli, rather than, say, environmental stimuli. These models are currently only conceptual, but the probability of horses responding in certain ways can be assessed using rein-gauge and pressure-detection technologies. The minimum pressure or tension required to elicit a response (the lightness) directly reflects the likelihood or probability of a given response.

The German scale (Table 7.2), while commendable for its focus on looseness and relaxation in the earlier stages, does not address the acquisition of a basic attempt, or stimulus control, and therefore lightness of the pressure signals. In the German scale,

Table 7.2 Examples of some traditional and contemporary training scales for horses in equitation.

Item	The German training scale (German National Equestrian Federation, 1997)	Baucher's training scale (Faverot de Kerbrech, 1891)	Equitation Science shaping scale (McLean and Mclean, 2008)
1	Rhythm	To train and adhere to lightness	Basic attempt – the horse offers a basically correct single response (e.g. one step)
2	Looseness	To obtain obedience to the legs	Lightness – the horse initiates its response to a light cue immediately (e.g. one stride)
3	Contact and acceptance of the bit	To obtain straightness	Speed control – horse offers multiple strides; intra-gait variations elicited by the rider or trainer are persistent
4	Impulsion	To get the horse used to doing without help from the cues	Line control – the directional line chosen by the rider or trainer is persistent
5	Straightness	To collect and engage the horse	Contact – rein, leg and seat connection and the horse's head, neck and body posture are sustainable. In dressage, this includes the continuum from engagement to 'throughness' and collection.
6	Collection		Stimulus control – the horse responds every time it is cued and only when it is cued, with all the above qualities in new environments and circumstances. (Collection emerges from this level as a result of transitions and progressive alterations in the horse's physique)

straightness is designated to be trained after impulsion. Since impulsion requires bilaterally uniform power from the horse and straightness implies even power of the legs (a horse that is not straight is drifting), we challenge the German scale. Biomechanical studies suggest that straightness and rhythm are interdependent and as such should be adjacent on a training scale.

Stimulus Generalisation

Stimulus generalisation is an important learning feature of higher vertebrates. It allows animals, in the face of slightly different experiential circumstances, to offer a response that is likely to be appropriate. It is also advantageous in training because it facilitates the acquisition of a learned response in different circumstances. For example, when a horse has learned to jump a few narrow obstacles, it will soon jump other similar ones in very different contexts. However, in the beginning phase of learning the new task,

the reaction is context-specific, only generalising later. Horsepeople see this phenomenon frequently. For example, a horse that has just learned to enter a horse trailer, water jump or racing starting gates will generally hesitate when presented with a different version of the same object/event. However, after some exposures to different versions, stimulus generalisation may begin to occur and, in combination with increased consolidation of the responses to the rider's cues, the horse shows progressively less hesitation (Figure 7.10).

Under-saddle horses soon learn to go forward from the leg signals of riders of different leg lengths. In other words, the place where acceleration is evoked is a different region of the thorax but nonetheless effective. The reason generalisation occurs is that there are sufficient contextual similarities between the older known stimulus and the new one to elicit the response associated with the older stimulus as also demonstrated by Christensen *et al.* (2008(b)) (also Chapter 4, Non-associative Learning). Having sufficient

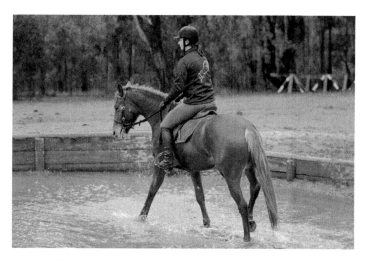

Figure 7.10 To generalise the stimulus of a water obstacle, a horse may need to have experienced going into several different water obstacles.

similarities is the important feature of stimulus generalisation for trainers to remember. Both stimulus generalisation and context-specific behaviours offer useful tools for the trainer. For the sake of efficiency, it makes sense to vary only one feature of an environment at a time, if possible, when attempting to generalise. The training of *piaffe* offers a useful example. In the beginning stages of *piaffe* training, most trainers attempt to elicit characteristically shortened steps. These will be highly context-specific at first, as the horse will associate not only the rider's signals but also the entire environment of the manège. However, the trainer soon wants the environment to be generalised so that the horse responds only to the rider's signals. It is, therefore, useful to train these early steps in just one place until the response is well under stimulus control and then begin to vary the place in small stages.

Principles of Training Arising from Learning Theory

The fundamental task of horse-training is to install desirable learned responses or habits. Habit formation results from the process of long-term potentiation and there are certain conditions surrounding repetitions that enhance the process. It is well known that repetitions that are too close can inhibit learning. There is some evidence that inter-trial spacings of less than 20 seconds are less efficient in classical conditioning of involuntary responses (Prokasky and Whaley, 1963), but this is largely unexplored in horse-training.

A further question arises: what is the optimal number of improved or correct repetitions for efficient learning? In answering this question, we must consider the problem of overtraining, which can render horses stale and unresponsive (van Dierendonck, 2006). New neural pathways cannot sustain repeated stimulation, partly because of the massive oxygen and glucose demands of brain tissue and partly because of their lack of maturation. So, training presents us with a dilemma. The more repetitions we can achieve, the more consolidated learning will be, yet if we do too many repetitions, learning and perhaps some welfare aspects may decline. However, we know that in naïve animals, learning can begin to manifest in a few repetitions (Skinner, 1938). So, this suggests that trainers should terminate practice after eliciting three to five consequentially correct, improved, or corrected responses. While it is an age-old maxim in horse-training to always 'end on a good note', it is likely to be more efficient to end on a short *train* of correct or improved responses.

Trainers sometimes call the grouping of repetitions a *set*. To maximise the number of repetitions, we can repeat this train of repetitions a second or third time, provided a sufficient time gap is left between the sets of repetitions. During the resting moments, it is important not to repeat the particular repetitions, but other learned responses can be expressed because these arise from different neural pathways (Figure 7.11).

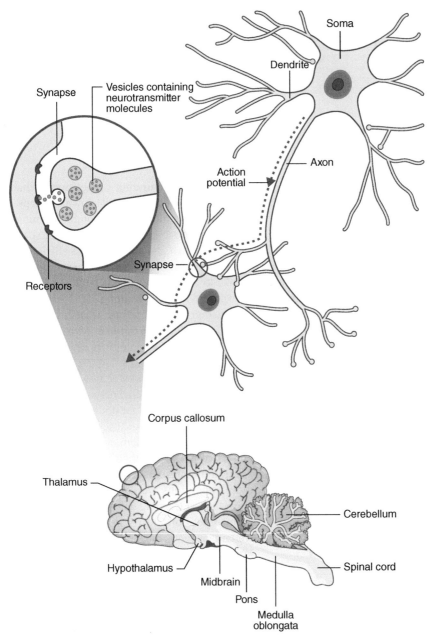

Figure 7.11 When a horse acquires a new learned response in training, specific neural pathways are activated. Repetitions strengthen these until habits begin to form. (Reproduced from *Equine Behavior*, copyright Elsevier 2004.)

The following sections give a detailed description of each of the 10 Training Principles (TP) introduced at the beginning of this chapter.

TP 1 Train According to Horse Ethology and Cognition

Ethology is the study of animal behaviour that provides information on how horses have evolved to live. It helps to explain natural equine social structures, including the complex dynamic social organisation, with a social order that determines access to resources. Horses need the company of their own species and readily form attachment bonds, so isolation is detrimental. They have evolved to walk and graze for about 16 hours per day and their digestive system and behaviours have adapted to this regimen.

Cognition refers to the ways in which animals process information about the world. Compared to humans, their prefrontal cortex is diminished, so horses may not recall events as we do. They excel at memorising and recognising stimuli that trigger certain responses, which is what keeps them safe. We must be careful not to overestimate equine intelligence (e.g. 'he knows what he did was wrong'), especially in an attempt to justify punishment. Equally, we should not underestimate equine intelligence by supposing that horses do not have emotions and feelings. Both over- and underestimating horses' intelligence can have negative welfare implications.

Training according to the horse's ethology and cognition means paying regard to the way horses have evolved, to their natural needs and to what motivates them. Although domestic horses have been bred in captivity for many generations, their social behaviour and social needs remain relatively unchanged (Figure 7.12).

(a)

(b)

(c)

(d)

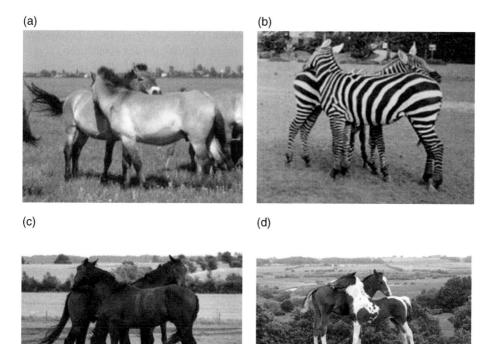

Figure 7.12 The behavioural repertoire of horses remains relatively unchanged by domestication. Grooming Przewalski stallions (a); Plains zebra stallions (b); Warmblood stallions (c); and foals (d).

TP 2 Use Learning Theory Appropriately

All training systems should demonstrate the appropriate use of learning theory, including both non-associative and associative learning.

Habituation is achieved when animals stop responding to events and stimuli as they become accustomed to them. Horses are innately fearful of the unfamiliar and often find the characteristics of various stimuli aversive (e.g. stimulus size/magnitude, novelty, proximity, and sudden appearance or occurrence). Movement, especially if an object's movement is erratic or is advancing towards them, may be hard for them to identify, even when the object is familiar.

Habituation refers to the process of response decrement in the horse, whereas desensitisation techniques refer to the methods applied to achieve habituation. Systematic desensitisation, approach conditioning, overshadowing and counter-conditioning are some methods of desensitisation.

Sensitisation occurs when an individual's response intensity is increased. If an individual experiences a series of arousing stimuli, sensitisation describes the likelihood that it will respond more quickly or with increased intensity to this or another stimulus presented soon after.

Operant conditioning describes training using rewards and consequences. There are four subsets:

1) *Positive reinforcement:* The addition of an outcome the horse values to increase the occurrence of a desired behaviour. Primary reinforcers can be any resource that horses naturally value. Examples used in training are food and touch. To be used as rewards in training, they must be issued to the horse immediately at the *onset* of the correct response. Secondary positive reinforcers must be linked to primary reinforcers, which often take the form of auditory stimuli, such as a clicker or a consistent vocalised sound issued when the desired response is offered.

2) *Negative reinforcement:* The removal of an event or outcome, which the horse wants to avoid, to increase the occurrence of a desired behaviour. Negative reinforcement can, and should, be very subtle. Pressure motivates horses but the release of that pressure is what trains them. Applying pressure for inter-gait and intra-gait transitions relies on the trainer beginning with a light pressure cue, followed by the maintenance or increase of the pressure and then the release. Good trainers always aim to reduce cues to light forms of pressure.

3) *Positive punishment:* Adding an event or outcome that is aversive to reduce the occurrence of a behaviour. Positive punishment has negative welfare implications so should be avoided. If used, it must be contingent and contiguous with the undesirable behaviour.

4) *Negative punishment:* Removing an event or outcome, which the horse values, to reduce the occurrence of a behaviour. Negative punishment is rarely used except for prompt removal of attention or food to suppress a behaviour. If delayed, it is ineffective.

Shaping is the gradual step-by-step building of behaviours. Each step should differ only slightly from the previous step so that it is as obvious as possible for the horse to trial (or offer) the correct/desired response. *Classical conditioning* uses cues (such as light tactile, voice or visual signals) to trigger and elicit behaviours. These cues must be timed with exquisite precision to coincide with the start of the desired behaviour.

Appropriate use of learning theory means paying regard to these learning principles in the training of horses. That said, even though a training method can be explained through learning theory does not necessarily mean that the method is ethical or safe. It is the responsibility of the trainer to always prioritise the welfare of the horse above any training goal.

TP 3 Train Easy-to-Discriminate Signals

Training sometimes places the horse in a difficult discriminatory dilemma. It must habituate to some pressures, yet respond to others. For example, the horse must habituate to low-pressure levels of rein, leg and seat contact, particularly in the sport of dressage. These low neutral pressures are known as *contact*. When the variety of gaits is considered in relation to their effect on a rider, random variations in rider contact confound the horse's ability to discriminate between contact pressures and signal pressures.

Numerous signals from the rider are used to elicit the responses of *go, stop, turn* and *sideways* and their subsets of *quickening* or *slowing* the steps, *lengthening* and *shortening* the steps and changing the gait (walk, trot, canter and gallop). In the competition dressage horse, the number of responses is further increased when other movements and postures such as *rein-back*, *lateral bend* and *lateral flexion* are added, altering the head-and-neck posture, *collection*, *straightening* the horse, lowering the hindquarters, as well as the movements of *turn on the forehand* (*walk*), *pirouette* (*walk and canter*), *shoulder-in* (*trot*), *travers* (*trot*), *half-pass* (*trot and canter*), *piaffe* and *passage*.

Despite the large number of responses, the limitations of the rider's interaction with the horse's body mean that there are insufficient sites on the horse's body in which to condition these responses. If a site is used to elicit several different responses, confusion can set in. For example, it is not uncommon for a rider's legs to stimulate horses from sites on the horse's thorax not only to *quicken*, *lengthen the strides, go sideways*, and *canter*, but also to *turn* (instead of using the reins, for example). When it is considered that the normal scope of sites that the rider's leg stimulates is within the range of 10 cm to perhaps 20 cm, it makes the accurate discrimination of these four responses a difficult task, and

the precise delivery of signals a great challenge for riders.

Similarly, across the range of equestrian disciplines, the bit in the horse's mouth is frequently used to elicit responses of *slowing, shortening the strides, turning the forequarters or hindquarters, head raising, head lowering, neck shortening,* straightening crooked necks and correcting tilting noses. The horse's back shows kinematics that are specific to each of the three gaits and these movements make the task of maintaining an even rein contact difficult in sports such as dressage, which demand these criteria. Thus, the discrimination challenge for the horse is further complicated. Unsurprisingly, rider position and balance are typically the chief focus of equestrian coaching.

It should be mentioned, however, that some signals are less distinctive than others. Consider the seat, for example. The norm in most equestrian sports is to use saddles to disperse the weight of the rider and under-saddle padding (e.g. numnahs) to diffuse the saddle pressure to avoid back soreness in the horse (Figure 7.13). The saddle itself is padded or sometimes nowadays filled with air. The effect of this, however, is to dilute to some extent the signals of the seat. Another problem with the seat lies in its complex three-dimensional oscillations throughout the three gaits (Fruehwirth, *et al.*, 2004). So, even in best practice equitation, other signals, such as rein and leg signals, are likely to be more easily discriminated by the horse. Riders seeking to use subtle signals can shrink rein and leg signals more easily than seat signals. This is probably the reason many riders believe that for downward transitions they do not use their reins at all but instead use their seat (yet, at the same time, they recognise that they are unable to relinquish rein contact). Perhaps the clearest use of the rider's seat, insofar as the horse's discrimination is concerned, is in its effect of maintaining a particular gait, speed and rhythm through its 'sweeping' and bouncing effect.

A solution to the disparity between responses and signal loci can be found in the

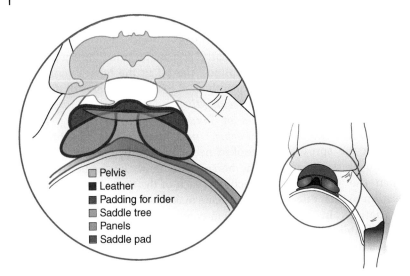

Figure 7.13 Whereas the reins and legs of the rider are in relatively close contact with the horse, the rider's seat is separated from the horse's back by layers of padding. This not only prevents back injury to the horse but also disperses signals from the rider. This compromise renders the rider's seat a less salient signal locus than the reins or legs.

various ways the signals can be combined from the following:

- the rider's legs can exert unilateral or bilateral pressure;
- the rider's legs can exert pressure from the upper leg (knee), calf and lower leg;
- the reins can exert tension on the mouth unilaterally or bilaterally;
- the reins can be raised, lowered, opened away from the horse's neck or closed toward the neck;
- the reins can also exert lateral tension on the horse's neck (neck-reining);
- the rider's legs can exert pressure that varies in duration (brief or more prolonged signals);
- the reins can exert tension that varies in duration (brief or more prolonged signals);
- the rider's seat can express variations in site, lateral distribution, speed and range of motion;
- spurs used as a light signal can be precise in terms of site; and
- verbal cues are sometimes used in equitation, although the use of the voice is forbidden in the sport of dressage (FEI, 2008).

These permutations emphasise the dual importance of rider position and training know-how in effectively achieving consistent responses in the horse.

TP 4 Shape Responses and Movements

The final desired responses required of horses in all disciplines are complex and each response, such as *go*, *stop* and *turn*, requires the trainer to recognise the earliest attempts by the horse to offer the correct response and then gradually shape them towards the goal response. Each stage should be consolidated to some extent before moving on to the next piece to be shaped. Trainers should, therefore, not expect perfect responses to emerge from the onset of training but should gradually shape the horse's responses by careful successive approximations towards the training goal. Each stage of shaping should consist of a precise response that is *identifiable* for both horse and trainer, then this is repeated and finally reaches consolidation. During the training of locomotion, developing steps, then strides, then the gait itself fulfils this requirement. A universal shaping scale is essential for acceptable modern horse-training in every discipline.

TP 5 Elicit Responses One-at-a-Time

In training, the rider's legs and reins acquire learned associations with retraction, protraction, abduction and adduction of the horse's limbs in the stance or swing phase of the various gaits. These associations will be gradually extinguished if signals elicit responses that are impossible to fulfil because the horse's legs are in positions that make responding difficult (Figure 7.14). Even more impossible is when the reins and the rider's legs attempt to stimulate responses simultaneously, as seen in some contemporary training methodologies as a way of producing what is known as engagement. The horse cannot simultaneously retract and protract the same limbs and so is placed in a confused state. The horse's reactions depend on his genetic predispositions as well as the duration and intensity of the opposing signals. Such confusion may lead to:

- lowered responding to the individual signals;
- acute stress resulting in raised muscular tonus and fearful behaviours;
- conflict behaviours, such as bucking, bolting, shying and rearing;
- frequent stress resulting in physiological and immunological deterioration;
- learned helplessness, where the horse tolerates pain with severe welfare compromises; and
- wastage where the horse is removed from the population (i.e. sent to the abattoir).

Pavlov (1927) described the situation that arises when two stimuli compete for salience. He defined the effects of this competition as resulting in 'overshadowing', where the more salient stimulus would outcompete the other. In the ridden horse, analogues of the overshadowing phenomenon manifest as habituation-like phenomena, where the horse may learn not to attend to the pressures of the bit (heaviness) and the rider's legs when simultaneously used during training (McLean, 2008). Anthropomorphically, the consequent dullness to the pressures may be interpreted as loss of 'willingness', 'laziness' or, when conflict behaviours arise, 'sourness', 'resistance' and 'evasion'. For our purposes in this text, we use the term 'overshadowing' to describe this parallel phenomenon, where one signal outcompetes another less salient stimulus.

It is now common for this important principle to be disregarded, even at the highest

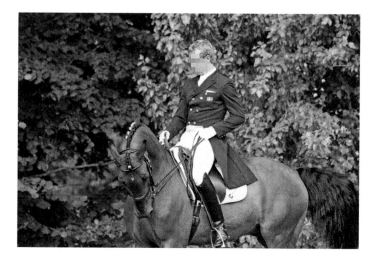

Figure 7.14 When both reins and leg signals are applied simultaneously, confusion sets in. Deterioration of one or both responses can also occur by overshadowing, which results in significant losses of responding to the reins or legs for *stop* or *go*. (Photo courtesy of EponaTV.)

levels of contemporary training practice; for example, the German National Equestrian Federation (1997) proposes that rein cues 'should only be given in conjunction with leg and weight' cues. Yet Decarpentry (1949), one of the great masters of French equitation, maintained the importance of separating rein and leg cues with the famous French maxim 'hands without legs, legs without hands'. This should be re-embraced as an important ideal that allows optimal learning and eliminates the potential for confusion for all equitation disciplines. Signals must be elicited singly and any set of signals should still be separated and elicited consecutively (Decarpentry, 1949).

TP 6 Train Only One Response per Signal

A horse cannot be expected to know the intentions of its rider. It makes sense to recognise that confusion can also occur when a single signal has more than one response associated with it. For example, in equitation, the stimulus of the single rein is the fundamental signal for the *turn* response. When riders attempt to bend the horse's neck laterally using the single rein, the horse can easily become confused between the dual response of either *turning* (changing direction) or *lateral flexing* of the neck: two responses from one signal. A similar confusion may result when both reins are used for altering the horse's head-carriage, because use of both reins together has an earlier fundamental association with *slowing*. McLean (2003) suggested that such confusions account for a significant number of conflict behaviours in the ridden horse and *ipso facto* add to behavioural wastage statistics.

Effective habit formation requires that a particular response must be elicited repeatedly. Discrete locomotory characteristics, such as the steps or strides of the horse, provide clear single units of responses that have an obvious beginning and end-point. Thus, it is useful for horse-trainers to be aware of the

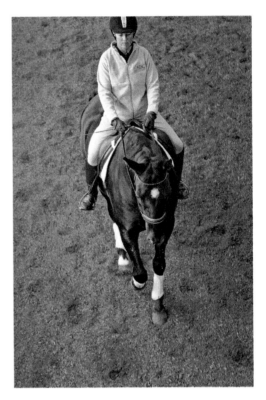

Figure 7.15 The rider should begin to signal the turn with the direct rein when the foreleg (on the side to which the horse is to turn) is leaving the ground.

biomechanical characteristics of the horse's locomotion during acceleration, deceleration and turning. Biomechanical studies suggest that, for example, when training basic (direct) *turn* responses, the most appropriate time to apply the signal for a *right turn* is when the right foreleg is beginning its swing phase (Maes and Abourachid, 2013) (Figure 7.15). Similarly the most appropriate time to initiate an indirect *turn* (where the rein closes toward the neck) is when the ipsilateral forelimb begins its swing phase. If riders focus on this moment to elicit a response, the horse's acquisition rate is optimal. Many riders learn to feel these optimal moments with their seat, and this timing should be an important part of equestrian coaching. Similarly, the optimal time to decelerate is at the beginning of the swing phase of one of the forelimbs.

Turns of the forelimbs require even more astuteness on the part of the rider, when it comes to eliciting an exact copy of a single response in early training. For example, a horse may *turn its forelimbs* by first either abducting the limbs or adducting the limbs. In dressage, the *turn of the forelimbs* requires abduction as the first reaction, but in any sport, training is expedited by reinforcing the same response each time. If the use of the rein is taken as the signal that elicits the *turn of the forelimbs*, then the rein should elicit an abduction of the same-side limb in the swing phase in which the limb moves to some extent laterally.

At the same moment, the opposite fore-limb in the stance phase propels the horse to that direction to a greater or lesser extent, depending on the signal strength. Trainers, therefore, need to be precise in eliciting and reinforcing the correct abduction response: signalling with the rein at the beginning of the swing phase of the limb. It follows that there are moments when such a turn is impossible: that is when the limb to be abducted is already in the stance phase.

On the other hand, *turns of the hind-quarters* (which lead to *leg-yield* and *side-pass*) should begin with an adduction, where one hindleg first crosses over the other (Figure 7.16). For the same reason as above, efficient training requires that the adduction response should be elicited at precisely the moment when the limb is about to begin the swing phase.

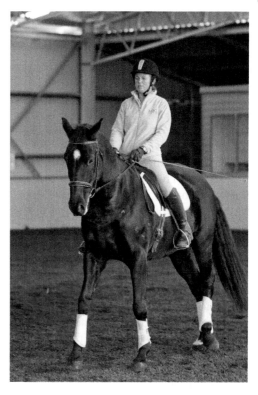

Figure 7.16 The rider should begin to signal the *leg-yield* with the leg signal when the hindleg (on the opposite side to which the horse is to yield) is leaving the ground.

TP 7 Form Consistent Habits

It is recognised among horsepeople that the horse should initiate a response to the rider's signals immediately. This does not necessarily mean that the response should be completed immediately, but simply requires that the horse begins responding without delay. Because any learned response has definable features in terms of action and duration, it follows that transitions should be completed within consistent time-frames. In different horse sports, the structure of these transitions from one locomotory state to another may differ according to the requirements of the particular sport. In sports such as reining, because of its origins in cattle mustering, certain transitions must be so abrupt that the horse's legs immediately complete their response to the rider's cue (e.g. the horse may skid to a sliding stop). Turns must also be powerful and fast. These rapid transitions also characterise polo, polocrosse, racing and, to some extent, show-jumping and cross-country jumping. In these sports, the transitions have a discrete structure with little room for confusion from that viewpoint.

On the other hand, in dressage and allied sports, transitions are not required to be completed abruptly, but instead should flow through a definable number of steps or time-frames. Anecdotal observation of horses that are successful at the highest level of dressage suggests that transitions are completed within a stride or two and within about 2 or 3 seconds. Yet contemporary dressage texts do not define the time-frame or step/stride sequence surrounding transitions, except to say that transitions should be within the rhythm of the strides (Decarpentry, 1949; Herbermann, 1980; German National Equestrian Federation, 1997). The absence of any clear prescription for transitions is an obstacle to the transmission of knowledge; and inconsistency in reinforcing responses is likely to present as a source of confusion in the horse. This also hinders the process of habit formation, which is a relatively protracted process of neural maturation to the point of consolidation. Forming consistent habits imposes a strong obligation to train responses, including transitions that are consistent in form and duration.

Given the characteristics of equine biomechanics and cognition, there are good grounds to suggest that the transitions can be consistently trained so that they become entities with definable aspects of locomotion and/or duration. For example, once the horse has learned a basically correct response to the rider's legs and reins, the alternating swing phases of both the horse's forelegs (in the walk and trot) can provide a definable framework to contain the three elements of the operant contingency: the discriminative stimulus (signal), the operant response and the reinforcer (release) (McGreevy and McLean, 2007; McLean and McLean, 2008). For example, during the development of acceleration, deceleration, abduction or adduction responses, the operant contingency can be exploited to align with the horse's forelegs. For the purposes of an example, let us assume that the left foreleg is the first to swing:

1) the light signal is applied to coincide with the start of the swing phase of the left foreleg;
2) the period of increasing pressure to motivate the response coincides with the swing phase of the right foreleg; and
3) the immediate removal of the pressure coincides with the start of the swing phase of the left foreleg.

When the horse has learned to perform the transitions within three beats, the middle

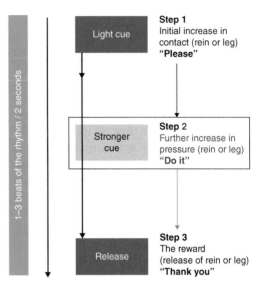

Figure 7.17 In horse-training using negative reinforcement, the operant contingency is expressed in this sequence: light signal, increasing pressure, release of pressure. In a short time, the period of stronger pressure is removed and the horse readily responds to light signals. The three beats can be thought of as *Please; Do it; Thank you.*

period of increasing pressure is no longer required and the light signal is extended (Figure 7.17). The transition remains in three beats of the forelegs, and so the sequence of signals is now as follows:

1) the light signal is applied to coincide with the swing phase of the left foreleg and is maintained with the swing phase of the right foreleg, and
2) the light signal is released to coincide with the beginning of the swing phase of the left foreleg.

So, during training of the transitions, the three elements of signal, pressure and release coincide with the three beats of the forelegs, whereas in the period following acquisition, the two elements of signal and release still coincide with the three beats of the forelegs. In this case, the signal continues for two beats of the forelegs, while release occurs on the third. Note that the transition occurs in two beats. We might ask why the light signal is not released after a single beat, but if that were to occur, then only one foreleg would be reinforced for the transitions. Given that the tempo of an individual foreleg at walk is about 55 bpm and at trot is around 75 bpm, a transition in these gaits is about 2 seconds in duration.

In the case of the canter, because the beats are so much faster (double the speed of walk beats), there is not sufficient time to carry out the three components of the operant contingency in alternating swing phases. Instead, in the canter, the three components of the operant contingency align with three canter strides (or the swing phase of the same foreleg). Having a different locomotory sequence surrounding the transitions in canter does not pose a cognitive challenge to the horse owing to its well-developed abilities to make associations (context-specific behaviours). Of greater significance is consistency on the trainer's part.

TP 8 Train Persistence of Elicited Responses ('Self-Carriage')

Because working and performance horses must respond to the rider's cues and sometimes continue responding for extended periods, it is important that they continue responding until signalled to switch to the next response. This principle is ubiquitous in horse-training literature and is described as 'self-carriage', meaning that the horse must maintain its rhythm and tempo, line and straightness, and head-and-neck outline.

Two centuries ago, Baucher described persistence of responding as a fundamental component of his training scale (Faverot de Kerbrech, 1891).

In equitation, it is considered that this persistence is partially maintained by the action of the rider's seat, which moves slightly differently in accordance with each gait's defining characteristics. The seat is also able to indicate to the horse that a shorter or longer stride is to be maintained, because of the concomitant shorter or longer movements of the seat during those strides. In-hand, persistence of forward movement is maintained by the visual stimulus of the stepping of the trainer. In the absence of such signals, riders and trainers must rely on the horse maintaining the correct response (i.e. keep trotting without constant cueing). If responses are continually elicited by 'nagging' with stimuli, habituation to signals may follow. It is proposed that trainers continuously test for self-carriage by completely releasing the reins or taking the legs away from the horse's sides for two steps in the walk and trot and two strides in the canter and gallop. In this short time-frame, the horse should not lose gait, rhythm, tempo, line, straightness or head-carriage. We recommend the use of this technique (known as the German technique of *Überstreichen*) as the test of self-carriage in all movements and gaits where possible both in training and in the execution of dressage tests (Figure 7.18). This could potentially serve to

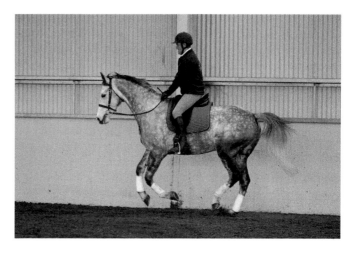

Figure 7.18 *Überstreichen* provides an important way of proving that the horse is in self-carriage, in any movement.

lower behavioural wastage in those horses that are held in forced frames (where the rider maintains relentless and intolerable rein tension) rather than the horse exhibiting correct learned responses.

TP 9 Avoid and Dissociate Flight Responses

Research indicates that fear responses are less prone to erasure than other behaviours (e.g. Le Doux, 1994). Fear responses range from hyper-reactivity to counter-predator behaviours, such as bolting, bucking, rearing and shying. So, if horses express these responses during their interactions with humans, these outcomes become more persistent. Therefore, it is important for reasons of safety for both horse and rider that such behaviours are neither provoked nor maintained. Fear and flight responses are therefore best dealt with using an error-free approach, where there is minimal risk for the horse to practise unwanted behaviours, or that stress levels increase above the level appropriate for training. This is important to consider before pressure is escalated. The example that we used earlier in this chapter, in which a horse refuses to enter a creek, can quickly turn into a dangerous situation if the horse's reluctance is caused by fear and the rider escalates pressure; fear reactions will be provoked and the risk that the horse will practise unwanted behaviour (flight and/or getting rid of the rider) is significant. In addition, it is likely that practising such behaviours has negative welfare implications leading to chronic stress, learned helplessness and behavioural wastage.

Horses that are unclear in their acceleration and deceleration responses, both in-hand and under-saddle, are at high risk for hyper-reactivity and conflict behaviours (McLean, 2005b), suggesting that re-training of basic responses must form part of the rehabilitation process of such 'problem' horses. Interestingly, how the horse responds to pressure signals in-hand and under-saddle serves as a diagnostic test that is predictive of conflict behaviours.

In re-training and prevention of undesirable fear responses, riders should use downward transitions to slow the horse's legs during these episodes, rather than simply ignoring them or accelerating. Current practices, such as round-pen techniques, lungeing, driving or chasing horses for any reason, are detrimental if they induce fear and elicit a flight response. Such responses are not difficult to distinguish, because they generally involve raised head-carriage, hollowed loins, short choppy steps and tendencies to quicken. We recommend that systematically inducing fear in horses should not be used in horse-training.

TP 10 Demonstrate Minimum Levels of Arousal Sufficient for Training

Learning requires arousal levels to be slightly elevated but certainly not beyond the point at which learning is inhibited. This has been described as the inverted-U relationship between learning and arousal, as reflected in the Yerkes-Dodson Law (Yerkes and Dodson, 1908; Mendl, 1999). The optimal arousal level for a specific task is related to how challenging the task is for the individual; simpler tasks can be performed successfully, even at high arousal levels, whereas challenging tasks are typically performed more successfully at lower arousal levels (Mair *et al.*, 2011; Starling *et al.*, 2013). Thus, there is a fine line between raised stress levels, sufficient for learning and responding, and higher stress levels that inhibit learning. Best-practice training using a paradigm of negative reinforcement involves applying this pressure gradient only to the level of optimal learning. Awareness and identification of this threshold are critical areas of study in equitation science. Trainers should be able to show that the horse is as relaxed as possible and central to this are two major components of psychological stressors, *predictability* and *controllability* (Weiss, 1972; Bassett and Buchanan-Smith, 2007).

Take-Home Messages

- The process of correctly applying learning theory to horse-training can be guided systematically by a set of ten training principles. Adherence to these principles provides a useful basis for optimal training.
- In the optimal use of negative reinforcement, for every learned response, there are three phases that progress through negatively reinforced operant (trial-and-error) learning, shrinking of the original pressures to the lightest versions and the installation of other unrelated cues (e.g. auditory or visual signals) via classical conditioning.
- Consistent outcomes from stimuli allow animals to have greater controllability (through operant conditioning) and predictability (through classical conditioning) of their environment, with a concomitant enhancement of their welfare.
- The timing of release of pressure is critical. Poor timing of release accounts for many behavioural problems in the ridden and led horse, which can manifest as conflict behaviours and descend into learned helplessness.
- Horse-riding and training is largely a process of negative reinforcement. However, positive reinforcement can certainly be used in conjunction with negative reinforcement (combined reinforcement) to increase training efficiency.

Ethical Considerations

- The simultaneous application of two or more cues results in overshadowing and, inevitably, habituation to the less salient cue as well as confusion. For this reason, optimal equitation should emphasise the separation of hand and leg cues.
- In competitive horse sports, performance success and equine welfare may clash. For example, the current focus on the head- and-neck position in dressage at the expense of locomotory responses is implicated in conflict behaviours.
- Regulatory bodies should consider mandating rein-tension meters or frequent testing for self-carriage (*Überstreichen*) by riders and coaches in all movements and gaits, during training and competition. This test would demonstrate which horses were exhibiting correctly learned responses and which were being held in a frame and therefore subject to reduced welfare.
- Punishment for non-compliance by the horse should be avoided.
- Negative reinforcement pressures should diminish rapidly to light cues.

Areas for Future Research

- An interesting area for future research is the relative salience of auditory, tactile and visual cues to horses. Studies on other species have shown that some associations are more readily learned than others.
- The duration of pressure-based signals in relation to stimulus intensity and in relation to individual perseveration tendencies is also an interesting area for future research.
- The use of combined reinforcement in equitation and the relative salience of positive, negative and combined reinforcement protocols in challenging situations need to be further explored.

8

Training

Introduction

For all animals, the world is full of competing and conflicting stimuli, so in the case of horses in training, certain stimuli can capture the horse's attention and consequently maintain control of its behaviour at the expense of other stimuli. For example, a plastic bag blowing past may compete with the rider's signals for control of the horse's behaviour. When the environment controls the ridden or handled horse, it will overshadow the animal's trained responses and the horse may freeze, baulk, accelerate, shy, rear or buck in response to the environmental stimulus *instead* of responding to the signals from the rider or trainer.

Learning theory allows us to recognise that some trained signals used in horse-training are diminutive versions of the initial pressure used to trigger a particular response, whereas others arise from previously irrelevant cues that come to be associated with negatively reinforced responses. For example, light rein and leg signals are discriminative stimuli that are usually derived from stronger rein and leg pressures in early training. Later in training, the horse may acquire some association of these fundamental signals with the rider's seat, posture or voice. So when the horse fails to respond to these later additional signals, trainers must revisit the earlier training that established the light signals derived from the original pressures. If the horse does not

respond to the light signal, the stronger more unpleasant one follows. Thus, the quality of the seat and position signals depends on the quality and consolidation of responses to stimuli from the rein and leg.

It is important to recognise that because horses are trained using negative reinforcement, they may, at times, be subjected to variable levels of discomfort. Like all animals, horses seek to avoid pain. If pain is unpredictable, inescapable and uncontrollable, horses may show increasing stress, manifesting as conflict behaviours. Thus, the aim of correct training is to diminish all painful interventions, such as strong or relentless bit or spur signals, until they are mild discriminative stimuli. This highlights the importance of self-carriage in creating a controllable *umwelt* for the ridden horse. When self-carriage and light signals are wholly predominant, they provide maximum controllability and promote the first stage of training: longitudinal flexion, which occurs when the poll lowers and the neck lowers and lengthens and the horse's nose is extended forward. To be scientifically correct, this posture should be termed 'longitudinal extension', since technically it involves more decontraction.

The timely use of negative reinforcement is a critical component of successful and ethical horse-training. Timing in this case refers to the application and removal of tactile pressures. For optimal outcomes, the

Equitation Science, Second Edition. Paul McGreevy, Janne Winther Christensen,
Uta König von Borstel and Andrew McLean.
© 2018 John Wiley & Sons Ltd. Published 2018 by John Wiley & Sons Ltd.
Companion website: www.wiley.com/go/mcgreevy/equitation

application of tactile pressures should occur at the beginning of a swing phase. Maes and Abourachid (2013) point out that during the swing phase, the limb is free of external mechanical constraints and the motor control is free to adjust the limb kinematics and dynamics. During the stance phase, mechanical proprioceptive constraints prevail. This suggests that rein signals should be applied at the onset of the foreleg(s) swing phase and leg signals should be applied at the onset of the swing phase of the relevant hindlimbs. Similarly, a pilot study suggested that the removal of rein tension should occur at the onset of the response (Egenvall *et al.*, 2012).

Longitudinal flexion and looseness are crucial features of traditional horse-training (Decarpentry, 1949; de la Guérinière, 1992; Hölzel *et al.*, 1995; German National Equestrian Federation, 1997). Even though the poll is required to be higher in later stages of dressage, such as collection, it is generally proposed that horses begin each training session in a lowered neck outline to induce relaxation (Hölzel *et al.*, 1995). When the horse is trained to maintain its own tempo and rhythm, is functionally straight in its footfalls, and its head and neck posture is consistent, it relaxes and exhibits the quality known as 'looseness' (Hölzel *et al.*, 1995). Its locomotory behaviour is now under optimal control of the rider. Consistency of signals and responses confers the greatest level of predictability.

In-Hand Training

Habituation and Familiarisation

Most domestic horses become familiar with humans early in their lives and may learn not to fear humans, either through individual learning or if they observe their mothers being handled from time to time (Henry *et al.*, 2005; Hausberger *et al.*, 2007b). With a foal at liberty, this process of gradual habituation is an important stage in early training and facilitates later foundation training.

Furthermore, Ladewig *et al.* (2005) suggest that the more similar a horse's foalhood is to its adult life (including handling and management procedures), the easier the transition will be for it to its adult domestic situation. Young horses living in social groups rather than in isolation are likely to be easier to handle (Søndergaard and Ladewig, 2004). Foals often initiate contact early, if they do not perceive humans as chasing them and, more subtly, provided that humans do not negatively reinforce flight responses. Given that horses are adept at learning via negative reinforcement, the latter scenario is not uncommon. For example, handlers should be very mindful that when they lay hands on the naïve foal and the foal runs or bucks to remove the hands, the very first lesson in escape learning via negative reinforcement is embedded. The best scenario is, therefore, to touch the foal (e.g. by scratching the tail region, which many foals find pleasant) and only remove the hands when the foal is immobile and relaxed; in this way, the first lesson about human contact is *not* to remove it.

Approach

Making physical contact with horses of any age for the first time may be facilitated by knowledge of learning theory. Contemporary approaches, such as the advance–retreat method (Wright, 1973), are based on the subtle use of negative reinforcement. Indeed, both successful and unsuccessful advance–retreat owe their results to negative reinforcement. For example, when used optimally, this method involves the trainer advancing towards the wary horse but stopping as soon as he detects that the horse is about to escape, at which moment the trainer takes a step back (Figure 8.1). The trainer then takes a couple of steps towards the horse and again stops and steps back *before* the horse does. In this scenario, the trainer gradually reduces the flight distance by negatively reinforcing the horse's immobility. If, however, the horse steps back and the trainer also steps back, the horse's retreat is now

(a)

(b)

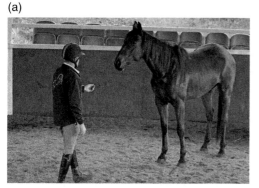 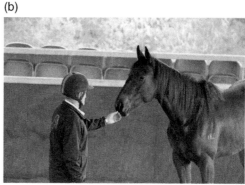

Figure 8.1 The advance–retreat method of catching horses is one of the more subtle examples of negative reinforcement. As the trainer approaches the wary horse (a), he makes sure that he retreats a step before the horse does. The trainer can then take two or more steps towards the horse before having to retreat a step and, thus, he gradually closes in on the horse (b). The retreating (removal) of the trainer negatively reinforces the horse's immobility.

negatively reinforced and the horse learns the wrong response – to step back at the approach of the human. This shows just how subtle negative reinforcement can be. For the horse's cognition, however, the process is abundantly clear.

Initial Contact

Many foals are weaned prematurely and abruptly at six months of age. This has been associated with a range of physiological and psychological responses, including development of abnormal behaviours, which may be reduced if foals are weaned gradually and/or housed with other foals and adults after weaning (Waran *et al.*, 2008; Henry *et al.*, 2012). It is currently unknown if weaning stress affects neophobia, training outcomes and the performance of horses. Many horsepeople begin training foals at weaning time, and this is often the time foals habituate to a halter and train to lead for the first time (Hausberger *et al.*, 2007b). Successful first contact with the foal can occur through allowing/encouraging the gradual approach of the foal or the human using advance–retreat. Experienced trainers generally recognise that if the foal runs and the trainer advances towards it or, worse still, rushes at it, damage is done to the foal–human

relationship. In effect, the trainer has negatively reinforced the foal's fear and the response may take disproportionately longer to repair because fear responses are acquired so rapidly. If the foal or young horse does not accept contact, food can be used to attract it to approach (e.g. by letting the horse feed from a bucket held by the trainer). The trainer's other hand can then gradually move closer to the horse's neck, and can be removed to reinforce immobility. Caressing the young horse at the base of the withers expedites relaxation and habituation to the trainer.

Leading and Control

To lead a horse, a lead-rope is generally attached to a headcollar, or reins attached to the bridle are used. Optimally, all equipment commonly used to lead the horse should be associated with thorough habituation. Training across all methodologies in-hand involves placing locomotory movements in all directions under stimulus control (Chapter 7, Applying Learning Theory). Therefore, the horse is trained to *go forward* (including upward inter-gait and intra-gait transitions), to *reverse*, *stop* and *slow* (including downward inter-gait and intra-gait transitions) and to change direction with the forelegs or hindlegs.

Shaping

The optimal use of learning theory prescribes that in-hand responses, including those listed above, are progressively shaped. The beginning of training entails motivating the horse to *go* and *stop* and *step back*, and rewarding any attempt in the correct direction. This is achieved through negatively reinforcing the desired reaction (by increasing the pressure and then releasing promptly the instant the horse responds). When the horse is responding to light signals, the next step is to reinforce an increasing number of strides. A stride is defined as a complete cycle of the repetitive series of limb movements that characterise a gait (e.g. all four legs at walk) (Back and Clayton, 2001). In all training, pressures should begin with the lightest versions, so that these act as discriminative stimuli and eventually elicit the transitions.

Further shaping involves maintaining the chosen directional line, whether it is a straight line (for acceleration and deceleration), or a curve (for turns). The final level of shaping in some methodologies involves reinforcing a consistent head, neck and body posture. These should be the last elements of the horse's basic foundation training to be reinforced, because limb movements are essential for control and safety, whereas the head and neck posture is of less critical importance. Regardless, when the horse's limbs are reliably under stimulus control, head and neck postures show fewer variations. Stimulus control is achieved when these shaped elements are consistently incorporated into the learned responses for acceleration, deceleration, turn of the forequarters and (especially under-saddle) going sideways in various environments that the horse may encounter and at any time (Table 8.1). In all training, it is most efficient to begin shaping the smallest unit of a learned response and then target the smallest improvements so that, in the end, the animal is achieving the targeted learned response.

Inter-Gait and Intra-Gait Transitions

It is often useful to train horses to shorten and lengthen steps in-hand, such as for the show-ring. Regardless of any competitive purpose, it is helpful to train such responses because they elaborate training, giving the horse a greater set of cues and responses, and longer strides encourage relaxation. To avoid problems in discrimination between stride length and stride tempo, temporal characteristics of the lead-rein tension may be altered to provide cues for longer versus faster steps (McLean and McLean, 2008). These temporal tension variations should

Table 8.1 An example of shaping a response, in this case forward: *go*.

Shaping component	Learned response	Effect
Step 1	Part of the correct stride from pressure	Horse steps forward
Step 2	A whole stride from signal	Horse steps a complete walk stride (4 steps in walk)
Step 3	Multiple strides from signal	Horse steps many strides
Step 4	Strides in the right direction from signal	Horse steps forward and maintains direction
Step 5	Strides with consistent posture from signal	Horse's posture is unchanged during forward locomotion
Step 6	Stimulus control	Horse goes everywhere and anywhere with above qualities

manifest as light signals, applied at the beginning of the relevant swing phase and removed at the onset of the correct response.

Fortifying Responses

Usually in horse-training it should not be necessary to increase pressure above the level that causes moderate discomfort. Thus, if a horse does not respond to a lead signal via the headcollar, halter or bridle, the signal should be accompanied with a supplementing signal, such as from a long whip. For example, if the horse does not step forward from the lead-rein, the whip can be used for tapping on the ribcage, ceasing the instant the horse offers a single step forward. It is important that the horse is not afraid of the whip and does not react when the whip touches its body. To habituate the horse to the whip, it is laid on the horse's body and is removed only when the horse ceases to react (Figure 8.2). Alternatively, to overshadow an adverse reaction to the whip, it can be laid on the horse's body and the horse is then signalled to move back then forward repeatedly until its reaction to the whip subsides (McLean, 2008).

During in-hand training, is it useful to use signals as similar as possible to those used under-saddle, as this reduces the possibility of confusion. So when the whip-tap is used to strengthen in-hand and under-saddle signals, the trainer or rider may tap the shoulder for turning, the sides for acceleration and the hindquarters for going sideways. The zones used for whip-tapping may differ between training systems but the main point is that the zones are used consistently and are easy for the horse to discriminate. Tapping the hindquarters for sideways rather than where the rider's legs press the horse's sides for sideways is common in dressage, because of the difficulty in accurately tapping the ribcage on two distinct sites for forward and sideways (Figure 7.6). In addition, discrimination can be further facilitated by shaping the training of the whip-tap for each of the three body sites in two ways: two taps for faster steps and one tap for longer steps.

While inducing mild to moderate discomfort should be sufficient to motivate the horse to perform the correct response, in everyday training there may be situations in the re-training of problem horses where

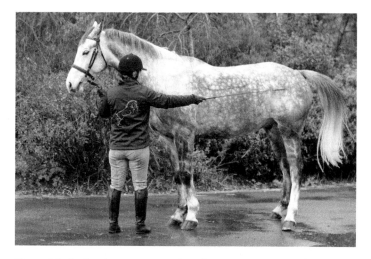

Figure 8.2 As visual cues can sometimes be given unintentionally and are, therefore, confusing for the horse, it can be useful to ensure that the sight of the whip or the approach of the whip is not a signal for movement. To do this, the whip is gently rubbed over the horse's body while simultaneously reinforcing immobility with the reins (overshadowing). This helps ensure calmness and responsiveness to the tapping of the whip as a useful signal.

skilled trainers need to escalate the pressure above this level. As long as the strong pressure is quickly removed and then diminished, this will not usually be a welfare concern and may be the only solution for horses that have developed dangerous behaviours.

Alternative Signals

Learning theory prescribes that there is a range of signals that can be used both in-hand and under-saddle. In other words, there are no necessarily correct or incorrect signals, as long as the signals are specific, consistent and easily discriminated.

Welfare considerations demand that every pressure signal should be reduced to very light pressures that are released as soon as the horse responds.

Managing Fear

Fearful, hyper-reactive responses should be very carefully managed. Dealing with fear responses is examined in detail in Chapter 13, Stress and Fear Responses. Most fear responses involve the horse quickening its legs and attempting to place distance between itself and the frightening stimulus. The increased distance reinforces the escape response. Different desensitisation techniques (Chapter 4, Non-associative Learning) can be useful to alter the horse's reaction to the frightening stimulus (Christensen *et al.*, 2006; McLean, 2008). On the other hand, flooding is sometimes used in foundation training (e.g. for habituation to saddle and girth). Some horses may quickly learn to accept saddle and girth pressure, but there is always a risk connected to the use of flooding compared to gradual habituation, especially if the horse succeeds in removing the saddle or girth – any response that led to this outcome will be negatively reinforced. Similarly, the horse may injure itself or others and it may associate the negative experience with other stimuli, such as the trainer or the training environment. Systematic desensitisation

to girth pressure is described in Figure 8.14. In cases of milder expressions of fear, careful management involves using downward inter-gait and intra-gait transitions to inhibit fear responses.

Rewards

Positive reinforcement in the form of primary or secondary reinforcement, such as clicker training (Chapter 5, Associative Learning (Attractive stimuli)), can not only expedite training, but may also serve to enhance the horse–human relationship (Sankey *et al.*, 2010(a),(b)). A convenient use of positive reinforcement, both in-hand and under-saddle, is to caress the horse's withers (Figure 2.5b). This may also be used in the format of secondary reinforcement where a specific utterance such as 'good boy' serves as the secondary reinforcer, as described in the previous chapter. The optimal use of positive reinforcement is shown in Figure 8.3.

Signals for Acceleration (Forward)

Training the horse to *lead forward* begins with operant conditioning (negative reinforcement) where increases in lead-rein pressure motivate the horse to move. The operant contingency begins with a cue of light lead-rein pressure *in the anterior direction* followed by a period of stronger pressure (Figure 8.6a), which is released when the horse offers the first sign of a correct or near-correct response (i.e. protraction of a forelimb). When the horse has acquired the learned response of a visible but not perfect step in the forward direction, the trainer then targets reinforcing a single walk stride (a step by each of the four legs).

This anteriorly directed pressure acts on the poll (and dorsal parts of the mouth when a bridle is being used) and, in a broad sense, signals all upward inter-gait transitions in-hand as well as the intra-gait transitions of faster steps and longer steps. Many trainers make it easy for the naïve foal or young horse to offer the desired response of walking forward when first cued by applying pressure

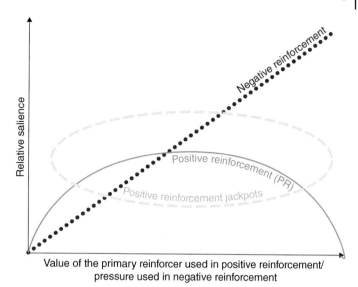

Figure 8.3 When positive and negative reinforcement are used concurrently, one may overshadow the other, depending on their relative salience. At low levels of negative reinforcement (rein tension/leg pressure) and high levels of positive reinforcement (jackpotting), positive reinforcement may be more salient, but as pressures increase, positive reinforcement may become less salient. This suggests that positive reinforcement is best used when negative reinforcement pressures have been converted to light signals.

slightly to one side instead of straight ahead (Figure 6.6). This lateral pressure causes a slight loss of balance, so the horse steps to the side and the pressure is released. Through shaping, the horse learns to lead straight (Table 8.2).

While the lead-rein itself, lightly pressured in the anterior direction, offers a clear classically conditioned cue for initiating forward steps, trainers sometimes unwittingly use a variety of cues. These range from voice commands to the trainer's steps, which can initiate and maintain the horse's mobility (Figure 8.4). Provided the voice is used in a precise, standard and predictable way, it can be very effective and is marred only by the likelihood that the horse is constantly subjected to words uttered by people and may previously have learned to ignore them. Effective users of the voice in animal-training tend to adopt voice characteristics that are used only for training.

It is important that specific cues are used to elicit mobility responses. These may be in the form of voice commands, hand signals or rein cues. Trainers who use their steps to elicit movement may face difficulties and even some conflict behaviours, unless they have trained the horse to respond to a 'stay' cue. Otherwise, for the horse to discriminate when the steps of the human are meant to be a cue and when they are not can be

problematic, because it relies on the horse learning that there are 'exceptions to the rule', which is cognitively challenging (Figure 8.4). For example, when the trainer moves around the horse during care and maintenance, the horse is generally expected to remain immobile, yet the trainer's steps cue the horse to move. The horse may then be punished for doing something it was cued to do. To solve this dilemma, some methods advocate that the trainer adopts specific postures when cuing the horse to move. While this has some merit, it also becomes context-specific in that leading and non-leading postures of one person compared with another are not easily discriminated so that handing the horse over to another trainer may result in confusion and apparent non-compliance. Another problem arises when humans are inconsistent and ineffective in adopting the specific posture. However, the trainer's movement is not irrelevant, for it may provide the most reliable cue for *maintaining* movement in the horse once elicited by other stimuli, such as the lead-rein.

Lead-rein responses can be strengthened with a rhythmic whip-tap if the lead-rein signals fail to evoke a response. Horses can be trained to elicit various directional responses to specific whip-taps, so it is optimal to facilitate discrimination of the whip-tap signals. This is achieved by tapping in the same place

Table 8.2 Examples of stimulus–response characteristics of **in-hand** training.

Targeted response	Targeted biomechanics	Operant discriminative stimulus	Motivation	Reinforcement	Other associated and maintaining cues	Possible verbal cue
Upward inter-gait transition and faster limbs	Accelerating protraction (swing) and retraction (stance)	Prolonged (2 foreleg steps) anterior lead-rein signal	Anterior lead-rein pressure/whip-taps on ribcage	Release pressure on improved step	Trainer walking forward	'Walk on', 'trot on', 'canter', tongue click
Upward intra-gait transition: longer steps	Increased protraction (swing) and retraction (stance)	Brief (1 foreleg step) anterior lead-rein signal	Anterior lead-rein pressure/whip-taps on ribcage	Release pressure on improved step	Trainer lengthening steps	Tongue click
Downward inter-gait transition and slower limbs	Decelerating protraction (stance) and retraction (swing)	Prolonged (2 foreleg steps) posterior lead-rein signal	Posterior lead-rein pressure	Release pressure on improved step	Trainer slowing or stopping	'Whoa', 'stand', 'waalk', 'tro'ot'
Step backwards	Protraction (stance) and retraction (swing)	Posterior lead-rein signal	Posterior lead-rein pressure/whip-tap on chest or foreleg	Release pressure on improved step	Trainer stepping backwards	'Back'
Downward intra-gait transition: shorter steps	Decreased protraction (stance) and retraction (swing)	Brief (1 foreleg step) posterior lead-rein signal	Posterior lead-rein pressure	Release pressure on improved step	Trainer shortening steps	Brief 'whoa'
Turn forequarters	Abduction (swing), adduction (stance) then adductions	Lateral lead signal	Lateral lead pressure	Release pressure on improved step	Trainer turning	Usually not used
Turn hindquarters and go sideways	Adduction (swing), adduction (stance) then abductions	Two whip-taps on hindquarters	Whip-tap pressure on sides of hindquarters	Release pressure on improved step	Trainer stepping towards horse's hindquarters	'Over'

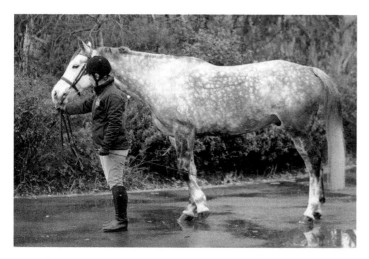

Figure 8.4 Horses are very adept at classical conditioning, so it is easy for a horse to learn to *step forward* when its trainer takes a step. Thus, the horse may appear to have learned to *step forward* from a light rein signal while in fact it has not, because in the past the light rein signal has been preceded by the visual cue of the moving trainer.

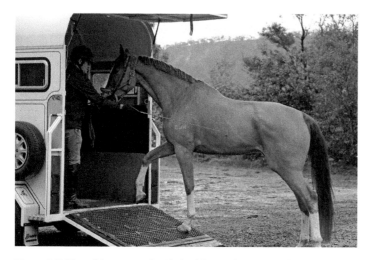

Figure 8.5 The whip-tap can fortify *lead forward* responses, because it is more difficult to habituate to the whip-tap than to lead pressure.

where the horse will be tapped under-saddle. From the standpoints of welfare and optimal training, the whip should not be used to punish a horse for non-compliance to the trainer's or rider's signals. The whip is as much a signal as any other stimulus and should be used simply to initiate responses (Figure 8.5). Whip-taps are used in two ways in negative reinforcement: by varying their frequency and magnitude. To tap rhythmically and increase the frequency of taps rather than increasing the magnitude is the most ethical method. Whip-taps should simply irritate the horse to react, not hurt him. The great usefulness of the whip is that it provides a larger range of aversive pressures than the lead-rein (or the rider's legs under-saddle), and within this range there is likely to be a specific pressure of whip-tap that will motivate most horses to react. Skilled trainers recognise optimal opportunities to enhance the response to lead signals through fortifying with whip-taps based on accurate observation of the horse's affective state (Chapter 7, Applying Learning Theory).

When stimulus control is achieved via the light signal or voice cue, the amount of negative reinforcement is dramatically diminished so the salience of the negative reinforcement is reduced to the point where a positive reinforcer can now be salient. Because the timing and delivery of primary positive reinforcers, such as food or caressing at the withers, can sometimes be impractical, appropriate use of a secondary positive reinforcer can maintain the transition.

In-hand, most trainers aim for several specific qualities (mentioned in the previous chapter) in the final product of a forward response, and these can be achieved by shaping. When the horse has learned to *lead forward* a single step, it is then reinforced for leading a number of steps from a single light signal. The next quality to be reinforced is to maintain direction. Trainers often negatively reinforce the direction by pressuring the lead-rein in the opposite direction of any drift. If the horse's head-carriage is too high or inconsistent, the horse may be motivated to lower its head from downward pressure, negatively reinforcing lowering the head with release from downward lead-rein pressure, and then shape this head-down response into

its leading forward response so that the horse leads with a consistent head height. When all the qualities of the response desired by the trainer are incorporated into the horse's leading forward response, the horse's forward responses come under increasing stimulus control as the response becomes consolidated. As described earlier, the horse can be trained to offer longer strides from a brief lead-rein signal applied for one step of the walk. If the horse fails to respond, the pressure is briefly raised for further individual steps until the longer steps are elicited from a brief light signal. From time to time, trainers may transiently increase the aversive pressure of the forward signals if the response wanes. However, in general, consistent responding can be optimally maintained by secondary positive reinforcement.

Signals for Deceleration

Slowing (deceleration) or stopping the horse is signalled by a light tension on the lead-rein, lead-rope or bridle reins, only this time *in the posterior direction* (Figure 8.6b). The pressure from the lead-rein in the posterior direction is perceived by the horse principally on its nasal planum or, in the case of a bitted bridle, in its mouth (as in under-saddle). So, there is a fundamental difference in direction between acceleration and deceleration signals. This posterior direction

(a)

(b)

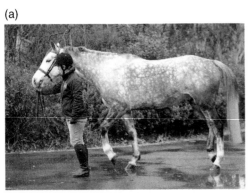 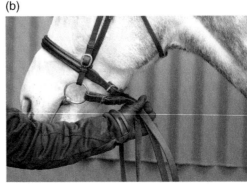

Figure 8.6 In-hand, the signal for going forward is lead-rein tension in the anterior direction (a), while for stopping, slowing and stepping back, it is posterior lead-rein tension (b). This difference is easily perceived by the horse.

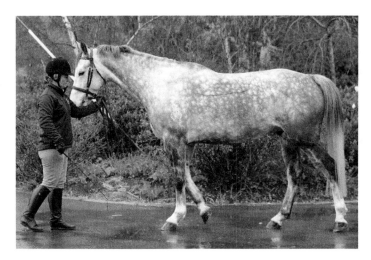

Figure 8.7 Training the horse to *step-back* in-hand enhances the *stop* and *slow* signals and provides a useful tool in re-training problems with the *stop* signals. This is because the neuromuscular coordination of stepping back is incorporated in all downward transitions to a greater or lesser extent.

signal is used to elicit all downward transitions, including slowing, shortening the steps, stopping and stepping backwards.

In early training and re-training, a basic attempt of slowing by the horse is initially reinforced. Then the trainer reinforces an entire stride of *step-back* (all four legs). The horse learns to associate the light signal with a subsequent period of stronger lead-rein tension and so learns to respond from the light signal alone (McGreevy and McLean, 2007). Maintaining a slower speed and remaining immobile are also part of the shaping process of the deceleration responses. As with the forward-leading responses, the slowing and shortening signals in-hand are usually further shaped so that they occur on a straight line and with a consistent head-carriage. To elicit shorter steps from brief lead-rein signals, tension is applied for a portion of a step. The tension should be removed when the horse responds and the signal repeated if it initiates longer steps again.

The slowing, shortening and stepping backwards responses can be thought of collectively because they all involve activation, in varying amounts, of protraction muscles in the stance phases and retraction in the swing phases of the steps of the transition. So training the horse to step backwards

simultaneously enhances the training of all the downward inter-gait and intra-gait transitions (Figure 8.7). Deficits in the step-back transition have been reported to be associated with deficits in downward transitions (McLean, 2005b). Like acceleration responses, the backwards response is triggered by escalating tension, beginning with light tension. The light tension acts as a predictor of a period of stronger tension and its subsequent release, so the horse soon learns to respond to the light signals.

In the event of the lead-rein not triggering a sufficient *step-back* response, the horse can be motivated with whip-taps on the horse's foreleg or chest, or by squeezing the *brachiocephalic* muscle (McLean and McLean, 2008) (Figure 8.8). Of course, the horse should initially be habituated to stroking with the whip so that it is not fearful of it. If the horse fails to respond, it makes sense to target a site that makes it most likely for the horse to offer the correct response to avoid prolonged tapping and confusion. The meta-carpal (cannon) bone of the horse's foreleg provides an obvious site because one of the horse's legs must retract in the swing phase to begin the *step-back*.

Ideally, when cueing *step-back*, the horse can either be tapped on the chest or on the

(a)

(b)

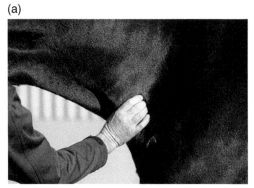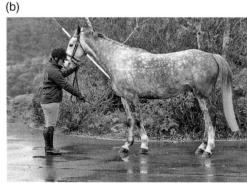

Figure 8.8 If the *step-back* response is difficult to elicit and tactile pressure (e.g. from a finger) is ineffective, it can be fortified by applying the light rein cue just before squeezing the brachiocephalic muscle (a) or just before tapping the metacarpal (cannon) bone of the foreleg that is likely to step first (b).

foreleg that is most anterior at any moment of immobility, as that will usually be the first to move. The foreleg can be tapped to ensure that the size and timing of the step is the required amount. If the horse reverses crookedly because of laterality differences in the diagonal couplets, then it makes sense to start with tapping one leg. It is important to choose a specific place on the foreleg for tapping, such as the front of the cannon bone, because other reactions may be required from tapping certain regions of the foreleg later in training, for example, lifting the legs higher. As with *forward*, it is vital to cease tapping as soon as the horse offers the first correct or near-correct response (depending on its experience with the learned response). The train of events should begin with light lead-pressure just before tapping the foreleg and should be contiguous with the whip-tap. Then, if the horse fails to *step-back*, the whip-tap can be used to evoke the response.

When the horse has learned to *step-back* from the light lead-rein signal, the response may come under the stimulus control of a discrete voice command, such as 'back'. When this or any other response arises from cues or light pressures, it can be reinforced from time to time using secondary positive reinforcement. Reinforcing responses on a variable schedule of reinforcement helps build resistance to extinction (Haselgrove *et al.*, 2004).

Stepping backwards can also be shaped. As soon as the horse steps back consistently from a cue or light lead-rein signal, a series of backward steps can be reinforced. Further shaping of the *step-back* is sometimes considered necessary to deepen the deceleration responses across the board of training and to assist in rehabilitating poor *stop* responses in horses with so-called hard mouths (McLean and McLean, 2008). The series of backwards steps can be trained to occur in a straight line. As with the forward leading response in-hand, the backwards steps can be trained to include a consistent head height by lowering or raising the horse's head just before deceleration signals are applied.

In-hand, the deceleration signals from the reins are virtually identical to those under-saddle, so it is not surprising that, in a young horse, the deceleration responses can be 'pre-trained' in-hand ready for use under-saddle. A horse with problematic deceleration under-saddle can also be at least partially rehabilitated in-hand (McLean, 2005a).

Signals for Turn of the Forelegs

Training the horse to turn its forequarters is not only essential for the obvious reason of changing direction but also useful in correcting tendencies of the horse to drift to one side or the other. Horses typically swerve and shy using their forelegs rather than their hindlegs (McLean, 2005a). This directional predominance of the forelegs over the hindlegs indicates that placing the forelegs under stimulus control is a major component in training straightness (where the hind-hooves step into the foretracks). It is likely that in-hand training of turns pre-trains the same response under-saddle; indeed, ridden and handled horses tend to show the same errors in acceleration and deceleration responses in-hand and under-saddle (McLean, 2005b).

Fundamentally, the turn signal initially learned by the horse in-hand is lateral pressure exerted on the headcollar or bridle of the horse (Figure 8.9). The effect of rein tension is to negatively reinforce lateral action of the forelegs conferred by alternating sequences of abduction and adduction (opening both forelegs then closing both forelegs) or vice versa. Because most horses are usually led using a single lead-rein attached to the underside of

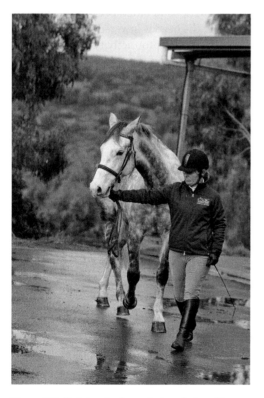

Figure 8.9 Training the horse to turn in-hand is useful in certain situations where the horse may veer to one side, such as when loading into a trailer.

the headcollar, there is generally no *discrete* lead-rein signal to turn the forelegs to either side, because the turn signals tend to merge with the acceleration or deceleration signals. If the horse is walking at the speed of the trainer or slower than the trainer, the turn blends into the acceleration signal of the lead-rein. If the horse is walking faster than the trainer, the turn signal merges into the deceleration signal. The negative reinforcement of the abduction/adduction sequence also *shapes* the turn response in terms of speed and direction.

A training whip can be used to negatively reinforce turns, especially in situations where the lead-rein pressure is not sufficiently clear or motivating. The horse is tapped rhythmically with the whip on its shoulder (more specifically, the flat deltoid area over the humerus), which is the ideal site. The whip acts as an additional signal that can support, strengthen and sensitise other signals, such as the lead-rein signal for the *turn* response. The horse should be trained to respond from the whip-tap alone (with no lead-rein signal) so that it has a clear learned response to turn from the whip-tap on either shoulder as well as from the lead-rein. Turning from the whip-tap can be useful in training the horse to load into a trailer, to help it maintain straightness.

Sometimes the horse may respond to the *turn the forelegs* signal by turning only the hindlegs or turning the hindlegs too much (i.e. stepping out of the line of the foretracks). In such cases, careful use of lead-rein pressures or mild whip-taps on the appropriate shoulder corrects the forelegs. Achieving biomechanically consistent turns is important, as it increases the efficiency of learning (long-term potentiation occurs more rapidly with identical responses) and, more importantly, lowers the potential for confusion and subsequent stress.

Signals for Turn the Hindquarters

Turning the hindquarters is significant in some disciplines, such as dressage and reining, so training the horse in-hand to move its hindquarters laterally is useful as pre-training for under-saddle work. It is also useful to be able to move the hindquarters in a range of daily management situations, including for 'parking in' (i.e. where the horse is signalled to stand next to a platform so the rider can mount) as well as in situations where the hindquarters have veered to the side, such as during trailer loading or training a young racehorse to enter starting gates. The hindquarter turn in-hand is, however, less important in terms of the totality of locomotory stimulus control than the more fundamental responses of acceleration, deceleration and turning the forelegs. When the horse is standing bilaterally symmetrical (upright), turns of the hindlegs tend to be effected by adduction before abduction (Figure 11.8). The sport of dressage follows this biomechanical predisposition in that turns on the forehand and leg-yield begin with an adduction step.

In some training methodologies, the cue for *turn the hindlegs* in-hand is often a touch or vibration of the fingers on the ribcage, while in others a voice command (such as 'over') is sometimes used. To elicit the response in early training, some trainers use whip-tapping on the hindquarters. To facilitate the horse's discrimination, the response is more easily achieved if the leg that is to be adducted is tapped around the hock area first. When the horse has learned to consistently adduct the tapped leg, the site of the whip-tap can be gradually moved up the hindleg to the lateral aspect of the rump (Figure 8.10). The subsequent shaping of the hindquarters response may include training the horse to respond to two light taps for faster steps and one light tap for a longer step, and transforming the signal to one or two vibrations of the fingers on the ribcage where the rider's leg would elicit the same response. In this way, the sideways response under-saddle can be pre-trained in-hand.

Some trainers also shape a *turn the hindquarters* response into a sideways response while going forward. This becomes an analogue of what is known as a 'leg-yield' and when this occurs, the trainer may shape various elements, such as leg-yielding in a maintained speed, line and head-carriage.

Head-Lowering

Many long-necked animals, including horses, show reductions in blood pressure and heart rate when the head is lowered, because of the effect of baroreceptor activity in the carotid sinus located near the fork of the carotid artery in the animal's neck. This is an adaptive effect that evolved to inhibit deleterious effects on the cell membranes of the brain when the head is lower than the heart. Many trainers have taken advantage of this effect to calm horses (Warren-Smith *et al.*, 2007(b))

(a)

(b)

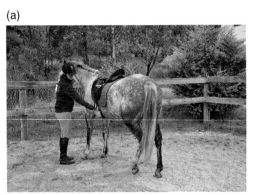 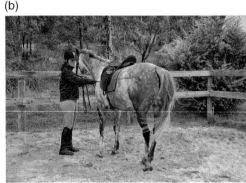

Figure 8.10 Stepping sideways (a) away from the whip-tap signal is facilitated by first tapping the horse's hock (where sideways is a more obvious reaction to the horse) and then (b) moving up the leg to the position of the rump. (Photos courtesy of Elke Hartmann.)

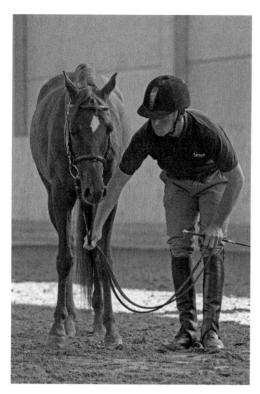

Figure 8.11 Training the horse to lower its head is a useful tool during in-hand interactions. It is important that this response is shaped gradually, beginning with initially reinforcing (release) for the smallest responses and gradually approximating the final targeted response where the horse will maintain its head lowered. (Photo courtesy of Elke Hartmann.)

(Figure 8.11). When anxiety is caused by environmental events (such as leaves rustling), calmness induced by head-lowering may also have an overshadowing effect. However, because a loss of calmness is frequently associated with poor use of negative reinforcement during acceleration and deceleration responses, lowering the head may give only temporary relief.

Lowering the horse's head is useful as a shaping component when training locomotory responses. A high head-carriage is typically associated with hyper-reactive states and, furthermore, an inconsistent head-carriage impedes the development of consistent reactions to acceleration, deceleration and turn signals. So, training the horse to lower its head and shaping this into the *go*,

stop and *turn* signals may facilitate calmness and consistency, hastening the acquisition of long-term potentiation for these responses.

Lungeing

Lungeing the horse often involves use of a round-pen where the horse may move freely or be connected to the trainer by a lungeing-rein attached to a halter, a lungeing-cavesson or bridle (Chapter 10, Apparatus). Training responses on the lunge and subsequently shaping them can be seen in the same format as other in-hand training (Figure 8.12). It is initially beneficial to train the naïve horse to walk in a circle that can gradually be increased in size. Slowing the horse is easily trained because the naïve horse is likely to offer slowing/stopping frequently and a verbal command can be given when the horse starts to slow. If stopping is then positively reinforced with food or wither scratching, the horse will quickly learn to respond to the verbal cue. The lunge can also be used as a tactile cue to slow the horse; however, it should be mentioned that the slowing signal predominantly pressures unevenly to one side of the horse's head, and so bears little resemblance to the slowing signals used in-hand. The lunge-line is used as a slowing signal by increasing vibrating/intermittent pressure and then releasing it when the horse offers slowing (negative reinforcement). The consistent and correct release of pressure will enable lunge-line signals to be rapidly shrunk to light versions. The lungeing whip is used to trigger forward reactions, and these can be brought under the stimulus control of voice commands. Variations of both the type and amount of deceleration and acceleration signals can be used to motivate and train faster and longer inter-gait transitions.

During lungeing, when the trainer in the centre of the lunge circle moves too far in front of the horse (so that the right angle represented by a line drawn from the human to the longitudinal axis of the horse via the horse's shoulder is increased) (Figure 8.13), the horse typically slows down. This is a typical ethological response to the horse

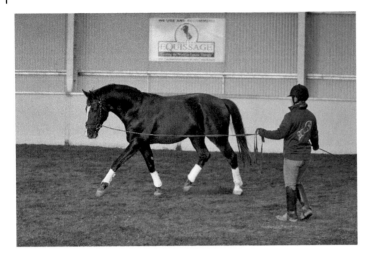

Figure 8.12 Lungeing is often used in training to assist in physical development, to help associate locomotory responses with signals, and to exercise a horse. Trainers should bear in mind that continuously lungeing a flighty horse can create associations between humans and the flight response that can be indelible.

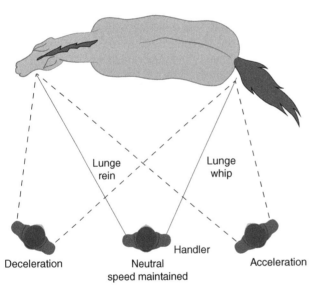

Figure 8.13 When the angle of the trainer's position opens or closes relative to the horse's shoulder, this may increase or diminish speed.

perceiving that its escape forward is thwarted. On the other hand, if this critical angle (of trainer to horse) diminishes to less than a right angle, the horse accelerates. Although lungeing procedures may use these ethological phenomena, most responses in the lunge are operantly and classically conditioned and the horse can basically be trained to accelerate and decelerate from any tactile, visual or auditory signal.

Fundamentally, flight responses should be avoided for ethical and safety reasons (Christensen, 2007) because of their rapid acquisition and resistance to erasure (Seligman, 1971; Le Doux, 1994). The horse should be trained gradually to increase and decrease its speed on the lunge and if it shows a flight response, it is important to slow the horse. It is a matter of good welfare that the horse is not put in a position of being 'chased' and expressing a flight response during lungeing. However, if the horse is quiet and consistently responding to the slowing signals (a good test!) or maintaining its speed, then lungeing is not detrimental. The same principles apply to round-pen work.

Under-Saddle Training

Foundation Training

When the time for foundation training arrives, the young horse is habituated to the appropriate equipment, such as bridle, saddle cloth, saddle and girth-strap pressure. This should preferably be done using negative reinforcement, systematic desensitisation and perhaps overshadowing, where the horse is first habituated to the saddle cloth with steps forward and back and the cloth is removed only when the horse stands still, so that immobility is negatively reinforced. An elastic girth can be used to habituate the horse to girth pressure by first rubbing the horse with the girth (Figure 8.14a), then gradually habituating it to the loose girth hanging beside it (Figures 8.14b,c), and to the human hand moving under its stomach and picking up the girth on the other side (Figure 8.14d). It is important at all stages to move forward so slowly that the horse is likely to show an appropriate response (standing still) that can be reinforced by removal of the hand and/or girth. This initial habituation should be performed in the company of other calm horses and in the stable or another place where the horse feels safe.

When the horse is habituated to the opening and closing of the elastic girth (Figure 8.14e), it can be signalled to move forward and to step back with the girth. Subsequently the horse can be habituated to the saddle. If initially habituated to the elastic girth, the horse is less likely to react aversively to the saddle girth. Following successful habituation, the horse then also undergoes gradual habituation to the presence of the rider either bareback or, after habituation,

with the saddle and girth. Regardless of methodology, habituation is facilitated by progressing very slowly so that the process of sitting up on the horse may have a dozen or so intermediate steps, such as habituating the horse to a human jumping up and down beside it, then jumping a bit higher until lying on the horse and then habituating the horse to the arrival of the trainer's leg over to the horse's off-side and then sitting up. For skilled horsepeople, it can be more efficient to habituate the horse to the rider bareback rather than saddled, to separate the mounting procedure from the habituation to saddle and girth pressure. An assistant handler can expedite training and render it safer. At the rider's request, the assistant should step the horse back and forward a stride from time to time as the quality of the *step-back* response positively correlates with the success of the habituation, and therefore the calmness of the horse and safety of the rider.

Some trainers drive the young horse in long-reins once it has habituated to the saddle and bridle (Figure 8.15). The disadvantages of this are that the young horse may perceive that it is being chased and develop a habituated mouth and hyper-reactive posture as it attempts to escape forward. It may also learn to associate some tension with horse–human interactions.

Signals Used Under-Saddle

Under-saddle, there are three points of physical interaction between rider and horse: legs, seat and reins. In early training, variations in acceleration, deceleration and changing direction are acquired primarily through negative reinforcement using rein tension and leg pressures and in optimal training the pressures reduce to lighter versions. There are many recipes for stimulating and training horses to perform; however, what is described here are examples of signals that are most easily discriminated by the horse. It is important to reflect that the number of responses required from horses exceeds the availability of easy-to-discriminate signals provided by a rider's reins, legs and seat.

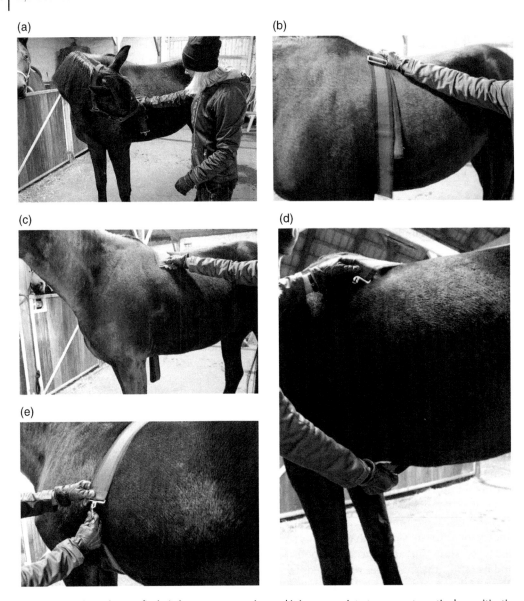

(a) (b) (c) (d) (e)

Figure 8.14 Some horses find girth pressure aversive and it is appropriate to use systematic desensitisation to habituate horses to the girth (see also Chapter 4, Non-associative Learning). The horse is initially habituated to stroking on the body and especially in the girth area with the folded girth (a). When the horse reliably fails to react to this stage, the girth is gradually made longer so the horse habituates to the loose girth hanging from its body, (b), (c). The trainer then habituates the horse to a hand moving under the stomach and picking up the girth on the other side without closing the girth (d). The girth should be completely removed at regular intervals at a moment where the horse shows appropriate behaviour (e.g. standing still, as the girth removal will then negatively reinforce immobility). It is preferable to have a second handler controlling the horse's movement to avoid the risk that the horse itself removes the girth by moving away, which will negatively reinforce an undesired response. When the horse reliably fails to react to closing the girth (e), it should be trained to *move forward* and *step back* while wearing the girth. Habituation to girth pressure is an important part of foundation training and should always precede mounting of the saddle.

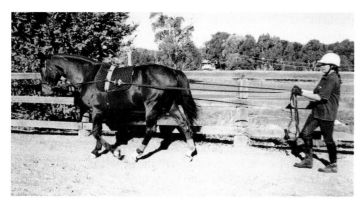

Figure 8.15 Long-reining the horse is sometimes a feature of foundation training. Because the trainer's hands are at a considerable distance from the horse's mouth, skill is required to ensure smooth and consistent delivery of rein signals. It is also important to ensure that the driven horse does not perceive that he is being chased or else fearful, hyper-reactive associations can be incorporated into training. (Photo courtesy of Greg Jones.)

Variations in magnitude of squeezing applied by the rider's calves may signal quickening of the horse's legs and gait changes. The lower portion of the rider's leg may be used to negatively reinforce longer strides. Pressure of a rider's single leg may signal sideways movements of the hindquarters. The rider's upper leg (femur) is often an acquired signal associated with turning the horse's forequarters or slowing. The rider's seat has less effect in terms of negative reinforcement, since there is a limit to which the rider can increase the forces of the seat. On the contrary, the seat is largely effective by classical conditioning: by association with the more powerful signals from the reins and rider's legs. Variations in the magnitude of the rein tensions may be used to signal gait changes, slowing the tempo and shortening the stride, while lateral movements of the reins may signal changes of direction of the forelegs.

Equipment

The Whip

The leg signals and seat signals for acceleration are typically supplemented with the use of the long whip, the riding crop and spurs. Whips should be used only as further signals

and not as a punitive stimulus that, as believed in some circles, forces the horse to *pay attention* to a previous signal. Both are wrong for welfare reasons and the second is wrong also because it relies on unrealistic cognitive expectations.

Spurs

Spurs should be used only to make a signal more precise (i.e. to refine the leg signals), not to inflict increasing pain on the horse's sides, so spurs should not be introduced until the horse's basic training is consolidated. Yet, it is not uncommon to see the use of spurs for young horses, for novice riders and for horses that are labelled 'lazy' (horses that have been inadvertently reinforced for not going forward, or horses that have habituated to leg pressure due to lack of reinforcement). So-called laziness should not be thought of as a personality disorder but rather as a behaviour with a significant learned component, or a behaviour related to pain.

Severe Bits

The action of a bit can be fortified by using a more severe bit. These tend to have an increased motivational effect through increasing pain; in other words, severe bits are effective because of their thinness, abrasiveness, corrugation, sharpness or via a lever effect. The lever effect is represented by the shank fixed onto the curb bit, which in physics is known as a 'first-class' lever (Figure 10.6). As mentioned previously, such equipment should not be used to induce pain, as the mouth of the horse is particularly sensitive. Only the mildest bits should be used and supported with additional signals in case the horse has learned not to respond to the discomfort induced by a mild bit.

It is crucial that riders recognise that the horse feels far more pressure inside its mouth from a curb bit than riders do in their hands, so 'feel' may be a rather inaccurate assessment tool. The importance of self-carriage (especially in horses in curb bits) and frequently testing for it by momentarily (for two strides) relinquishing the rein contact are of great importance for welfare reasons. This release for two strides is embodied in the German technique known as *Überstreichen*, and should be mandatory in all gaits and movements in dressage. The mandatory use of curb bits in equestrian competitions in the past decade has been the subject of popular debate and many countries are reconsidering the use of curb bits and, in some cases, removing the requirement altogether.

Posture and Position of the Rider

The posture and position of the rider is important because the horse can learn by negative reinforcement that he can alter the posture of the rider to his advantage. For example, he can reef the reins and pull the rider forward. Thus, a stable riding position has long been the focus of equestrian pedagogy. In addition, the ability of the rider to communicate efficiently with the horse via application of light signals and release of pressure at the right moment depends on a stable seat. If the rider is unable to adjust to the movements of the horse, he/she may rely on the reins to regain position, thereby exerting undue force in the reins (Heleski *et al.*, 2009). Variations in rein tension resulting from an unbalanced rider may

result in confusion and impaired learning. Furthermore, rein tension and the distance between the rider's hand and the horse's mouth have been related to the occurrence of mouth movements (Eisersiö *et al.*, 2013; Manfredi *et al.*, 2010). The presence of a rider also affects the horse's kinematics (Sloet van Oldruitenborgh-Oosterbaan *et al.*, 1995; Egenvall *et al.*, 2015) and the forces with which it impacts the ground (Clayton *et al.*, 1999). Research into impact forces at trot shows that the vertical oscillation of the vertebral column of the rider's body is subject to momentum and continues to descend until well after the reversal in the dorsoventral movement of the horse's back (Terada *et al.*, 2004) and these impacts have flow-on effects on the rider.

Riding level influences the rider's posture and significant differences in specific waveform parameters and phase shifts have been reported for professional riders and beginners (Münz *et al.*, 2014). Coordinated contractions of the rider's muscles not only stabilise the rider but also synchronise with the horse's motion and, furthermore, can influence the horse's performance. So the musculature of experienced riders coordinates with the rhythm of the horse's strides and each gait is characterised by a corresponding cyclic pattern of the rider's biomechanics (Engell *et al.*, 2016). It has been shown that, at the sitting trot, novice riders tend to grip with their legs, using their *adductor magnus* muscles to maintain posture, because they have not yet developed coordination between the *rectus abdominis* muscles (commonly known as the 'abs') and *erector spinae* muscles (the longitudinal back muscles), which is integral to the postural skills of experienced riders. Studies show that there is a brief but consistent burst of activity in the rider's *trapezius* muscles (shoulder blade) that possibly contributes to stabilising the rider's head and neck during the impact phase of the horse's stride (Terada, 2000).

Increased intra-abdominal pressure in the rider's torso, due to *rectus abdominis* contraction during the mid-stance phase at trot, has also been documented, suggesting that the tightening of abdominal muscles assists

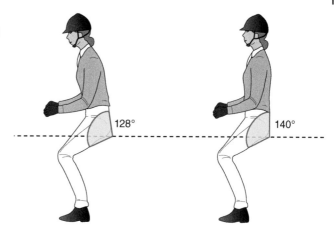

Figure 8.16 As riders become more experienced, they tend to be able to sit more upright and their limb-torso angles open.

128°   140°

in swinging the pelvis forward as the horse's dorsoventral oscillation reverses direction during mid-stance and begins to rise (Terada *et al.*, 2004). In addition, Engell *et al.* (2016) showed that trunk, pelvis and head kinematics of elite riders differed when riding with an active rider posture versus sitting passively in trot, but there were considerable individual variations. Similarly, Terada (2000) showed that there is considerable variation in the range of motion in hips and shoulders in experienced riders at trot. This may be explained by physical differences among riders or differences in coaching. Whichever, it also suggests that while successful dressage equitation demands certain essential biomechanics, other aspects, such as the movements of the rider's hips and shoulders, allow for some deviation from the norm.

Novice riders tend to lean forward to compensate for the horse's motion, which sends the rider's trunk forward and back (Figure 8.16). Terada (2000) reports that experienced riders adopt an almost vertical trunk orientation with a backward tilt of an average of 4 degrees. However, oscillations of the trunk occur in rhythm with the stride in the walk, trot and canter (Engell *et al.*, 2016; Lovett *et al.*, 2004).

Equestrian coaches have long focused on teaching their pupils to maintain their arms in a stable position beside their body. It is difficult to keep track of many body parts at one moment and human arms have shoulder joints, elbow joints and wrists that all provide different ranges of motion and, thus, can impede the acquisition of perfect balance if they are unstable or variable. Studies suggest that experienced riders maintain a more consistent distance from wrist to the horse's mouth by adjusting the angles of their shoulder and elbow joints to compensate for the rocking motion of their bodies (Terada *et al.*, 2004).

Inter-Gait and Intra-Gait Transitions Under-Saddle

Under-saddle, longer and shorter strides are often required in addition to faster and slower ones (tempo changes). In a similar format to in-hand training, faster and slower strides are usually trained and consolidated to the point where they can be elicited by light signals before longer or shorter strides are trained. Faster and slower strides as well as gait changes usually involve pressures for two steps of the horse's forelegs. The purpose of the pressure for the second step is to ensure that the correct tempo of the gait is achieved. However, when the horse has acquired the gait and tempo changes from light signals of the rider's calves, the signal duration is shortened to just one step. Lengthening and shortening signals involve brief pressures from the distal part of the lower leg applied briefly at the beginning of the swing phase of a particular limb. Later in the horse's education, longer and shorter steps are cued by brief seat cues that are acquired because of their early association with the rider's leg pressures.

Signals for Acceleration

Acceleration is the result of retraction of limbs in the stance phase and protraction in the swing phase (Figure 11.2). The fundamental signals for going forward under-saddle are provided by pressure from the rider's legs just behind the girth region (i.e. where they hang vertically down the horse's sides) (Table 8.3). For optimal acquisition, the ideal moment to issue an acceleration signal is at the beginning of the swing phase of one hindleg footfall (which coincides with the beginning step of the contralateral swing phase). In the early stages of training the response, the release should occur at the end of that step (Warren-Smith *et al.*, 2005a). As with all responses acquired by negative reinforcement, riders often resort to using the entire lower leg to motivate the naïve or poorly trained horse to *go forward*. Ideally, this pressure is preceded by light pressure of the calves, and so these discriminative stimuli become the light signals in optimal training. This is typically accompanied by a 'sweeping' seat signal of similar duration, which later achieves stimulus control. Cues for increasing intra-gait speed can be differentiated from those for upward inter-gait transitions by pressure differences: by increasing the amount of leg pressure and differences in associated seat posture for upward inter-gait transitions. Further shaping of the acceleration responses entails eliciting an entire stride of the chosen gait from a light signal of the calves. Multiple steps are then reinforced followed by the maintenance of directional line and body straightness and, finally, head and neck posture.

Longer steps are cued using brief pressure of the rider's legs for a portion of a single step and repeating until the horse learns to lengthen (Figure 8.17). Should the horse quicken, the rider generally slows it with the reins and repeats the longer step signal.

Under-saddle, the brief leg signals for longer strides often accompany an associated brief 'shoving' seat signal, which also eventually maintains the longer strides.

Longer steps are often established early in the horse's training, because they assist in lowering and lengthening the horse's head and neck to promote relaxation. Lowering and lengthening of the cervical vertebrae are intricately associated with the lengthening of the stride. This biomechanical feature confers the first and most vital stage of training in many traditional dressage and reining methods: *longitudinal flexion* (Figure 8.18), characterised by lowering of the poll, and lowering and lengthening of the neck. Many training methodologies advocate this as the first major step of training, because it promotes looseness of the musculature (Hölzel *et al.*, 1995; German National Equestrian Federation, 1997). However, many trainers ignore this and use straps and pulleys to force the horse's head down, causing both physical (Heuschmann, 2007) and mental (McLean, 2005a) damage to the horse.

Horses may drift off-line for several reasons, resulting in asymmetry (crookedness) (Chapter 11, Biomechanics). First, the rider may be sitting eccentrically, causing the horse to drift (Figure 8.19). Or the horse may simply drift of its own accord, especially if it is morphologically asymmetric, young and not going sufficiently forward (uneven propulsion). Horses may also be inadvertently reinforced for doing so. The accelerating signal of the single leg of the rider can straighten a horse's unilateral bulging ribcage (the beginning of crookedness and drifting off-line). Thus, the accelerating leg signal equalises the propulsion of both hindlegs, resulting in straightness.

On the other hand, it is important that the horse does not habituate to the whip as a signal. Trainers must be careful how they use it in training. For example, by the requirements of negative reinforcement, they should be clear to continue and perhaps increase tapping frequency until an improved response emerges, and then to be vigilant to immediately cease tapping at the

Table 8.3 Examples of stimulus–response characteristics of under-saddle training.

Targeted response	Targeted biomechanics	Operant discriminative stimulus	Motivation	Reinforcement	Other associated cues and maintenance	Verbal cue
Upward inter-gait transition and faster limbs	Accelerating protraction (swing) and retraction (stance)	Prolonged (2 steps) squeeze of rider's upper calves	Increased calves pressure/whip-taps on ribcage	Release pressure on second improved step	Accelerating seat	'Walk on', 'trot on', 'canter'
Upward intra-gait transition: longer stride	Increased protraction (swing) and retraction (stance)	Brief (1 step) nudge of rider's legs (lower calves)	Stronger nudge of rider's lower leg/ whip-tap on ribcage	Release pressure on first improved step	Shoving seat	Rider clicking tongue
Downward inter-gait transition (including step-back) and slower limbs	Decelerating protraction (stance) and retraction (swing)	Prolonged (2 steps) rein signal	Increased rein pressure	Release pressure on second improved step	Decelerating seat	'Whoa', 'stand', 'walk', 'trot'
Downward intra-gait transition: shorter stride	Decreased protraction (stance) and retraction (swing)	Brief (1 step) rein signal	Stronger brief rein pressure	Release pressure on first improved step	Bracing seat	'Whoa'
Turn forequarters: direct turn signal (opening rein)	Abduction then adduction	Opening rein signal (hand away from wither) or light rein squeeze	Increased opening rein pressure/whip-tap on shoulder	Release pressure on second improved step	Rider's shoulders turn and associated seat/leg effects	Usually not used
Turn forequarters: indirect turn signal (neck-rein)	Abduction then adduction	Closing rein signal (hand towards wither)	Increased closing rein pressure/whip-tap on shoulder	Release pressure on second improved step	Rider's shoulders turn and associated seat/ leg effects	Usually not used
Turn hindquarters and go sideways	Adduction then abduction	Prolonged signal of rider's single leg on ribcage	Increased leg pressure/whip-tap on hindquarters	Release pressure on second improved step	Altered seat weight distribution	'Over'

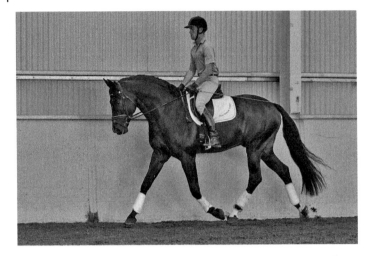

Figure 8.17 The difference between the so-called working gaits and the lengthened gaits is seen in the overtrack of the foretracks by the hindhooves.

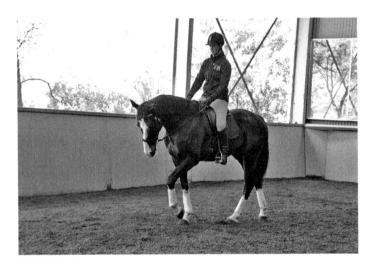

Figure 8.18 Longitudinal flexion is an important stage of daily training in the warm-up phase, because it stretches, loosens and therefore relaxes the horse.

precise moment of the improved response. Therefore, in the early stages of training, a series of whip-taps may be required to motivate forward, and then the horse rapidly learns to respond to only one or two very light taps. Optimally, the use of the whip-tap under-saddle should be an analogue of its use in-hand and it should be used on the same three sites as outlined earlier in in-hand work (Figure 7.6).

Because we are describing the training of the whip as a signal, but not as an instrument of punishment, it is of value not only to train but also to check regularly that the horse can respond correctly to whip-taps alone (without the rider's legs). When trainers deal with so-called lazy horses, they tend to use the whip-tap in tandem with leg signals. However, if the horse is trained to respond to the whip-tap alone, so that it goes from halt to trot from just two light taps of the whip, it also becomes simultaneously sensitised to the leg signals for the same response. This response may soon wane in a less forward-motivated horse. Nevertheless, if the trainer remains alert to any losses of responding from the rider's leg signals and reverts to using the whip-tap without legs for a series of transitions, the periods of poor responding to the rider's legs diminish.

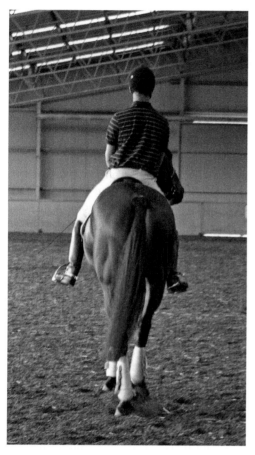

Figure 8.19 When riders sit asymmetrically, it becomes difficult for the horse to maintain its own symmetry and balance and typically results in the horse drifting and becoming crooked in its vertebral column, especially at the base of the neck.

Jumping

Jumping is a further extension of achieving complete stimulus control of forward locomotion: training the horse to go everywhere it is signalled. Beginning with small obstacles, perhaps cross-rails, the horse is trained to *go forward* and maintain an even rhythm and consistent line. This is generally done at the trot where errors can more easily be seen and corrected. When the horse has learned to maintain a consistent rhythm and line, the obstacles are changed (different form or different height), or the gait is changed (perhaps to a canter). It is optimal to change only one aspect at a time and train it. It is also optimal

when changing the height or width of the fence to do so very gradually, as the horse may baulk if changes are too sudden. Excessive changes in height or width (i.e. increments greater than 10 cm) are commonly known as over-facing.

When a horse is overwhelmed by an array of novel stimuli, he may baulk. While most obstacles in jumping courses are of a standard breadth (around 3–4 m) allowing the horse to negotiate the left, right or middle of the obstacle, there is some variation that increases the degree of difficulty for certain competitions. Eventing horses are required to learn to jump narrow obstacles, which may be only slightly wider than the horse's body. Context-specific aspects of learning deem that the horse must learn to attempt to negotiate significantly narrower obstacles. It is anthropomorphic and largely unsuccessful to presume that once a horse has learned to jump an obstacle, it will jump anything it is presented with. It requires significant generalisation to apply the same jumping response with different contextual features, such as a narrow fence.

The parabolic shape of the horse's jumping effort (Figures 11.14 and 8.20), and the approach speed, prescribe certain characteristics in the take-off point for jumping obstacles. A rounded fence shape allows a horse to take-off closer than a square topped, box-shaped fence. Fences that slope from ground level away from the approach side at low angles provide the closest take-off point, which may be just centimetres from the base. In a rushing horse, when the approach speed increases there is generally an associated lengthening of the stride, hollowing (lordosis) of the back and the parabolic shape becomes broader at the base of the jumping effort. The horse is more likely to knock a rail. Typical stride speeds in successful show-jumping horses are within the narrow range of 105 to 115 strides per minute (average 110), whereas in a sprinting racehorse the stride speed may exceed 150 strides per minute (McLean, unpublished data). While further investigation is merited, it appears that the average show-jumping speed of

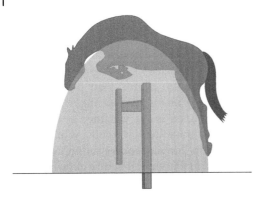

Figure 8.20 The parabolic jumping shape that characterises correct jumping technique results from the translation of forward locomotion to vertical thrust. Therefore, the take-off moment is critical in maintaining velocity and rhythm.

110 strides per minute provides optimal power for the jumping effort. The progressively overriding effect of the horse's mass at higher speeds tends to inhibit vertical lift, which explains the lower but longer jumping efforts of event horses and steeplechasers who tackle obstacles at greater speeds.

The jump effort is also modifiable by experience and learning. The horse learns to associate various approach speeds and take-off points with the type of obstacle. When horses refuse at obstacles, turning away from the obstacles and reductions of the horse's effort (e.g. stopping) negatively reinforce the refusal. Thus, refusing is rewarded and may become habitual. Delayed punishment techniques are inappropriate and are misinterpreted by the horse; instead, the horse becomes hyper-reactive and the jumping environment may trigger flight responses and losses of *stop* responses. The most appropriate solution is to lower the obstacle and re-train the horse over obstacles that are low enough not to require re-presenting, and therefore removing the reward of turning away or stopping (McLean and McLean, 2008).

Signals for Deceleration and Stepping Backwards

As with in-hand work, deceleration under-saddle comprises slowing, shortening the steps, stopping and going backwards. The fundamental signal learned by negative reinforcement is provided by bit pressure via rein tension. Optimally the deceleration response occurs in just a single stride and from a rein signal progressively lighter and shorter in duration. When the horse is going forward, the optimal moment to increase rein tension is at the beginning of the swing phase protraction of a foreleg. This also corresponds to the beginning of the contralateral foreleg beginning retraction in the stance phase. During this phase, the leg(s) diminish propulsion and begin bracing against the direction of movement so that the deceleration is active and energy-consuming. Of course, a horse may slow down gradually without any braking effort, as we may see in trail-riding scenarios. However, in equestrian sports, both upward and downward transitions are trained to be offered within a short time-frame (McLean, 2003), which requires an energy-expensive effort.

In terms of the muscles involved, active stopping, slowing, shortening and stepping backwards result from active protraction during the stance phase and retraction in the swing phase. Therefore, biomechanics suggest that training a horse to *step back-wards* should assist and enhance its *stop* response. Many training methodologies (particularly reining) embrace this observation and integrate steps backwards as part of their training methodology to improve the lightness of responding to the reins. The *step-back* response itself undergoes shaping so that when the horse has learned to *step-back* without delay from light rein tension, multiple steps backwards, called *rein-back*, are trained. The persistence signal (or keep-going signal) for *rein-back* that dressage riders often use is moving both legs back (without any medial squeezing of the calves or lower limbs) about 10 cm or leaning forward slightly. Persistence in other movements may be signalled by the action of the seat (Chapter 7, Applying Learning Theory, and see also later in this chapter).

Once the horse has acquired the fundamental signal for deceleration (light pressure via both reins), it later learns other associations, such as a bracing motion of the seat that terminates its sweeping motion towards the front of the saddle, via the process of classical conditioning. Some trainers, particularly jumping trainers, use closing the knees to signal deceleration, which again is learned by classical conditioning. Although the reins provide the only operant reinforcement for the deceleration responses under-saddle, it is worth considering the cognitive difficulty presented by this signal for the horse. The reins are physically distant from the part of the body that is intended to respond: the legs. This difficulty places considerable onus on the trainer to be aware of the actual leg movements that are to be reinforced. In shaping the deceleration response, the trainer initially reinforces a basic attempt, which may consist of any slowing, shortening or backward step. The next aspect to be shaped is an entire stride of the gait, so that the release of rein tension occurs as the horse offers the complete stride from a light version of the pressure signal. Multiple steps are also shaped, as well as shortening the steps, from a brief rein signal (pressured for a portion of a step). Finally, maintaining straightness and incorporating a consistent head and neck posture are trained. Shaping the rein responses is important and challenging: there are more conflict behaviours associated with rein responses than those with the rider's leg responses (McLean, 2005b).

At liberty, most of the horse's weight (around 60%) is carried on its forelegs, so deceleration places considerable force there. However, dressage practice revolves around the balance of the horse–human entity, with the putative aim of transferring weight to the hindquarters of the horse. As described in Chapter 11, Biomechanics, this involves a lowering of the horse's croup which, in best practice, requires a heterogeneous closing of the joint angles of the hindlegs (Podhajsky, 1966). Biomechanically, this places more involvement

of the hindhooves in deceleration. This occurs when the deceleration response involves a minimum of intermediate steps, which is characteristic of a highly trained horse (Argue and Clayton, 1993a,b).

Where learning theory is incorrectly used in training, the horse's tongue often retracts to escape unrelenting pain (Figure 8.21) and then is sometimes seen to droop flaccidly out of the mouth. This response may become habitual as soon as the bit is inserted into the horse's mouth. This is not uncommon in dressage and racing horses, where strong bit pressure is often maintained, even though it may be causing constant pain. Most likely the tongue drops out of the mouth because of tongue fatigue (the difficulty of sustaining the retraction) and there may well be a component of learned helplessness. In some horse-racing countries, it is legal to tie the tongue inside the mouth, which should be questioned and, instead, the reason for the behaviour addressed. It is imperative that lightness is the goal, unconditionally and throughout training. While moments of pressure may well be required to acquire certain responses, the horse should be free to travel in self-carriage.

Once again, we face the problem of the horse's ability to discriminate between the signals for alterations in stride speed and length: slowing and shortening. As with the acceleration signals, the problem is solved by using a consistent set of different rein tensions. For slowing the horse, including downward inter-gait transitions, the rein signal is usually more prolonged and is released immediately when the horse shows the desired downward transition. For shortening the stride, the rein signal is relatively brief. The rein signal for downward inter-gait transitions is the same as for slowing, except that it is slightly but perceptibly stronger. In addition, there are associated seat signals for downward inter-gait transitions, such as smoothly emphasising the bracing seat for a couple of beats of the rhythm. For the intra-gait transitions of shortening the steps, the bracing seat is stronger and brief.

(a)

(b)

(c)

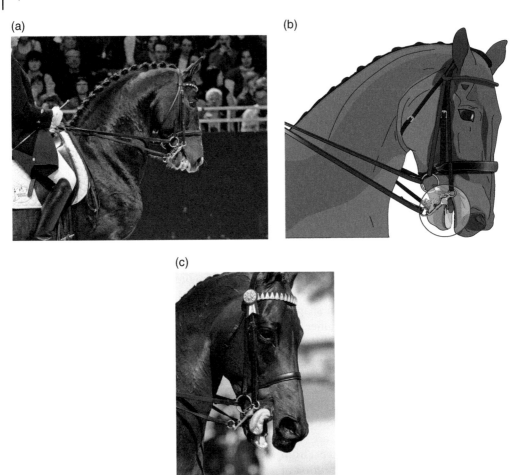

Figure 8.21 In best practice, the tongue should sit underneath the bit in a relaxed way. Relentless pressure across the tongue can restrict blood flow to the end of the tongue (a), a condition known as ischaemia that is characterised by the tongue's blue colour. (Photo courtesy of Minna Tallberg.). (b) When the horse's tongue remains permanently retracted, it is a sign that the horse finds the bit aversive: mouth pressure is too strong and unrelenting. (c) When the tongue cannot escape highly aversive bit pressure by retraction, it may droop in a seemingly paralysed way. (Photo courtesy of Julie Wilson.)

Correct early training results in a horse maintaining its own rhythm, line and outline, culminating in a posture known as 'on the bit' (Figure 8.22). Sometimes a horse may constantly lean on the bit and the rider notices that the reins are heavy. While some consider that leaning on the bit is something the horse does deliberately, a more likely explanation suggests that such a horse has developed this habit because of poorly timed, insufficient or absent negative reinforcement of the decel-

eration responses. In such cases, most horses accelerate when the reins are released, which places the horse in a confused state where the release of the reins that should reinforce slowing now elicits the opposite response: acceleration.

Although it is common in many equestrian disciplines to insist on a rounded outline early on, this can lead to confusion and conflict behaviours when the horse is still requiring pressure from the rider's legs, yet

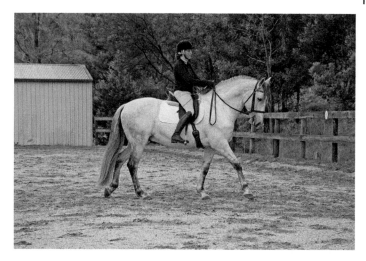

Figure 8.22 A horse under-saddle develops a rounded neck outline through longitudinal, lateral and vertical flexion. From this position, the horse gradually develops collection, where the poll is at its highest point and there is increased arching of the neck.

the rider is increasing tension in the reins to achieve a rounded outline. Because the muscles that provide acceleration are opposed to the ones that provide deceleration, the signals must never clash and should be separated, as outlined in the previous chapter. While it is common for riders to be taught to use leg pressures during all downward transitions, it must be recognised that this practice is inherently confusing for horses. If transitions are trained to be completed within the cycle of a single stride, the activity of the hindlegs remains and the rider's legs are obsolete at this moment.

Signals for Turning the Forelegs

Turning the forelegs typically facilitates changes of direction in equitation and results from consecutive abduction and adduction. In correct training, abductions and adductions are symmetrical: both forelegs open or close to the same degree, so that the horse's body is precisely upright and not leaning to one side. When turning, horses are trained so that the hindlegs also turn and follow the same path as the forelegs. However, when the forelegs are abducting, both hindlegs are adducting, so on curved lines this involves what is considered in dressage as *bend* along

the vertebral column, although, as described in Chapter 11, Biomechanics, the amount of vertebral bending is minimal in horses (Jeffcott and Dalin, 1980). Turns may begin with either abduction or adduction. That said, some sports, such as dressage, insist on abduction as the first response of a turn. Regardless, it is important that one or the other is *consistently* chosen to be elicited for the beginning of any turn to facilitate optimal long-term potentiation.

Light tension through the right rein is the fundamental signal for turning right, whereas tension through the left rein is the main signal for the left turn. It is common to find that riders bring both hands slightly towards the right for a right turn or both slightly to the left for a left turn. When relatively greater pressure is applied via the rein that moves *away* from the horse's neck, it is known as a *direct turn* (Figure 8.23a). Conversely, when relatively greater pressure is applied via the rein that comes *closer* to the horse's neck, it is known as an *indirect turn* (Figure 8.23b). When both turns have been consolidated, the reins are used together, where they move either left or right to a greater or lesser extent, depending on the horse's level of training. In cases when the horse's neck is laterally bending too much, or when the horse is drifting

(a)　　　　　　　　　　　　　　　　　　(b)

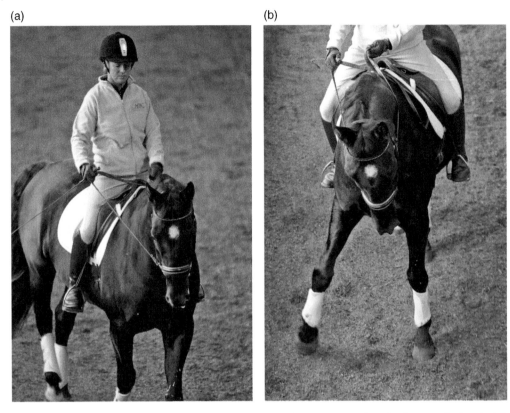

Figure 8.23 These photographs show the (a) direct and (b) indirect turn signals. In both cases, the hands shift towards the intended direction, but in the direct turn, the opening rein (moving away from the midline) is pressured, while in the indirect turn, the closing rein (rein moving towards the midline) is pressured.

one way or the other, or the horse is vertically tilting one way or the other, the indirect turn is remedial. In best-practice training, both direct rein and indirect rein tensions are intended to negatively reinforce the turn during swing phase.

Following the initial training of the rein signals, the horse learns to discriminate the shift in the rider's position as he turns his shoulders towards the new direction. These postural signals are conditioned stimuli that have been acquired secondarily through the process of classical conditioning. Some trainers also use leg signals to turn, or use leg signals concurrently with rein signals. Both present difficulties for the horse from the viewpoint of discrimination (i.e. the leg is also used in the same place for acceleration), and because the horse is asked to respond to the cues at the same time. The first may be

difficult in terms of discrimination, as there may be other responses elicited by the legs in the same location (e.g. up gait, faster, longer and bend). The second is difficult because of signal salience – which signal should the horse pay attention to? One or both signals may therefore undergo habituation. Concurrent leg and rein signals also present cognitive and biomechanical challenges, because only one leg or diagonal couplet will be in swing phase at any one time.

In foundation training, training the *turn* response begins with increased pressure on the single rein relative to the contralateral rein. The *turn* response is negatively reinforced until it is elicited from very light pressure. Usually, the trainer maintains somewhat less tension through the opposite rein to prevent the horse learning the obvious yet incorrect response of bending its neck. When

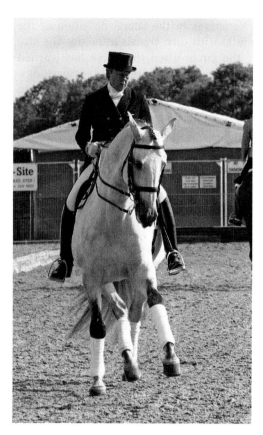

Figure 8.24 When the horse is moving on curved lines under-saddle in dressage, lateral flexion is required. This entails laterally flexing at the atlanto-occipital joint, as well as the joints surrounding C1, C2. (Photo courtesy of Kyra Kyrklund.)

the horse has learned to turn from light rein signals, further shaping of the *turn* response involves training the horse to maintain its speed and step length, maintain its line and straightness, and maintain a stable head and neck posture. Yet, more shaping occurs in dressage where the horse is trained to turn with lateral flexion (Figure 8.24): the horse turns its head and looks in towards the direction of its turn, and also tends to arch its neck to some extent. For this reason, lateral flexion, along with longitudinal flexion, is a key component of training roundness and being on the bit. Lateral flexion is facilitated by flexion of the cervical vertebrae at the atlanto-occipital junction, as well as C1, C2,

and diminishing distally. When lateral flexion is consolidated as a shaped component of the *turn* response, it is considered a precursor to what is known as lateral bend (described in Chapter 11, Biomechanics).

Typically, when horses shy, they suddenly change direction with their forelegs and this action is generally followed by forward acceleration. Horses frequently learn to shy and these responses are then inadvertently negatively reinforced when the rider momentarily and inadvertently releases rein and/or leg contact and position. Such reinforcement can be so powerful that the horse becomes increasingly likely to react to features of the environment. So, placing the horse's direction under the stimulus control of the rider is of primary importance. While many trainers correct drifting by negatively reinforcing the chosen direction using their legs, others prefer to use the reins. Because the forelegs are predominant in any alterations of direction (e.g. horses shy using their forelegs), it is preferable to interpret drifting primarily as a loss of stimulus control of the forelegs. Therefore, since losses of line are associated with losses of straightness (where the hind-hooves no longer step into the foretracks), placing the forelegs under stimulus control is a vital component in shaping straightness of acceleration and deceleration responses.

Many movements have turn responses incorporated into them, for example, lateral movements such as leg-yield, half-pass, shoulder-in and pirouette in dressage, and side-pass in reining, all owe their quality, in part at least, to the correct training of *turn* responses. If the abduction in the swing and stance phases is not symmetrical, these movements can become poor and diminished or the horse may even appear lame. For example, if the swing phase leg is seen to lose its momentum or falter, the stance phase limb reciprocates and an unevenness of step occurs.

For changes in direction, it is important from the horse's discrimination viewpoint that either the forelegs or hindlegs are targeted. For example, when the reins are used to train the horse to turn its forelegs, care

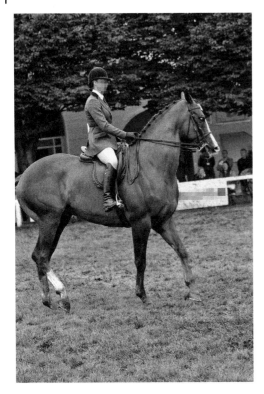

Figure 8.25 When the horse falls-in or falls-out, its head and neck are carried to one side, which becomes the concave side, while the horse drifts towards the convex side.

should be taken to avoid the horse turning its hindlegs from those signals.

Another problem arises when a horse makes random turns in the form of drifting right or left during locomotion. On circles, this is known as falling-in or falling-out when the horse drifts off the line of the circle (Figure 8.25). Other more subtle problems arise when horses abduct or adduct their forelegs asymmetrically. For example, during a turn right, the right foreleg abducts in swing phase and simultaneously the left foreleg abducts in stance phase. Any asymmetry results in losses of an upright posture and balance where one foreleg deviates less than the other. Problems of this sort are most clearly seen in lateral movements, such as half-pass, where the horse may appear to travel sideways in small inexpressive steps or, worse, it may show alterations in rhythm that appear as lameness.

Variations in the lateral deviation of the rein(s) with turn signals influence the size of the circle when the horse has learned proportional signal–response associations. Some trainers supplement a poor turn response using a single whip-tap on the outside shoulder at the beginning of abduction/adduction in the swing phase, just after the rein signals are issued. In this way, the rein response for turn can be classically conditioned in re-training.

Signals for Turning the Hindquarters and Lateral Movements

Under-saddle, turning the hindquarters without forward motion merges into going sideways when the horse is moving forward. Because the hindquarters largely drive the horse forward, they are not as involved in changes of direction as with the forequarters; instead, they are involved in changing line. Therefore, training sideways movements begins with training the hindquarters to step to the right or left from a standstill (known as turn on the forehand). Then, when moving forward, this is transformed into what is known as leg-yield. In dressage, lateral movements that involve turns of the hindquarters include travers, renvers and half-pass (Figure 8.26). Dressage requires that all lateral movements result in the horse going forward to some extent, but in other equestrian pursuits, such as reining, or working equitation, the horse may be trained to go completely sideways (full-pass) as well as sideways while going forward (side-pass). Clearly, in all sideways movements there is also an involvement to some extent of turning the forelegs.

Sideways movements are negatively reinforced by the rider's single leg. The discriminative stimulus is the light leg signal, which should coincide with the acquisition of an immediate response (McLean and McLean, 2008). Further shaping of sideways movements involves the horse persevering in going sideways and maintaining a consistent line. In dressage and reining, the postures of the horse's head and neck are also shaped.

whereas most lateral movements prescribe a lesser amount of crossover.

The typical signal for the sideways movement of leg-yield is light pressure of the rider's single leg. Generally, this single-leg pressure is applied farther behind (about 10–15 cm or 4–6in) the girth than the normal *go* signal. However, some trainers simply train sideways from the application of a single leg signal at the same place as the *go* signals. The horse's resultant struggle to discriminate between these signals emphasises the importance of rider position and training. The correct moment to issue the leg-yield signal is at the onset of the swing phase of the ipsilateral hindleg.

Sideways movements can be fortified by the whip-tap on the horse's hindquarters. Because the whip-tap is also a signal, it is important that the horse learns to respond to the whip-tap on the hindquarters alone so that the whip effectively fortifies the sideways reactions. When horses have habituated to the sideways signals and, thus, fail to respond sufficiently, the signals can be re-installed by classical conditioning where the leg signal is applied and contiguously followed by the whip-tap (once again used and pre-trained as a signal, not as a punisher).

Other Signals

The Rider's Seat as a Signal

It is generally accepted that once signalled to respond, the trained horse should 'go on its own'. Thus, if the horse is signalled to trot, it should ideally keep on trotting until signalled to do something else. However, the horse is likely to slow down after a while and the rider must re-apply the light leg signal before the horse will trot on. It is important that riders do not maintain responses through constant cueing (e.g. 'nagging') with their legs, because this will lead to habituation and conflict behaviours. The same is true for any constant use of signals where associated responses are not forthcoming. For example, riders often click with their tongues incessantly, which

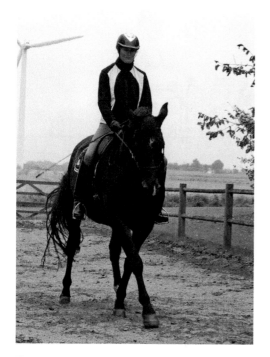

Figure 8.26 During lateral movements (including side-pass in reining), the sideways movement is conferred by consecutive abductions and adductions of the forelegs and hindlegs. To maintain balance, abduction of the forelegs can occur only during adduction of the hindlegs when the horse is going forward.

Like turns of the forequarters, turning the hindquarters is conferred by consecutive adduction and abduction of the hindlegs. Adduction may occur first or second at liberty, but in dressage and reining, it is required before abduction, which is the opposite of the forelegs. Horses are not inclined to abduct the forelegs while abducting the hindlegs – this would present a significant balance problem. So, if abduction occurs in the forelegs, this is accompanied by adduction of the hindlegs and vice versa. When turning the hindquarters to the left, the right hindleg adducts in the swing phase, while the left hindleg adducts in the stance phase. The amount of adduction required in equestrian sports is a function of the amount of sideways movement required. Full-passes and steep half-passes require that adduction occurs to the extent that the hindleg crosses the contralateral hindleg at the hock, dilutes the negative reinforcing effect of those signals, or they may overuse the term 'good boy' or other verbal praise which, if not connected to a primary reinforcer (e.g. food), diminishes the value of the praise as a secondary reinforcer.

The principle of training the horse to persist in its responding of speed, direction and posture is widely known and is embodied in the concept of 'self-carriage': the correctly trained horse should maintain his speed, line and head/neck outline without constant signalling from the reins or rider's legs. It is also possible that the rider's seat has an important function in maintaining responses. In early acquisition of the seat signal, if the horse slows down, the rider applies a leg signal. Through associative learning, the horse learns that a given change in the rider's seat precedes a leg or rein cue and so the well-trained horse will 'keep going' with minimal cueing from the rider.

Because the horse's back moves in a distinct way in each gait, the rider is obliged to move his or her seat slightly differently in accordance with the defining characteristics of each gait. For example, in the walk, the seat 'sweeps' forward and back as well as dipping a little forward at the most forward point as the horse's belly swings from one side to the other. When the walk is longer the seat movement is longer, and when the walk is shorter the seat's excursions are also shorter (Figure 8.27). If the rider's seat is slower, faster, shorter or longer in its action than the movement of the horse's back, then the horse's locomotion is disturbed.

Similarly, during a rising trot, if the rider increases or decreases the magnitude of the rising, then the horse's mobility is affected. Finally, if the rider's seat is not centrally balanced or if during the rising trot the rider lands in the saddle in different places, the horse's rhythm may be disrupted. On the other hand, if the horse randomly alters its own rhythm or tempo, and the rider can maintain the original rhythm and tempo of the gait, then the horse is likely to resume the correct tempo. For this reason, the action of

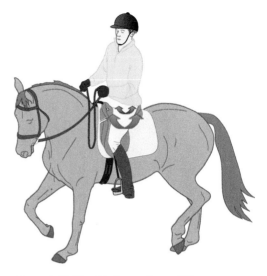

Figure 8.27 The rider's seat shows different characteristics with different gaits and stride lengths. For example, it has a long sweeping motion for longer strides (green arrow) and moves only a small amount for shorter strides (blue arrow).

the rider's seat is a chief focus of equestrian coaching. The correctly moving seat of the rider in each gait may provide a unique signal that can be operantly conditioned, to some degree, to maintain the locomotory activity.

During rising trot on a circle, equitation theory prescribes that the rider rises as the outside foreleg begins the swing phase and the seat intercepts the saddle at the start of the stance phase (Figures 8.28 a,b). This loads the diagonal pair of abducting outside foreleg and adducting inside hindleg with more weight and lightens the inside foreleg to facilitate turning.

At canter, the rider's seat 'sweeps' forward and back, maintaining the tempo and stride length of the canter by lengthening/shortening or quickening/slowing the seat. There is also a lateral dipping of the seat towards the leading foreleg at its moment of maximal reach. This results in a slight asymmetry in the rider's seat movement that reflects the asymmetry in the gait itself. The seat is lighter in jumping because the rider's feet in the stirrups support more of the weight than in non-jumping equitation. In addition, the jumping rider may have a more forward-leaning upper

(a)

(b)

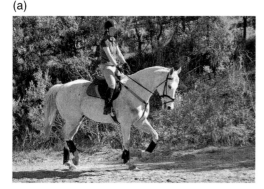 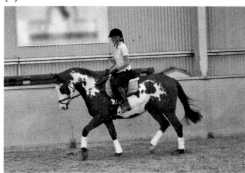

Figure 8.28 During the rising trot (i.e. when the rider rises within the beat of the trot), optimal balance is believed to occur when the rider rises (a) and falls (b) as the outside forelegs and inside hindleg undertake their swing and stance phases. Correct equitation involves refining this synchrony.

body posture to counteract the shorter stirrups and greater accelerations.

The rider's seat is considered an important source of signals. If we were to rate the operant pressure-based signals according to their salience, we would note that signals issued to the horse's mouth have the highest degree of salience, because this is most likely the most sensitive tissue, followed by signals issued to the horse's back and sides. Furthermore, the rider's legs are against the horse's sides, whereas the saddle and cloth separate the rider's seat from the horse. We would conclude that the horse's back receives more dispersed signals (because of the presence of a saddle and a cloth) than the ribcage does from the rider's legs (Figure 7.13). This dispersion plus random and accidental alterations in weight and pressure from the rider in the various gaits (which vary according to skill level) make the seat a difficult cue to train and maintain in consistency. Thus, a considerable degree of habituation to the seat signals may occur for all but the most elite riders. The consequential effects on the horse's perception of seat cues means that a tiny rein signal would be as salient as a strong seat signal. Therefore, when a rider feels that he is using his seat rather than the reins (especially with the lever effect of a curb bit), he is probably unaware of the differential perception of these signals by the horse. This is demonstrated when the reins are released and the horse is signalled to stop with the seat alone: in most cases, the horse will show no response or a diminished response to the seat. Therefore, as signals for inter-gait and intra-gait responses, those from the seat are most likely to be used in conjunction with subtle leg or rein signals. Nevertheless, in situations of optimal rider skill, it is plausible that small adjustments to the rider's seat can be perceived as signals.

Western horses show powerful downward transitions from the seat alone, where the reins are entirely looped. These horses are ridden in curb bits with a high degree of lever action (Chapter 10, Apparatus), so rein tension is related to a high degree of aversiveness. By classical conditioning, the seat becomes the discriminative stimulus and comes to elicit such responses by itself. The aversiveness of the curb rein also determines how long the seat remains a distinct discriminative stimulus without fortification from the reins. Clearly, when the operant conditioning is powerfully reinforced, a relatively benign discriminative stimulus achieves a high degree of salience.

Gait Signals

Generally, signals for upward and downward inter-gait transitions are the prolonged and slightly greater magnitude signals of the rider's calves and reins, respectively – they are like the signals for quickening and slowing but are of greater magnitude. These stronger signals are derived, logically, from the signals for faster or slower, since each upward gait involves the legs going faster by around 20 beats per minute: typically, the greater the speed change, the stronger the signals. So, a halt-to-trot signal is similar to, but stronger than, a halt-to-walk signal. The upward inter-gait transition to canter involves the same type of prolonged signal, but it also has a unique signal and preparation, because it is an asymmetrical gait with leading and trailing forelegs and hindlegs. The leading leg is said to be on the inside because cantering and galloping quadrupeds universally tend to ensure that their leading forelegs are on the inside of their curved line. Therefore, the rider's signals are:

1) light signal of the inside rein;
2) inside leg in the normal position (girth region);
3) outside leg a few centimetres behind the girth (Figure 8.29).

The inside rein is the preparation and the outside leg is the cue to canter (although later in the horse's education the cue is the rider's inside leg, or both legs). Remember that the single rein is the primary turning signal (see *Signals for turning the forelegs*, above) and should have stimulus control of the same-side foreleg. For canter, the inside rein signal stimulates lateral flexion (an integral component of turn). The turn rein signals the leading leg, as the leading leg is associated with the turn. In some methodologies, the presence of the rider's outside leg behind the girth serves as a signal in conjunction with the seat in maintaining the canter.

Canter to Canter (Flying Change)

One of the later gait-change signals the horse learns is for the flying change. When changing lead from canter, the first leg to initiate the new canter configuration is the horse's *outside* hindleg; the change occurs following the period of suspension. For this reason, the fundamental signal for the flying change is the rider's outside leg. The difficulty for novice riders attempting their first flying changes involves the timing of exactly when to apply the signal in the ephemeral suspension phase. This is a good example of the utility of the school horse in enabling riders to learn more complex and precise aspects of equitation.

Horses are often reluctant to change from one leading leg to another under-saddle. This is partly because it is common to train counter-canter (where the leading leg is the outside foreleg) before flying changes (Figure 8.30), and this unfortunately necessitates inhibiting flying changes to a greater or lesser extent. To train flying changes, some trainers use counter-canter on a small circle (perhaps only 15 m in diameter) to motivate a flying change, because of the difficulty and effort of counter-canter on small circles. Others may use lateral movements, such as half-pass, towards a wall to motivate the change and still others use a pole on the ground where the horse canters over the pole and the change is signalled at the take-off stride before the pole. The pole is gradually removed, whereas the place is kept the same and success arises because of the

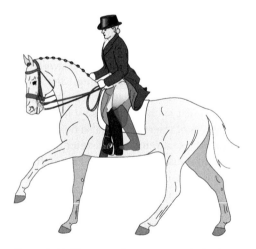

Figure 8.29 The canter is an asymmetrical gait characterised by leading foreleg and hindleg. The signals for canter require indicating to the horse the appropriate leg to lead with, and this is made possible by the altered outside leg position (farther back).

(a)

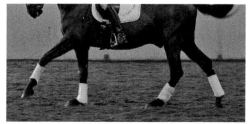

(b)

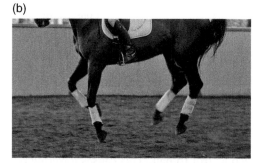

(c)

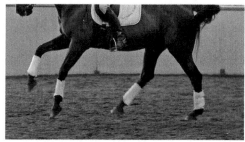

Figure 8.30 When the horse does a flying change (of leading leg), all four legs alter from leading/ trailing to trailing/leading, (a) and (c), during the moment of suspension (b). Skill is required to elicit this successfully at the optimal moment.

context-specific nature of the horse. The whip-tap on the outside hindleg can more effectively replace the rider's outside leg if it fails to elicit a change or the change is 'late behind' (the hindlegs change after, rather than at the same moment as the forelegs).

A canter is distinct from a gallop not only for differences in speed but when the uni-diagonal pair of legs separates to two individual leg beats while still retaining the moment of suspension. There is no specific signal for the gallop, partly because this moment of conversion from canter to gallop is not easily recognised. In some languages (e.g. French), there is no distinction between the words for canter and gallop. The prolonged pressure of the rider's legs in the canter configuration is the signal for the increased speed of the gallop.

Movements

When horsepeople fully grasp the profound significance of the four basic responses of *go*, *slow*, *turn* and *sideways*, they quickly appreciate that the so-called 'higher movements' consist of two or more of the four basic responses in a specific sequence (Table 8.4). Therefore, once the basic responses are properly trained, the horse is generally able to perform at least a single step of a movement. Following this, the movements themselves require gradual shaping so they progress from a step to a stride and so forth. It follows that when movements fail, trainers should go back to repair faults that will be evident in the basic responses. The critical importance of separating the delivery of the signals when training or eliciting the higher movements cannot be over-emphasised, because of the possibility of confusion and negative welfare implications. Every composite movement in equitation is optimally elicited by closely spaced, yet separated by footfalls, single signals. For example, before the horse has learned to maintain piaffe and passage without continuous signalling, these movements may be elicited from rein and leg signals a single step apart. This separation coincides with the sequence of the various leg movements, diagonal pairs and different gaits surrounding the movements. In all cases, the optimal effect is achieved when rein and leg signals occur at the onset of the relevant swing phases. For such reasons, the higher movements are the province of experienced and skilled riders, since only an experienced and correctly trained horse can respond to such closely spaced consecutive signals.

Some movements have precursors, for example, half-pass is a movement that involves several components. The horse has

Table 8.4 The basic responses that produce the movements in dressage.

Movement	1st response component	2nd response component	3rd response component	Timing of signals
Shoulder-in	Reins for *turn of the forelegs*	*Go* response from the inside leg		Consecutive
Travers	Indirect rein *turn of the forelegs* including bend	*Turn hindlegs*		Consecutive
Renvers	Indirect rein *turn of the forelegs*			Consecutive
Half-pass	Shoulder-in components	*Turn hindlegs*		Consecutive
Pirouette (walk and canter)	Shorten stride	*Turn forelegs*	*Turn hindlegs* a small step	Consecutive
Piaffe	Shorten	Lengthen		Within the stride
Passage	Shorten	Lengthen		Within the stride

to go sideways, but with the added features of laterally flexing and bending into its turn direction, and leading with the foreleg. Thus, the half-pass is traditionally trained subsequent to the movement known as shoulder-in. Shoulder-in itself is a mixture of *turning the forequarters* and continuing to *go forward*. So, the establishment of shoulder-in sets up the leading forequarters, bend and flexion for the half-pass. With these characteristics, the only additional signal that the rider is required to issue for the half-pass is the sideways signal of the outside leg.

In training all movements, trainers should recognise the importance of the principle of the exclusivity of signals (Chapter 7, Applying Learning Theory) and attempt to evaluate their training and deconstruct movements to their base components. They may then find that tension, hyper-reactive behaviours, dullness or conflict behaviours that appear in their work from time to time will disappear.

Higher Steps – Collection

It is generally recognised in dressage circles that the collected outline is not something that is trained *per se*, but is an emergent property of the process of engagement where the hindlegs step one hoofprint closer to the forelegs, which is first seen in transitions such as trot to halt. This causes lowering of the hindquarters during intra-gait transitions. German riding traditions describe this quality with the term *durchlässigkeit*, which translates as *throughness*: that quality in a horse that permits the signals (primarily the rein signals) to influence the hindlegs (USDF, 2002). Here, the desirable response is that hindlegs participate in slowing the horse by reaching forward to grip onto the ground more, which also lowers the hindquarters. In the development of collection, the steps of the horse are shortened, the poll raised and the steps become higher. Piaffe and passage also develop from elevated shortening of the stride of the collected trot.

Piaffe, being on the spot, represents the ultimate collection of the trot, whereas in passage, the horse moves forward with shortened higher steps than in the collected trot (Figure 8.31). Piaffe also differs from passage and collected trot, in that it has no period of suspension (German National Equestrian Federation, 1992). As the musculoskeletal system of the horse adapts to the stresses of the progressive biomechanical features of lowering the croup, the horse's physique alters with its topline musculature becoming more pronounced and its movement developing cadence: a rhythmic pause at the highest and lowest points of the step.

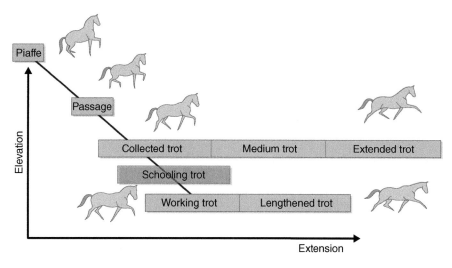

Figure 8.31 This graph shows the increased collection and simultaneous shortening of the stride as the horse becomes more educated towards piaffe.

Take-Home Messages

Horse-training is considered optimal and most likely to succeed when trainers:
- target a discrete biomechanical action, such as retraction, protraction, abduction and adduction;
- use easily discriminated signals;
- use a separate signal for each response;
- use the operant contingency correctly;
- place the horse under the stimulus control of the trainer/rider;
- reinforce the first correct or near-correct response;
- gradually shape the response by adding one quality of a response at a time;
- reinforce transitions and movements using a variable schedule of positive reinforcement;
- dissociate from all training any expressions of flight response;
- keep stress levels to the minimum level required for training.

Ethical Considerations

- The whip and spurs should be used only to make signals more precise and never as a punishment, or in the erroneously held belief that they serve to make the horse attend to a preceding signal.
- The enforced use of curb bits and spurs in FEI dressage and reining competitions directly reduces horse welfare and should be reconsidered.
- Particular attention and care should be given to shaping the rein responses, because there are more conflict behaviours associated with rein responses than with the rider's leg responses.

9

Horses in Sport and Work

Introduction

Every sporting discipline or field of work creates a different set of challenges for the horses involved, as well as for breeders, trainers, grooms and riders. This chapter not only explores the attributes of horses that excel in each of these contexts, but also examines the way in which the application of learning theory can be customised to each discipline. Likely sources of conflict are also described for each discipline and the lessons to be learned from a particular pursuit are discussed (Table 9.1).

A number of significant changes in the rules and structure of organised horse sports have emerged in response to concerns for horse welfare. For example, in some countries, such as Norway, whips have been banned from horse racing, and arduous elements of eventing prior to the cross-country phase have been removed, chiefly because of concerns about horse exhaustion. It will be interesting to see how welfare concerns shape the future of some of these sports. Certainly, equitation science is poised to contribute substantially to the debates that surround any proposed changes.

Performance Sports

Dressage forms the focus of many discussions throughout this book and so will be given only brief coverage here. The word 'dressage'

comes from the French 'dresser' – to train (animals). With an emphasis on accurate execution of standard tests, dressage demands that all the horse's locomotory responses are under stimulus control. The subjective judgment of dressage leaves it open to criticism from both competitors and some scientists. Furthermore, since points can and should be deducted for a perceived lack of submission (although we encourage you to consider whether, to gain marks in this domain, the horse must *submit* to signals or simply *respond* to them) and signs of resistance, it is not surprising that some elements of the welfare lobby are setting their sights on dressage. Practices during the warm-up, including hyperflexion, have come under sustained surveillance and some criticism, because they fail to align with what is considered acceptable in the competition arena itself (Figure 9.1).

The problem here is that if the competition is all about training and producing inherent equine athleticism on demand, any training practices that fall outside the traditional appreciation of a powerful horse bearing a rider are questioned. While some biomechanical benefits from hyperflexing the neck may be possible under certain conditions, there are numerous studies also showing detrimental effects on both biomechanics and horse welfare (König von Borstel *et al.*, 2015). Clearly, if the horse cannot sustain this position without rein tension, the practice is not likely to be wholly beneficial. From an ethological viewpoint, relentless tension

Equitation Science, Second Edition. Paul McGreevy, Janne Winther Christensen, Uta König von Borstel and Andrew McLean.
© 2018 John Wiley & Sons Ltd. Published 2018 by John Wiley & Sons Ltd.
Companion website: www.wiley.com/go/mcgreevy/equitation

Table 9.1 Summary of the ethological and learning challenges offered by various sporting and working contexts.

Work or sport	Ethological challenges	Learning and cognitive challenges
Dressage and equitation	Showing display behaviours out of context	Discriminating between physically similar tension and pressure cues from riders
	Suppression of signals to conspecifics	Learning to respond to *stop* and *go* signals that are almost simultaneous
Show-jumping	Jumping obstacles that they would naturally go around	Learning to ignore novel colours and structures. Sizing-up on-approach previously unseen obstacles for both their height and width
		Learning to retain clean jumping style, even when they have learned that fences fall when hit
Eventing	Combinations of the above two rows with speed and stamina	Combinations of the above two rows plus balancing the demand for boldness, fitness (for the jumping elements) with steadiness (for the dressage). Learning to judge if an obstacle can be brushed safely or not
Racing on the flat (Thoroughbreds, Quarterhorses and Arabians)	Socially facilitated hyper-reactive responses	Maintaining learned response when fatigued or response is impossible
		Responding to jockey before and during flight response
Steeple-chasing and hurdling	As for all forms of racing (see above). Arriving at a fence simultaneously rather than with self-selected companions	Traversing obstacles and landing on unseen terrain. Learning to jump cleanly in gallop and when fatigued
	Socially facilitated launching at fences	
Harness racing (pacing and trotting)	As for all forms of racing	Learned inhibition of upward inter-gait transition (to canter)
		For pacers, if not inherently gaited, the need to modify 2-beat gait to lateral couplets within the constraints of the hobbles
Endurance	Entering unfamiliar areas. Sustaining speed despite fatigue	Combining attention to the rider and the novel challenges of the environment. Also, remaining calm can represent a challenge to some horses, especially Arabians, most of which are predisposed to reactivity. Negotiating entirely novel terrain
Gymkhana and mounted games, including tent-pegging, polo and polocrosse	Being among conspecifics that often travel at speed but in different directions	Learning the significance of various items of apparatus that cue 180-degree turns, changes of leg and abrupt halts
Stockwork, cutting and campdrafting	Approaching other herbivores at speed	Learning to take cues from both the cattle and the rider
		Anticipating the movements of the bovine protagonist
Reining	As for any horse working in isolation	Discrimination of classically conditioned positional cues from rider
Hunting	As with steeple-chasing	Learning to remain under stimulus control, despite socially facilitated cues that can prompt bolting

(Continued)

Table 9.1 (Continued)

Work or sport	Ethological challenges	Learning and cognitive challenges
Driving	Tolerating constant unseen auditory and physical presence to the rear. In teams (multiple configurations), there is a potential for socially facilitated bolting	Habituating to carriage and other pressures on the body while remaining responsive to rein and voice signals. Reliance on rein tension as the chief means of communication by the human. Learning to maintain gait and rhythm without persistent cues
Draughthorses and logging horses	As with driving. Sometimes working alone without presence of conspecifics for several hours per day	As with driving, although voice cues are often the chief means of communication. In this case, horses need to learn the voice cues that may in practice not always be introduced according to the principles of classical conditioning
Breed and hack classes	Remaining calm in company, a challenge exacerbated by hyper-reactivity triggered by conspecific displays and high-energy diets	Responding to cues from riders, some of whom may be unfamiliar (e.g. judges who ride) and trainers in novel contexts
Side-saddle classes	As for all breed and hack classes (see above)	Learning to respond to unilateral leg pressures from rider when sitting to the side and then resuming responses in normal (astride) riding
Rodeo	Repeated counter-predator responses	Learning that the process is finite Unrelenting pressure from belly strap
Police work	Approaching humans who are behaving unpredictably	Sustained habituation to multiple, random cues as found in crowds. Learning to recognise those physical stimuli that come only from the rider
Horses in mining	Barren environment	Learning to respond to auditory cues from the trainer and discriminate them from incidental conversations. The absence of a peripheral view (because of being in a tunnel) and of any depth to visual field (because of being in the dark)
Trail-riding	Sometimes walking in single file in an enforced, rather than natural order	In hired horses that are exposed to many changes of rider, learned responses are likely to be fewer. Navigating novel terrain
Vaulting	Remaining at a calm canter without change in rhythm or pace for an extended period	Habituation to multiple stimuli, including vaulters running towards and around the horse. Learning to ignore pressures from the vaulters while remaining responsive to lunge and voice cues by the trainer as well as cues by the rider during compensation training
Gaited horse classes	Maintaining a certain gait at a speed that normally dictates a transition to a slower or faster gait for energy efficiency	Discriminating between physically similar pressure cues from riders

leads inexorably to all sorts of problems, not least habituation, and the tendency for the horse to begin to travel with its neck too short. At elite levels, the rules of competitive dressage require that riders wear spurs and use a double bridle, even though absolute lightness is valued in principle. These apparent contradictions are explored in Chapter 16, The Future of Equitation Science.

At the outset of training, *show-jumping* relies on the rider being able to make horses jump on cue. After that, most trainers expect

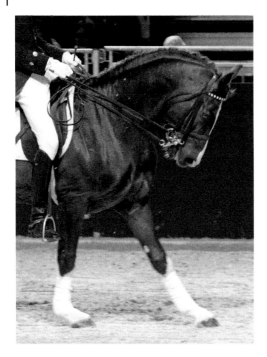

Figure 9.1 A horse being hyperflexed. (Photo courtesy of Julie Taylor/EponaTV.)

a talented horse to use the obstacles themselves to gauge an appropriate take-off point. For responses to be predictable, the horse must be under stimulus control. Of all the critical qualities that must be under the rider's control, we propose that speed and line are paramount in show-jumping. The informed rider takes the opportunity to walk the course and map out the number of strides between obstacles, the take-off and landing spots for each fence and, as necessary, where time can be saved. These judgments contribute to success in show-jumping, in addition to a rider knowing his or her horse's idiosyncrasies (e.g. which jumps they are likely to be unfamiliar with or wary of).

Horses have evolved to save energy (Reilly *et al.*, 2007). Therefore, if given the choice, they generally avoid extra locomotion and instead prefer to return to their social group or housing (Lee *et al.*, 2011; König von Borstel and Keil, 2012). They will take detours around ground-based obstacles (Górecka-Bruzda *et al.*, 2013) and jump only if they have no other option (Figure 9.2). Jumping obstacles for sheer *joie de vivre* has not been

recorded in free-ranging horses. In the domestic context, loose jumping (jumping without a rider) can give the illusion of the horse exercising a choice to jump, but we should never overlook the effects of guiding rails, arena walls, jump-wings and the trainer's whip. That said, we *may* be breeding horses that are less fearful to the extent that some happily jump if there is a jump in front of them. Breed-specific data on this possibility would be extremely valuable.

When training horses over fences, trainers are giving horses opportunities to learn what they are capable of. This involves training them at slower speeds or gaits, such as trot, as well as with variables such as increasing the jump's height and appearance. Applying the principles of shaping, it makes sense to change only one variable at a time when training. While gradual shaping is the goal, over-facing horses by failing to observe a gradual increase and instead presenting them with obstacles that are too high is a real possibility. Horses that run out have sometimes learned to do so because the rider turns the horse away after coming to a halt at a fence. Both the halt and the turn away are reinforcing (Chapter 8, Training). It is highly likely that the horse will repeat this response in future, even if it involves some pain in the mouth and sides as the rider attempts to suppress the response. Loss of line and subsequent steering failures also contribute to these evasions (Chapter 13, Stress and Fear Responses).

A popular way to train show-jumpers is to sensitise them to very light leg pressures and put them in a mildly controlled flight response. Show-jumpers often seem to have habituated to a holding rein and this may be why their riders can be inclined to change bits often or use more severe bits to give them the feeling of more-controlled power. Proponents say they want the horse to 'draw' to the fence, so if they release the reins the horse will go a bit faster, even though this acceleration is minimal. They say that horses jump better this way than when in perfect self-carriage in terms of rhythm and tempo. In the light of this

Figure 9.2 If given the choice between taking a straight way to a food reward with a small (up to 50 cm) obstacle and a detour, most horses will take the detour rather than jump or walk over the obstacle (figure amended and redrawn with permission by Aleksandra Górecka-Bruzda).

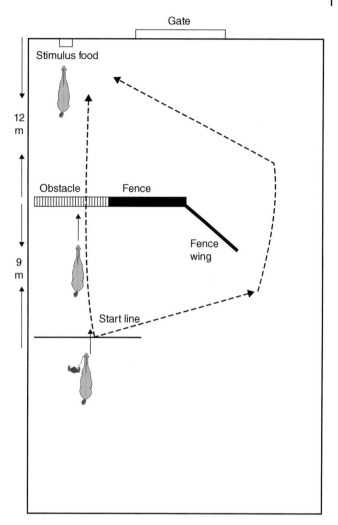

approach and the horse's adoption of a mild flight response, we can see why, during training, show-jumping riders prefer to use a running martingale more so than in other sports, such as dressage. This is because when the horse shows a mild flight response it tends to raise its head and become hollow in the back. In addition, the horse needs to raise its head to obtain stereoscopic vision of the obstacle, an important means of judging spatial relationships. The martingale tends to keep the head lower. One of the drawbacks is that the sensitivity to rein tensions required for slowing and turning can deteriorate if the reins are used for head-carriage but not slowing.

We have to wonder what might be going on with horses described as 'loving their jumping'. These horses do not maintain the rhythm and speed set by the rider's signals. Instead, they are under stimulus control of the fence itself, so they require few leg signals from their riders. By maintaining a tighter grip on the reins, riders usually end up detraining the *stop* response. The horse no longer responds to the more subtle signals of the reins, because it has become habituated to constant tension. Horses may approach fences at increasing speed and give the impression of keenness when, in fact, they are simply rushing. Training horses to be under stimulus control of the rider's rein, leg and seat signals is an important feature of a well-trained jumping horse (McLean, 2005a). It is likely that these horses have experienced some pain from either the rider's hands or from hitting the top rail and then learned to run away. From this, they soon perceive the fence as stimulus for acceleration.

Horse trials or eventing, as it is sometimes known, combines the precision and obedience of dressage with the scope and athleticism of show-jumping and the stamina and so-called boldness of the cross-country phase. This combination emerged from military riding schools as a test of all-round obedience. The level of feeding and fitness required for successful performances in the cross-country phase can lead to horses that are highly reactive. This constitutes a serious challenge in the dressage phase.

Welfare concerns about horses injuring themselves on the solid fences of the cross-country course (Figure 9.3) prompted a modification of fences in Fédération Equestre Internationale (FEI) competition. More technical fences (such as arrowheads and apexes) intended to test accuracy, also served to slow horses down. So, modern courses are characterised by these challenges rather than just big galloping-on fences. Frangible pins have been added so that jumps collapse on substantial vertical impact. All of this has led to a decline, in turn, in the popularity of rangy Thoroughbred types in favour of horses with a higher proportion of Warmblood in their pedigree.

The problem of solid fences is pivotal for the sport, because the rider knows (better than the horse) that the fences are potentially lethal. This means that the rider's confidence and ability to ride according to their own plan rather than the horse's immediate preference is largely what is being tested. Fence design will most likely continue to be moderated until fatalities of both riders and horses cannot be reduced any further without the discipline becoming a form of long-distance show-jumping. It is worth emphasising that despite extensive debate about rider deaths in eventing, the effects of course design and the demands of time limits, insufficient focus has been given to training the horse to maintain its speed and be under stimulus control by the rider. In contrast to horses that are under stimulus control, those that rush at solid fences and take off when at erratic speeds are at risk of flipping over the fences. The recent shifts towards more emphasis on collected movements in dressage tests, as well as the move towards more technical cross-country courses (e.g. inclusion of very narrow obstacles that can be easily avoided by the horse and thus require very precise riding), appear to be steps in the right direction.

However, eventing is one of the equestrian disciplines that is still broadcast fairly frequently on television, and the influence television spectators have on the sport via the economic importance of television should not be overlooked. Event organisers are highly dependent on sponsorship linked to television broadcasts, and the need to fulfil the television audience's desire for exciting competitions to remain attractive to television

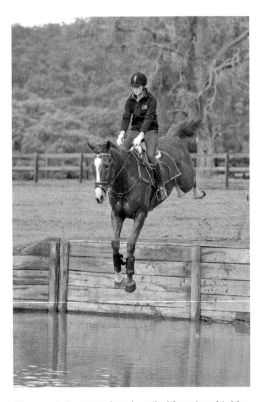

Figure 9.3 Eventers that show 'boldness' are highly prized.

may lead to time allotments and course designs that are suboptimal in terms of horse and rider safety. Some non-horse sports, such as biathlon, have entirely changed their competition format to retain the interest of television audiences (Heinecke, 2014), and similar attempts to remain attractive to television can be expected from the organisers of eventing. Whether these changes are always in the interest of horse and rider welfare remains to be seen.

Racing

At first glance, traditional Thoroughbred racing appears to be all about speed. But, most notably in non-sprint races, checking speed during the race is an integral skill if there is to be some energy left for the finish. Training the racehorse to accelerate at gallop and in the presence of other horses is a critical skill, but it must also be trained to decelerate from light signals in order to manoeuvre during the race. Some horses are said to be field-shy, in that they are disinclined to enter a cluster of galloping horses or sometimes to gallop close to others. So the acceleration and deceleration responses must be trained almost unconditionally to be under the stimulus control of the rider. Similarly, if the horse turns more poorly one way compared with the other (or if it turns poorly both ways), it will tend to drift. Drifting in racing is called lugging and, though very common, it has deleterious effects on speed. The resultant drifting as a result of poor steering tends to increase the distance to be covered, shorten the gallop stride and tire the horse. Lugging creates accusations of interference with other horses. This tendency is likely to be predisposed in horses with an innate motor or sensory bias to the left or the right (McGreevy and Rogers, 2005) and begs further study.

Around turns, racehorses are biomechanically inclined to using their inside lead, for example, using the left lead stride pattern when running counter-clockwise around a track (Adams, 1979). On straight sections of the track, where they can lead with either leg, they show a preference for one stride pattern over the other, unless injured or fatigued. A study of Thoroughbreds, Arabians and Quarterhorses racing in the USA, where horses race around an oval racetrack in a counter-clockwise direction, showed that 90% preferred their right lead stride pattern and 10% preferred the left (Williams and Norris, 2007).

Heterogeneous features in the surfaces used for racing can cause limb injuries (Fredricson *et al.*, 1975). Most horses lead with the right leg when cantering and galloping to the right (i.e. in a clockwise direction) (McGreevy, 1996)), but fatal injuries on US racetracks are more likely to involve the left limb (Peloso *et al.*, 1996). In any epidemiological assessment of this sort, it is critical that the direction in which horses are raced is factored in. Any lateralisation seen may not necessarily be an effect of training to work in one direction, since kinematic differences between the left and right limbs have been reported in 8-month-old Standardbreds that have yet to be trained (Drevemo *et al.*, 1987). Nevertheless, training and racing can influence asymmetries since it has been shown that, when moving around a turn, Thoroughbreds strain the outside forelimb consistently more than the inside forelimb (Davies, 1996). This may reflect the extra abductive and retractive power required of the outside limb in canter and gallop on curved lines.

Most racehorses in training have little opportunity to canter (or gallop) in one direction spontaneously (i.e. without a rider), because they are stabled or kept in training pens that deny them the space to pick up sufficient speed to canter. However, prior to training and whenever they are turned out to pasture, they may demonstrate such a bias. Since the direction of racing for gallopers varies from track to track and state to state in many countries, including the UK, the USA and Australia (e.g. clockwise in New South Wales and counter-clockwise in Victoria), and also vary from country to country (e.g. counter-clockwise in Singapore and clockwise in Hong Kong), the relationship between motor biases and competitive success and wastage through injury may be important. The screening of individual horses for left and right motor bias may allow trainers to select horses more carefully for racing or other work.

Preparing racehorses focuses chiefly on cardiovascular parameters, but physiological conditioning may be of no avail if behavioural conditioning is neglected. It is important to acknowledge that having horses' locomotory responses under clear stimulus control translates into effective acceleration. This demands that all riders must deliver acceleration signals (chiefly those from the legs and whip) effectively. They must continue applying pressure until the correct response emerges, and stop when it does. Teaching personnel about learning theory would enhance racing success. While leaving the starting gates at speed is an important feature of a successful racehorse, simply increasing arousal in anticipation of the start is counter-productive. There is compelling evidence that horses that *lose* races tend to be more aroused and require greater control in the parade ring/mounting yard than winners (Hutson, 2002). Conversely, the calmer a horse is before the race, the more it will perform to its potential. For example, horses that are difficult to load into starting stalls are likely to perform far more poorly than their cardiovascular indicators at home have suggested (Figure 9.4). It is recognised that nervousness in the parade ring may be a consequence of poor leading responses (McLean, 2003), so training to walk in-hand can have a significant impact on performance. Some of the more important dependent variables are summarised in Table 9.2.

The social dynamics within a group of racing horses have yet to be explored. Do they jostle for the lead? Or do they jostle for safety? It is unlikely that horses have evolved to want to lead the herd, given that this is a vulnerable position that exposes them to potential threats. Understanding the cognitive aspects of horses during racing informs us about what is meant by the 'will to win' (Figure 9.5). Perhaps a Thoroughbred has been

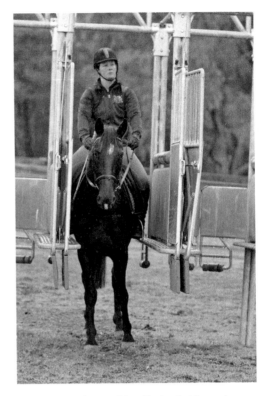

Figure 9.4 A Thoroughbred being habituated to starting stalls.

selected to be reinforced for running for its own proximate benefits over and above leading. Or perhaps it is a characteristic of horses in general to find running reinforcing. What does the finishing line represent to them? It is likely that with repetitions, horses learn to 'know' something about the finishing line, given that the rider changes his or her behaviour immediately after crossing it. That said, it seems unlikely that horses have evolved to have a concept of such a goal, but how does this align with the evolutionary advantage of outrunning a predator or a conspecific (during play)?

It is important to recognise that current selection pressures in breeding only partially reflect those that created the original breeds. The modern show-ring is the only environment in which conformation prevails in importance. Historically, breeding for different types of work would have placed more emphasis on behavioural tendencies than on conformation. There is some evidence of

Table 9.2 Some of the features of a racehorse's behaviour and presentation that can be used to predict poor performance (i.e. not winning).

Location	Variable	Extent to which this variable predicts poor performance
Stalls	Weaving and repetitive head movements	********
	Kicking	*****
	Pawing	**
Saddling enclosure/ parade ring	Crossover (figure-of-eight or grackle) noseband	********
	Gaping mouth	****
	Twisting neck	***
	Nose roll (sheepskin noseband)	***
	Third metacarpal bandages	***
	Other bandages	**************
	Pacifiers (meshed eye protection)	**
Mounting yard	Slow gait	********
	Fast gait or circling	*****
	Bucking	*****
	Balking	****
	Courtship behaviours	***
	Ears pointing laterally or backwards	**
	Defecating	**
	Flicking ears	*
Track	Late	********
	Conflict behaviours	****

Source: Adapted from *Watching Racehorses*, with kind permission of Geoffrey Hutson.
Asterisks are used to depict the extent to which each variable predicts poor performance.

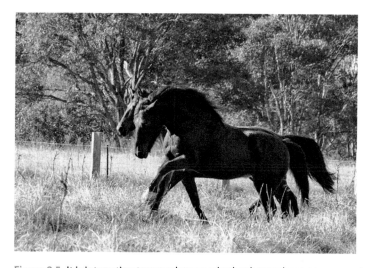

Figure 9.5 It is interesting to speculate on whether horses have any concept of racing.

links between morphology and neural tissue (Evans and McGreevy, 2006), a finding that may predict behavioural tendencies. Selection for work shaped the horses considered typical of many breeds. We propose that, generally speaking, equine trainability and ease-of-habituation are characteristics that negatively correlate with each other. The horse that habituates rapidly becomes insensitive to pressure signals and therefore fails to discriminate between cues that differ only slightly in their location or intensity. These horses are not likely to excel in dressage or indeed most performance sports, but may have a place as mounts for novices, assuming that they do not habituate to bit pressure and become unstoppable.

The hyper-reactivity of Thoroughbreds is beyond dispute. They have been selected almost entirely for speed and the tendency to respond to the opening of the starting stalls and stimuli (hands, heels and whip) from the jockey, which is why Thoroughbreds, in general, are not considered safe carriage horses. Imagine the weekly human death toll that would have been associated with using such a reactive breed in the shafts of horse-drawn vehicles.

While some breeds are more reactive than others (e.g. Graf *et al.*, 2014), some diets further increase reactivity (most notably in foals) (Nicol *et al.*, 2005). These are the diets most often fed to the most reactive breed of horse, the Thoroughbred. The mixture of breeding and feeding contributes to most of the dangers associated with racehorses. The other factor is social facilitation. One horse's flight response can trigger a flight response in conspecifics. From the authors' long-term experience in legal cases, the Thoroughbred seems to have aggregated a larger human toll than any other breed.

Steeple-Chasing and Hurdling

When raced over fences, Thoroughbreds are favoured for 'boldness' or 'bravery'. Outstanding steeple-chasers or hurdlers could alternatively be labelled 'oblivious to danger' or 'having a poor sense of self-preservation'. Perhaps this reflects habituation or the horse learning that the threshold of aversiveness for environment is lower than the signals from their backs – so they go where they are pointed. As if jumping fences at speed is not dangerous enough, there is the additional challenge of jumping among a large gathering of other horses. This creates a further hazard: social facilitation on approach to a fence can trigger a premature leap, with horses landing on top of a fallen or falling horse or rider. In Australia, this dangerous tendency is called 'half-lengthing'.

Harness Racing (Pacing and Trotting)

The relative calmness of Standardbreds reflects selection not only for different gaits (trotting and pacing) but also for steadiness in a horse that is to be worked in *harness*, an aversive set of stimuli that may equate to being chased from behind. The calmness of Standardbreds reflects the selection of horses that are sensitive enough to accelerate easily but do not run readily when being chased. This lowered flight response makes Standardbreds great trail horses, especially suitable as beginner mounts. The pace is innate for some horses (e.g. a large proportion of Icelandic horses), but can be acquired by others. The progeny of pacers almost always pace, whereas only some 20% of the offspring of trotters are innate pacers (Cothran *et al.*, 1987). These findings correspond to the recent findings on the genetic background of gaitedness in horses (Andersson *et al.*, 2012). While the genetic predisposition to gaitedness is mandatory for a horse to show gaits other than walk, trot and canter/gallop, not all horses with a genetic predisposition to gaitedness show these gaits, or show them in a uniform rhythm (e.g. two-beat rhythm for pace). Instead, horses may show variations with shifts in rhythm towards one or the other gait, and they may be able to alter rhythm flexibly. Besides the need to prevent horses from falling into a distinct gallop (which leads to elimination from a harness race), it is, in part, due to this ability to alter rhythm on a virtually continuous scale that such a large amount of equipment is permitted and used in harness racing to keep horses within the desired two-beat rhythm of either pace or trot (Figure 9.6).

The use of blinkers (Figure 9.7) and sheepskin nosebands in racing and harness racing is interesting from a technical perspective, since the wearer may be less distracted by

(a)

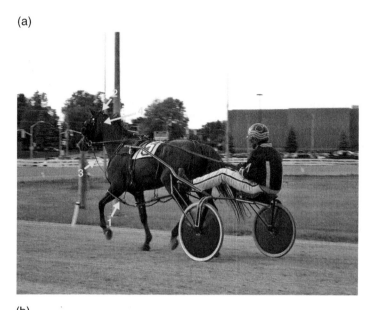

(b)

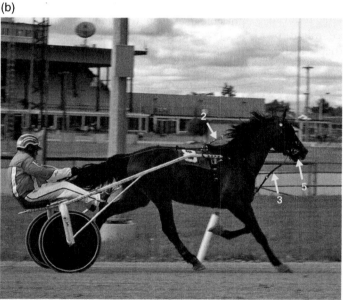

Figure 9.6 Harness-racing horses wearing hobbles to prevent changes in rhythm away from a pace (1 a), an over-check (2 a and b) enforcing a high head position that makes it difficult for a horse to fall into a gallop, a tie-down (3 a and b) to stop the horse from a too-high head carriage, ear plugs connected with a cord to the driver (4 a) that are used as an 'acoustic whip' by being pulled when approaching the finish line, and a tongue tie (5 b), ostensibly to prevent dorsal displacement of the soft palate.

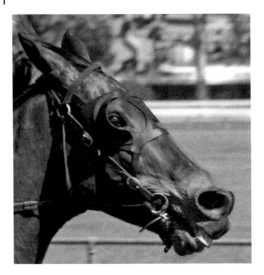

Figure 9.7 A racehorse wearing blinkers to modify its flight response and reduce distraction by other horses. (Photo courtesy of Sandra Jorgensen.)

lateral and ventral stimuli and the ground, and perhaps even its own forelegs. Reduced distractibility, at least in the first few outings, may not always equate with calmness, and it remains to be seen whether these devices are always calming. Given the high incidence of claustrophobia among horses, the reduced ability to maintain surveillance might be potentially threatening. Or perhaps, in this case, 'out of sight' *is* 'out of mind'.

Other Forms of Racing

Racing in other breeds, such as Arabians and Quarterhorses (originally developed for stock work and now represented in both reactive racing and unflappable pastoral lines), follows the same training strategies to achieve swift acceleration and straightness in response to pressure cues and shares a focus on producing young sprinters. This provides a platform for an interesting ethical discussion. The emphasis on youthful performers is fuelled chiefly by the industries that seek to encourage breeding by valuing the next great star, rather than longevity in individual horses. A high turnover of racing horses is in the interests of the breeding industry. However, if veteran races attracted significant prize money, there would be greater incentives to keep horses sound for longer, resulting in enhanced welfare for the racing population. Horses would not be rushed into racing as early as possible, which would allow more time to be spent in foundation training (breaking-in) of young stock, an outcome that would probably make retired racehorses more useful and valued as riding horses. Indeed, with Icelandic pace-racing horses, which are generally started under-saddle at the comparably old age of around 4 years, and which are generally trained not exclusively for racing, but also for riding and showing in other gaits, there seem to be few problems in finding another occupation for the horses after their racing careers.

In the case of **endurance racing**, the need for stringent welfare controls was accepted almost from the outset. Riding horses to exhaustion would never have been considered a sport otherwise, so veterinary checks (gates) are a fundamental element of the sport. Successful competitors select and produce horses that recover quickly from the physiological load that long-distance work creates. Enforcement of the rules governing the sport does a great deal to prevent unsuitable and poorly prepared horses being entered for competition, but even at the highest level, horses can succumb to exhaustion (EFA, 2003). And although riders in other equestrian sports may say that the gaits of the endurance horse are not ideal (a big trot is preferable to a slow canter for endurance horses) (Figure 9.8), the horses engaged in endurance riding seem to have a long working life.

Has this left us with ethical double standards when we compare traditional racing with endurance racing? If racing codes were emerging for the first time in the present day, what steps would be taken to ensure horse welfare? Would riders be allowed to whip horses that simply *could not* respond because of fatigue? These questions are explored further in Chapter 14, Ethical Equitation.

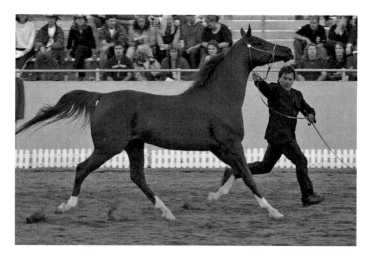

Figure 9.8 Arabian horse showing a big trot that is a characteristic of an endurance horse. (Photo courtesy of Julie Wilson.)

Mounted Games

Polo and **polocrosse** have emerged from the ancient traditions of Chinese, Persian and Japanese mounted ball sports and the equally ancient pursuits of '*buskashi*', involving the mounted dispute over decapitated goat carcasses (by Pashtuns) or the Tibetan tradition of hitting a recently bludgeoned muskrat. They rely on considerable horsemanship and balance, because the rider must be able to lean out of the saddle, wrestle other riders and execute hairpin turns at great speed all the while aiming to obtain or retain the team's possession of the 'ball'. From the horse's perspective, the challenges in this sport are considerable. Strong signals from the rider, and severe bits and bridles are commonplace. In addition, neck reining can lend itself to potential confusion (Figure 9.9) for the horse if the two rein signals (contralateral neck pressure and ipsilateral rein tension) are applied concurrently. The challenge for the discerning rider is to ensure that only one rein signal is given for the turn response. A single rein signal can be delivered with far greater clarity. Through a process of habituation, this means that signals tend to get stronger. Against this backdrop, many polo stables exercise horses (as many as four per mounted rider) in-hand

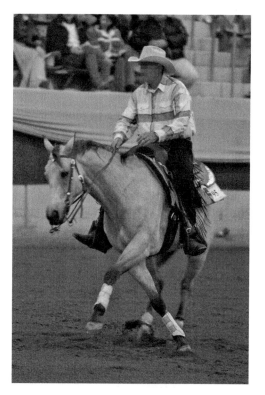

Figure 9.9 Neck-reining turn. (Photo courtesy of Julie Wilson.)

simultaneously. This may maintain cardiovascular fitness and may even have reinforcing properties for the horses if they are a stable social group, but does little to maintain shaped responses. The wastage in polo and, to a lesser extent, polocrosse is significant, but it is more likely a product of trauma than behavioural issues.

Games such as ***gymkhanas*** and ***mounted games*** organised by pony clubs are designed to foster horsemanship and develop riding skills with far lower potential for confusion, habituation and trauma than the adult versions of mounted games, polo and polocrosse. Sometimes the ability to deliver signals with clarity is thwarted by the specific challenge of the activity but, as with the military and mounted police tradition of tent-pegging, the ability to maintain control of the horse while riding with one's centre of gravity to one side is highly valued.

Stock Sports

The uniquely Australian sport of ***camp-drafting*** (Figure 9.10a) similarly has a history based on utility in cattle farming. Camp-drafting involves separating (cutting out) a calf from a group and moving it into a small yard, called a *camp*, herding it through gates and around pegs in clockwise and counter-clockwise directions. The turns are facilitated by neck-reining but there is an added complication from other animals – the targeted calf and its herd-mates. The genetic trait of some horses to show 'cow-sense' (target, chase and show agonistic behaviour towards an errant bovid) is a fascinating phenomenon (Figure 9.10b), although possibilities to alter it via selective breeding appear to be limited due to low heritability of this trait (Kieffer, 1968, cited in Hintz, 1980). In Africa, however, it is not uncommon to see equids, such as zebras, chasing wildebeest, so this predisposition may possibly exist in the genome of the horse. It would be interesting to see what other behavioural traits are linked to this tendency and whether they can be harnessed for more traditional activities (Figure 9.11). Could cow-sense, for instance, be associated with boldness in jumping or even in work as a police horse?

Reining competitions are now recognised by the FEI and can be seen as the Western (American) version of dressage. With its voltes and sorties (evolved from bull-fighting), reining is said to reflect the status of dressage at the end of the Middle Ages, the period in which Spanish conquistadors took equitation to the Americas. There is arguably more self-carriage in Western riding than in modern dressage, since the rein contacts are lighter. It carries with it the same theoretical requirements for training reliable responses to subtle signals in self-carriage. As the sport matures, it will be interesting to see how equitation science develops technologies that assist in the refinement of training and improvement of welfare.

(a)

(b)

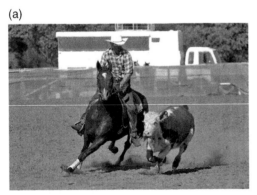
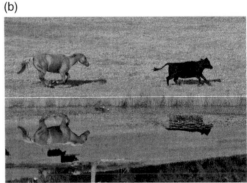

Figure 9.10 (a) Camp-drafting. (b) Cow sense is an innate trait found in some stock breeds, such as the Quarterhorse. (Photos courtesy of (a) Julie Wilson and (b) Nic Ward.)

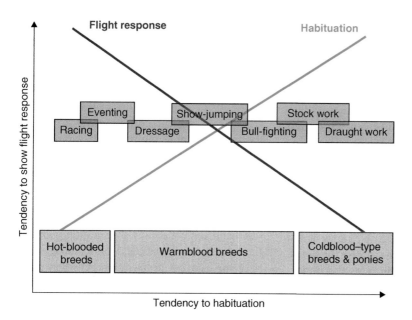

Figure 9.11 Horses typically used for different tasks and of different breed types seem to have different tendencies to show flight responses and to show habituation when faced with a potential threat.

Gaited Horse Classes

Several horse breeds possess the ability to perform, in addition to the walk, trot and gallop (and possibly pace in the case of Icelandics), an additional 4-beat gait. These breeds include, for example, the Icelandic horse, Rocky Mountain horse, Tennessee Walking Horse, Missouri Foxtrotter, Peruvian Paso and Paso Fino, and the additional gait is known by breed-specific names such as tölt, rack, running walk, foxtrot or paso (fino/corto/largo). Depending on the breed and sometimes also the speed of travelling, the rhythm can be either regular (e.g. an ideal tölt in the Icelandic horse) or irregular (e.g. a foxtrot in the Missouri Foxtrotter) 4-beat rhythm, but in all cases, there is at any time at least one hoof on the ground, so there is no suspension phase. For this reason, these gaits give the rider a very comfortable feeling, compared to riding at a similar speed at trot.

There are breed-specific classes, namely for Icelandic horses, in which exhibits are judged on either speed and/or quality of the gait. Besides the desired rhythm, valued attributes often include the range of limb motion, posture and/or the ability to alternate speed without loss of rhythm. Therefore, these horses need to be under good stimulus control for the *stop* and *go* response. However, these horses are generally capable of performing the rack or its equivalents only with a fairly high head posture, so there is considerable temptation for riders to attempt modifying head posture by rein tension, (i.e. to guide the horse into a rack rather than a trot), resulting in conflicting signals for the *stop* and 'head high' response.

Selective breeding has produced horses with a remarkable range of limb motion in several of the gaited breeds. Given that gaited horses are often small breeds, commonly ridden by adults, and are regularly exhibited on hard surfaces to better showcase their gaits, it is perhaps unsurprising that, despite their sturdiness, approximately half of these horses end their riding career because of musculoskeletal disease (Björnsdottir *et al.*, 2003), a proportion that is comparable to rates observed in many Warmblood or Thoroughbred populations.

Hunting

The use of horses in hunting has undergone some fundamental changes over the years, because of the introduction of barbed-wire stock fences and the development of drag hunts (in which the hounds follow a prepared trail). The ability to keep horses under stimulus control is tested in this context, because travelling at speed in the company of conspecifics is extremely arousing for horses. Maintaining speed is important, but occasionally a rider makes the frowned-upon misdemeanor of overtaking the master (a sure sign of being out of control), because their horse will not slow easily. This emphasises the importance of a reliable slow response. Working against this for many years was the traditional hunting seat, which saw riders leaning back in the saddle as they jumped, a technique that was thought to spare the horse's legs from injury. However, it also reliably increases the chances of jabbing the horse in the mouth, which can habituate it to bit pressure.

Driving

When horses pull any item (a plough, cart or carriage), low reactivity may be highly desirable from a safety perspective. It is clearly preferable to select and recruit horses that do not bolt in response to these challenges, but are sufficiently sensitive to signals and keep going.

An analysis of the cues given to driven horses provides some fascinating insights for equitation scientists. In driving, it is possible that some habituation to rein tension arises because of the driver's distance from the horse's mouth and so the sensitivity of the training is easily compromised. The signal to *go forward* comes from either the whip, the voice (by classical conditioning) or from the reins (slapping the rump). In contrast to the ridden horse, which receives cues from the rider's and legs, there are no ongoing signals for driven horses to maintain speed and rhythm. This is critical because the absence of 'keep going' cues from the seat increases the need for consistent acceleration signals. Inconsistency in these cues would increase the need for frequent deceleration cues that ultimately would increase the likelihood of habituation to oral pressures. These problems may be offset by it being far easier, in the driven-horse context, to control speed and line without interference, as the carriage is stable while the rider on a horse's back moves a lot and thus may produce redundant cues (Figure 9.11).

Horses being driven as singles, in tandem, or in unicorn formation, may receive signals from either side equally. In contrast, asymmetry is of particular significance when horses are driven alongside one another. Asymmetry in horse use reflects the tendency for one horse (the most responsive) to be the lead horse and to be placed on one side of the team rather than the other. This means that the work required of the horse and the direction with which it may pull laterally against the other horses in its team is unbalanced.

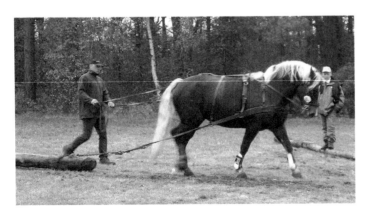

Figure 9.12 In draught work, horses must persist in a given gait in the absence of 'keep going' pressure signals.

While carriage driving can be broadly divided into dressage and cross-country courses that value accuracy and stamina, the larger driving shows have other classes that focus on different aspects of training. For example, reinsmanship classes are primarily judged on the work of the driver or whip. Here, the driver must work the horse at a walk, slow trot, working trot and strong trot and may be requested to back his or her horses and vehicles or execute a figure of eight. This class is judged 75% on the driver's posture, overall appearance, rein- and whip-handling, and horse control; 25% of the score is awarded for the condition and fit of the harness and vehicle and neatness of attire.

Meanwhile, in drive-and-ride classes, a single horse or pony is driven first and then worked under-saddle at a walk, trot and canter. They are judged 50% on 'performance, manners and way of going under-saddle'. The same person need not show the horse/pony in both sections of the competition. Similarly, in combination hunter classes, a single horse is shown under harness, then ridden over a hunter course of at least four fences. These classes are judged 40% on 'performance, manners, way of going and suitability' in harness, 30% on these qualities under-saddle, and 30% on performance over fences.

Showing: Breed and Hack Classes

Also known as **hacking**, showing classes are designed to showcase the horse's various aesthetic qualities. Classes include riding codes, best-dressed, best rider, hack classes, side-saddle classes, hunter classes, equitation classes, exhibition, breed classes, type classes and colour classes. As can be seen from Table 9.1, the ethological, cognitive and learning challenges in the show-ring are similar for those for other codes that focus on gaits and executing set displays (e.g. dressage).

The morphology and gait of the horse may take priority over its compliance and athleticism. This potentially sends the fate of pure-bred horses in the same direction as that of pure-bred dogs, since it places selection pressure on qualities that may not align directly with health and welfare and thus can precipitate the emergence of inherited disorders (McGreevy and Nicholas, 1999). Classes that value the horse's compliance when ridden by unfamiliar judges are extremely important for maintaining useful breeding lines. Conversely, the introduction of (in-hand) classes in which horses are not required to canter (e.g. for Arabians) has reduced the selection pressure on quality at all gaits and, thus, may permit the inheritance of a poor canter (Figure 9.13). The use of

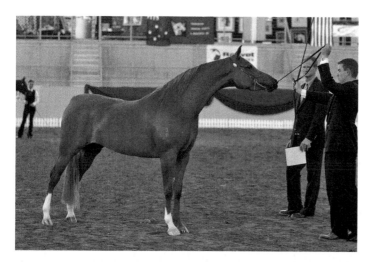

Figure 9.13 An Arabian being shown in-hand. Too much emphasis on in-hand appearance in the show ring may signal a departure from selection for an optimal riding horse. (Photo courtesy of Julie Wilson.)

psycho-pharmaceuticals to moderate the behaviour of horses fed high-energy diets merits scrutiny by governing bodies, as do any interventions that alter the arousal or tail carriage of horses in show contexts (Chapter 14, Ethical Equitation).

Rodeo

Spurs and cinches/bucking straps in rodeo are irritants that evoke flight responses in the same way that whips make horses run faster on the racecourse and whips/spurs make horses jump fences in show-jumping. However, just because all these forms of horse-use rely on negative reinforcement does not make them all as acceptable as one another. The emphasis in any negative reinforcement paradigm should involve the use of minimal pressure. Ethical equitation requires subtle cues that are released as soon as the desired response is offered, but it is difficult to see this maxim being adhered to in rodeo practices. The demand in rodeo for a sustained flight response of at least 8 seconds violates this requirement. The animal is stimulated to perform counter-predator responses until the strap is loosened. Its counter-predator responses may be helpful in removing the rider, which brings at least some reinforcement.

Animals that can do nothing to improve their welfare are said to be susceptible to learned helplessness. If choke chains on dogs always strangled for at least 8 seconds, even though the dogs had immediately stopped pulling on the lead, would we find them acceptable? This raises a very interesting ethical question about duration versus intensity. Is a dressage horse held with tight mouth pressure daily for an hour really any better off than a rodeo horse required to undergo sustained pressure around its abdomen for a matter of seconds once a week or fortnight?

Ethological and veterinary opinions have led to some countries banning the use of the flank strap, the spurs in bronco riding (bareback and saddle bronco riding) and the

so-called wild horse racing (in which unbroken horses are roped, brought to the ground, mounted and then sent forward over a set distance).

In rodeos, horses may be housed in groups, an approach founded in convenience but with the potential to enhance welfare when contrasted with the isolation housing systems traditionally used for most performance horses. Rodeo horses are required, as part of their work, to produce exaggerated counter-predator responses. Indeed, Schonholtz (2000) points out that some horses are purpose-bred for a heightened counter-predator response (e.g. one line of buckers accounted for 30 horses used at the US National Rodeo Finals in 1996). While this is claimed by some to be evidence for the increasingly humane treatment of rodeo animals, it may simply indicate that hypersensitive horses can be bred. This means that selected animals are simply less likely to habituate to being ridden and they continue to find the procedure aversive. So, purpose-breeding seems an unconvincing justification for the use of selected rodeo animals on welfare grounds.

Work

Mounted police perform a wide variety of duties, ranging from park and street patrols to parades, escorts, training demonstrations and crowd control at special events (Figure 9.14). In all these contexts, horses work in pairs and are required to remain calm and have their locomotory responses under stimulus control, regardless of extraneous stimuli (the critical characteristics of aversive stimuli are discussed in detail in Chapter 6, Associative Learning (Aversive stimuli)). The pairs in which they work usually comprise experienced, comprehensively habituated horses and less-experienced conspecifics. The role of police in crowd management involves controlling the movement of pedestrians, dispersing riots or conducting arrests so, at all times the horses must be under the rider's control and not

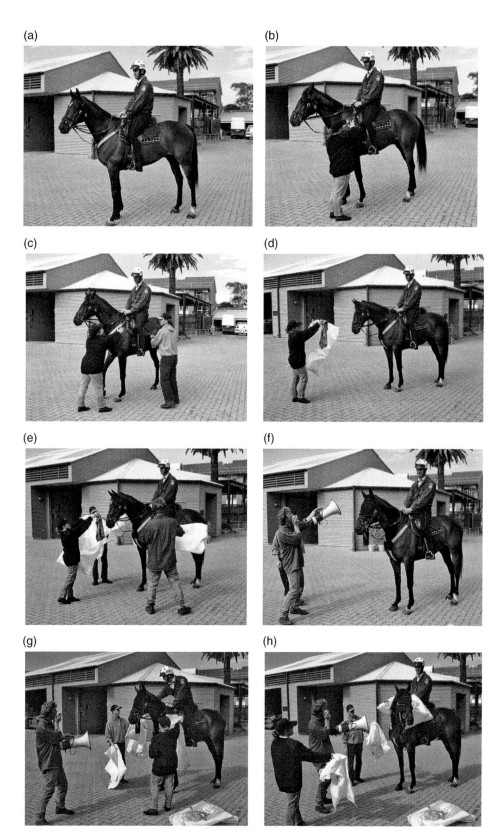

Figure 9.14 A police horse being habituated to crowds.

react to stimuli from the environment. The horse must learn to be as relaxed as possible and remain under stimulus control in the face of physical pressure from a noisy, pushy crowd, and to push pedestrians when directed to do so by the rider. Police horses are particularly well-trained in sideways responses, since this moves them laterally as if they were a mobile, equine barrier.

Crowd-control training begins with step-by-step habituation. Each new factor, such as a banner or a loud noise, is introduced to the horse either when it is stationary, or by over-shadowing. Only once the horse appears to have become accustomed to the changed conditions, is it prompted to respond to simple, established signals (e.g. *walk* and *halt*) under novel circumstances that are fabricated. The horse thus becomes habituated to responding despite the new stimuli. Further potential distracters are introduced in the same manner, until the horse can work in a wide range of situations.

The use of horses in **tourism** includes trail-riding and carriage-driving in urban contexts. With **harness** horses, long working hours have a critical effect on the availability of water and food during these periods. As with all horses working in urban contexts, those that have been hand-fed by passers-by are at risk of learning to nuzzle hands and pockets for food and, if not muzzled, may eventually become so-called muggers or even biters. Hard surfaces underfoot also predispose horses to concussive musculoskeletal disease such as ring-bone (Higgins and Wright, 1995). Providing shelter from sun and precipitation is important for horse welfare, but overwork and the prevalence of poorly fitting harness are perhaps paramount.

Ponies used underground in **mining** activities were said to take some time to adjust to the light and to moving stimuli when brought back above ground. Blinkered, and often stabled underground for months on end, they were not used to seeing much other than miners, ponies and the inevitable rat. Nowadays, at least in the Western world, few, if any mining ponies are still put to work, but reliable data from developing countries are scarce, and so, worldwide there may still be a considerable number of ponies working underground.

The exposure of trail-riding horses to incompetent riders is a concern for both welfare and behavioural reasons. Typically, their *go*, *stop* and *turn* responses are poor but they tend to have deeply ingrained following responses based on an ethological tendency to remain in the social group. Poor timing and failure to provide relief from pressure are likely to lead to habituation and the emergence of conflict behaviours. Clearly, hired horses are high risk for trialling undesirable responses and developing behaviour problems. The extent to which they can be remediated and indeed spared abusive handling depends largely on the frequency and quality of any supervision by the hirers and their staff. Operators who allow horses to be ridden without supervision place their horses at risk of inappropriate training that can amount to abuse.

Vaulting

The sport of vaulting differs from other equestrian sports in that one, two or a team of eight athletes closely interact with the horse, while the horse must pay attention to cues from only the trainer, who guides the horse via lunge, voice and whip signals. Throughout the performance, which takes approximately 15 minutes for a team performance, the horse is required to canter on a circle on the left rein, while the vaulters jump on and off the horse to perform acrobatic figures and manoeuvres with up to three vaulters on the horse simultaneously (Figure 9.15). Ridden compensation training is important for vaulting horses, due to the strong focus of working on just the left hand.

The vaulting horse is equipped with side-reins to restrict head movement, which is important because vaulters often base their manoeuvres on the horse's neck. That said,

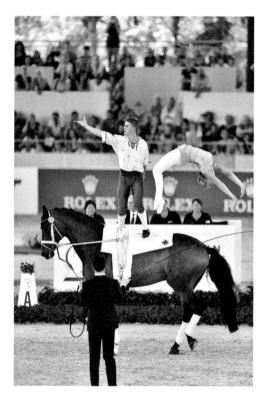

Figure 9.15 Vaulting horses need to learn to distinguish between pressures exerted by vaulters, to which they need to habituate, and pressures used as cues by the trainer or a rider during ridden work. (Photo by im|press|ions, www.kaiser-impressions.de).

vaulters may sometimes touch the side-reins inadvertently or purposefully rely on them for support. Vaulting horses must habituate to these pressures while remaining responsive to the lunge and a rider's rein cues during compensation training.

Conclusion

The breadth of equestrian sporting activities and ways in which horses have been made to work for us serve to emphasise the species' tremendous behavioural flexibility. The qualities of breeds that specialise in various domains include their ability to meet the particular ethological, cognitive and learning challenges that these activities present.

Take-Home Messages

- Negative reinforcement is used in all examples of the horse at work and in sport.
- Despite the enormous variety in horse sports and equine work, four basic responses are required in almost all of them: *stop, go, turn the forequarters* and *turn the hindquarters*.
- Foundation training these basic responses allows horses to be trained with a customised plan that is specific to the discipline they are intended for, but also means that they can be re-trained for secondary work when their first career is over.
- Behavioural conditioning (improving the responsiveness) of racehorses is often overlooked in pursuit of cardiovascular fitness.

Ethical Considerations

- Welfare is often a reflection of horses' usefulness to humans, so should sport-horse organisations place more emphasis on ensuring that sport-horses remain useful throughout their careers, not least by remaining under stimulus control (rather than succumbing to undesirable habituation)?
- Should sentient beings be exposed to complete novices who are not simply learning to ride but are also learning to balance?
- Can competitions that use horses (and therefore aversive stimuli under a negative reinforcement framework) ever reward welfare above all else?

Areas for Further Research

- Evidence of communication among horses competing as a group has yet to be explored.
- Will an on-board device that measures fatigue and exhaustion ever be developed for riders to use and competition judges to check?

10

Apparatus

Introduction

The horse is as behaviourally flexible as any of the domestic species. This means that it tolerates suboptimal conditions and so makes itself vulnerable to welfare insults. For an animal that has evolved to spend up to 16 hours a day grazing in the open and to expend considerable effort to avoid becoming trapped, the consequences of confinement and restraint for our convenience can be profound. The observation that horses do not vocalise when in pain further contributes to welfare insults, as humans may simply overlook that a device is causing discomfort or pain.

This chapter examines the various techniques and devices we use to contain and restrain horses. It asks how equitation science can be used to explain the effects of these traditions and innovations. It explains how equitation science can question items used solely because of tradition, and highlights potential problems in training that emerge from the use of force rather than behavioural conditioning.

Stabling and Feeding

We stable horses for our own convenience: it makes them easy to catch and to keep warm and clean, but stabling obliges us to hand-feed. Dried foods are favoured because they are easy to store and transport, and concentrated cereals deliver nutrients in a form that more than meets the working horse's needs. Most horses bloom in coat and condition when fed at above their maintenance requirements and, for some breeds, show judges are quick to reward owners who present animals with unhealthy amounts of subcutaneous fat (Figure 10.1). Unfortunately, many young horses are routinely overproduced to give the impression that they are well-grown for their age. In contrast, for other breeds, such as those commonly used as sports horses, the other extreme may be favoured. Judges may reward lean, muscular horses, while pasture-reared horses that typically present with a larger abdomen due to adaptation to digest larger volumes of feed, may be penalised for their appearance. Thus, by their preferences for horses that better match their notional ideal, judges may encourage housing and management practices that can be unhealthy for horses. The emergence of young horse championships in many disciplines also encourages levels of growth and training that may be too advanced and rushed.

Unfortunately, high-energy feeding can also trigger oral stereotypies, gastric ulceration and hyper-reactivity and, if feed is not reduced in anticipation of a smaller workload, some horses may be predisposed to develop exertional rhabdomyolysis (Valentine *et al.*, 1998). Explosive energy under-saddle often aligns poorly with training goals, because calmness underpins clarity during response

Equitation Science, Second Edition. Paul McGreevy, Janne Winther Christensen,
Uta König von Borstel and Andrew McLean.
© 2018 John Wiley & Sons Ltd. Published 2018 by John Wiley & Sons Ltd.
Companion website: www.wiley.com/go/mcgreevy/equitation

acquisition. Confinement in a stable is far removed from the horse's natural environment of cursory grazing. Stabled horses can become so excitable when they emerge from

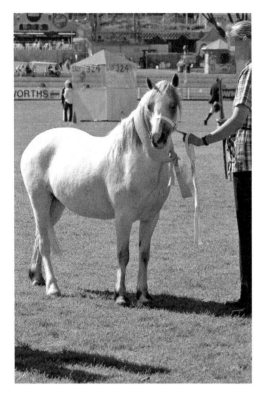

Figure 10.1 Animals of certain breeds are often clinically obese yet, in the show-ring, their owners are frequently rewarded for creating this condition. (Photo courtesy of Sandy Hannan.)

confinement that they are prone to injure themselves in a frenzy of activity known as the post-inhibitory rebound (Figure 10.2). Indeed, horses that receive shorter amounts and irregular turnout are more prone to health problems of the locomotory system compared to horses that receive longer and/or more regular turnout (König von Borstel *et al.*, 2016a). Although we struggle to measure it, many horses seem to find pleasure in free exercise (Kiley-Worthington, 1987) and can find physically restricting environments stressful. That said, research to date has failed to find evidence that horses enjoy exercise in typical training environments, as preference tests have revealed that most horses avoid jumping (Gorecka-Bruzda *et al.*, 2012) or riding altogether, if given the choice (König von Borstel and Keil, 2012). However, it is also important to note that there are clear individual differences in the preferences for amount and type of exercise. For example, in a study by Gorecka-Bruzda *et al.* (2012), trained sporthorses were more willing to jump over an obstacle than leisure horses were.

When mares confined for urine collection were released after six months in standing stalls, they showed a post-inhibitory rebound in locomotion (Houpt *et al.*, 2001), indicating that they were compensating for exercise deprivation in the same way that crib-biters show more of the behaviour after a period of

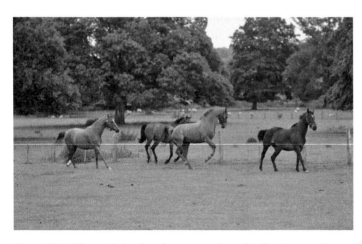

Figure 10.2 After periods of confinement and overfeeding, horses show a post-inhibitory rebound of locomotory responses.

deprivation (McGreevy and Nicol, 1998). So the heightened motivation for movement and indeed general activity (Mal *et al.*, 1991) can translate to unusually athletic manoeuvres and some injuries when confined horses are turned out. In addition, the bones of confined youngsters are less dense than those of mature horses, and this may predispose them to fractures and other harmful effects on the musculoskeletal system, which is generally compromised by confinement (Bell *et al.*, 2001; Hiney *et al.*, 2004).

Confinement reduces spontaneous exercise, normal sensory stimulation and access to preferred conspecifics. It also imposes relative darkness. Horses in a dark stabled environment have demonstrated a preference for a lighted environment by learning to turn on lights by means of an operant device (trial-and-error learning; Houpt and Houpt, 1988). Being at pasture may be sufficiently enriching to account for data showing that training takes less time in pastured horses than in stabled horses (Rivera *et al.*, 2002). We know that horses make good associations with stables, because that is where they are fed and usually where they find conspecifics. Their inability to assess the long-term consequences of confinement is revealed by their willingness to enter stables for short-term gains. The same might be said of entering a float (trailer) that brings with it the added aversiveness of being on a moving platform and in a confined space. Indeed, anecdotal evidence suggests that even after they have endured traffic accidents in floats that have overturned, some horses still enter a new float seemingly willingly.

Apparatus used to Distribute and Apply Pressure to Horses

A range of saddlery items (tack) are discussed in this chapter, but this does not imply that the authors necessarily approve of their use or suggest that they are humane. Some might just as well appear in Chapter 12, Unorthodox Techniques. Our approach to the following discussion of equipment in horse-training assumes that the reader is conversant with learning theory as described in Chapters 4 to 7.

Welfare is compromised by excessive pressure from apparatus. Pressure is a measure of the force exerted over a surface area and is usually expressed in Pascals (Pa) or pounds per square inch/grams per square centimetre. For example, the pressure of rider and saddle is the combined weight divided by the area of the horse's back with which they are in contact. Therefore, with any piece of tack, the broader the area that touches the horse, the less discomfort it causes and the less rewarding is its removal. Essentially, all training places the horse in a discriminatory dilemma – it must respond to some pressures while habituating to others. When the stimuli to which it must habituate are too challenging, the horse may be at risk of learned helplessness. In addition, physical damage due to repeated, overt pressure can include skin lesions or muscle atrophy. Specific attributes of the interface between the human and the horse that can also compromise welfare include bits made of twisted or longitudinally ribbed (so-called bladed) metal or chain.

Saddles, Treeless Saddles, Saddle Pads, Girths, Cinches and Surcingles

The premise of a saddle is twofold: to support the rider's position and to distribute the rider's weight across the musculature on either side of the horse's thoracic midline. The tree (rigid or semi-rigid framework) within a traditional saddle prevents the rider's weight from pinching the horse's back or, particularly, its vertebral column.

The still-evolving design of saddles remains purpose-driven. The traditional *'selle à piquer'* held the rider firmly and deeply in one place, with his or her legs descending ventrally directly as they do in a modern dressage saddle. Earlier saddles from various equestrian pursuits prompt riders to adopt a so-called chair seat in which the rider's legs are carried forward. They place the rider so that he or she sits on the horse's back, whereas in dressage the rider's weight goes directly down to the seat-bones and then to the feet. Jumping saddles have knee rolls that provide a forward buffer and are designed to be ridden with short stirrup leathers that tend to place the legs forward again. Racing saddles are tiny (weighing as little as 280 g) and the current trend is for stirrups to become ever shorter.

Saddle-fitting is becoming more scientific as pressure-detection technology becomes more refined, which has allowed humans to meet the needs of the horse for comfort during its athletic work. While saddle pads generally appear to be unable to compensate for grossly ill-fitting saddles (Kotschwar *et al.*, 2010a), certain types may help to decrease maximum pressures with well-fitted saddles (Kotschwar *et al.*, 2010b). However, the more padding a saddle includes, the greater the potential loss of what is known as 'feel'. The more widely the rider's weight is distributed across the horse's back, the less easily discriminated by the horse are precise signals from the seat.

Saddle pads are used to give unbalanced young riders rudimentary support, but they offer no protection to the horse's back. Treeless saddles are undergoing something of a renaissance because, without any rigidity, they are thought less likely to pinch. However, results from studies comparing pressure measurements in treeless saddles with regular saddles are inconclusive. One study showed similar pressure distributions for treeless and traditional saddles (Latif *et al.*, 2010), while another recorded a less uniform pressure distribution with the treeless saddle on Icelandic horses (Ramseier *et al.*, 2013). Generally, treeless saddles may be less likely to support and distribute the rider's weight as successfully as a well-fitted traditional saddle and so may be considered inadequate for performance sports that involve jumping and other high-impact gaits or manoeuvres, where there is a high-speed descent of the rider into the saddle on landing or stopping. Ideally, treeless saddles will undergo rigorous empirical comparisons with traditional and cutting-edge designs (such as the so-called cantilevered saddle that flexes at the pommel) using pressure-detection technology to determine how the rider's weight is distributed at various gaits.

Saddles are now available with a wide variety of types of padding and even pneumatic cushions. In some instances, the angle of tree can be adjusted to suit horse backs of different widths, a potential boon to owners of horses that fluctuate in weight with the seasons. There are also innovations in tree design, moving away from the traditional front branch in favour of a curved fibreglass mould, in order to avoid pressure over the scapula when the horse is in motion. Straps prevent saddles from slipping: girths around the thorax, surcingles for both saddle and thorax, cinches or cinch-straps for the abdomen, breast-plates for the base of the neck and pectoral region and cruppers for the tail-head. If any of these are too tight or in contact with damaged or highly sensitised tissue, counter-predator responses may ensue (e.g. girth-shy horses are described in Chapter 13, Stress and Fear Responses).

Bits, Bridles, Reins and Nosebands

The horse's mouth never evolved to accommodate a bit and there is no convenient space in the buccal cavity waiting to be filled by one. When the tongue is depressed by a bit, it does not fit in the narrow inter-mandibular space, so many bits press the tongue against the bars of the mouth (Figure 10.3). Fluoroscopic studies show that the bit rests on the tongue, rather than on the bars of the mouth as was originally believed. The regular snaffle bit is designed to apply pressure broadly across the tongue and, some believe, also the upper palate. Jointed bits tend to form a peak as tension increases in the reins; these are said to have a nutcracker action across the tongue and into the upper palate. In contrast, double-jointed snaffles are thought to reduce the tendency for the joint to travel dorsally when the reins are under tension (Clayton, 2005). Proponents claim the shape of the entire bit aligns better with the internal mouth shape. The tongue normally fills the oral cavity, so the bit sits on it but can easily press up on the bony, hard palate.

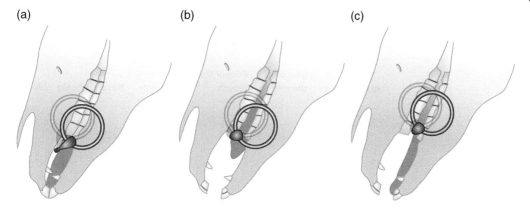

(a)   (b)   (c)

Figure 10.3 Fluoroscopic studies have revealed where the bit lies: (a) in the normal case; (b) when the tongue is retracted; and (c) when held between the molars.

When the horse relaxes the muscles of the tongue, the bit can simply indent the upper surface of the tongue. This relieves any bit pressure against the palate (Clayton, 2005). Certain types of bits may be associated with a reduction in swallowing frequency (Manfredi *et al.*, 2005), possibly by restricting the tongue movements necessary in deglutition.

The multiplicity of bits now on the market strongly suggests that bit designs are used to overcome training and performance issues, many of which probably reflect some deficits in training or riding.

Horses can be easily trained to pull against harnesses, breast-plates and collars in contact with well-muscled areas, such as the shoulders and pectoral regions, but are reluctant to fight pressure from bits in the mouth (especially if they touch only in small areas, as in the case of thin, bladed and twisted bits). When used only occasionally, chains in the curb groove or in the mouth are likely to have a strong effect, especially in the short term. Bridles and bits of different basic design contact only small anatomical sites and the severity of their action is described in Table 10.1. It must be emphasised that the severity of action depends on various physical features of the equipment, such as tightness of the curb chain, the thickness of the bit and the length of shanks (Figure 10.4).

Unrelenting pressure from a bit can prompt a horse to trial evasions (as described in Chapter 13, Stress and Fear Responses).

Unorthodox bits apply pressure with greater severity or to different parts of the mouth. Even though they can, and sometimes do, sever the tongue (Rollin, 2000), saw-chain bits (so-called mule bits and correction bits) are readily available to riders unable to produce a response in their horse with a milder bit. High rein tensions are commonly observed during riding with regular snaffle bits (5–22 Newton (N), depending on gait, discipline and local riding culture) (Kuhnke *et al.*, 2010; König von Borstel and Glißmann, 2014; Eisersiö *et al.*, 2015). However, horses' voluntary acceptance of rein tension is generally considerably lower than these values (mean tensions of 10 N in entirely naïve horses, and 6 N in the same horses after brief experiences with bits (Christensen *et al.*, 2011b). Older, more experienced horses tolerated mean tensions of 2–3.5 N (Kubiak *et al.*, 2016) with maximal tensions, ranging between 30 and 40 N, being tolerated for only brief moments in attempts to gain a food reward (Christensen *et al.*, 2011b, Kubiak *et al.*, 2016). Considering all these observations, the move to allow more severe bits for maintaining control over a horse seems quite alarming.

In some equestrian cultures, hackamores and bosals are the preferred means of controlling the head; in others, they are used more often when traditional bits have proved ineffective. It is also worth noting, that horses' tolerance levels of pressure with various

Table 10.1 The anatomical sites of negative reinforcement in which bridles and bits of different basic design can act. The severity of action (implied by the degree of shading) would depend on various factors, such as the tightness of curb chains, the thickness of the bits and the length of shanks.

	Lips	Tongue	Bars of the mouth	Roof of the mouth	Ventral mandible	Nose	Cheeks	Poll
Head-collar/halter								
Bitless bridle								
Dually halter[a]								
Hackamore[b]								
Bosal[b]								
Unjointed snaffle								
Jointed snaffle								
Running gag[c]								
Dutch gag								
Curb bit without curb chain					*			
Curb bit with curb chain[d]					*			
Bit and bridoon								

a Increases the effectiveness of a standard halter by additional pressure on the maxillary and mandibular regions.
b Works outside the buccal cavity, by compressing the nose and/or mandible.
c The aversiveness of the bit is increased by pulling it towards the ears.
d Transforms bit into fulcrum, thus increasing its aversiveness.
* Depends on the presence of a joint.

bitless bridles is like that shown with single-jointed snaffle bits (Kubiak *et al.*, 2016). However, with bitless bridles that amplify tension by reduced contact surface or leverage effects, horses' pressure-tolerance levels decline (Kubiak *et al.*, 2016). If changing or increasing mouth pressure is unsuccessful, riders and trainers may resort to an alternative or additional means of making the horse adopt the desired shape by applying pressure to other parts of the head. Typically, other 'training' devices employed include curb bits with chains, gags, draw-reins, side-reins, balancing-reins and chambons (Figure 10.5). Such devices generally use shanks that amplify the tension on the rein by lever action and so can create a misleading impression of mildness (Figure 10.6). The length of the shank magnifies the leverage through the bit. Unfortunately, the tendency is to develop a reliance on these extra pulleys, rather than to use them solely for re-training.

Most naïve horses respond to humans as they would to a predator. They move away

bodily or posturally to avoid physical or psychological pressure. While successful modification of these basic evasive responses can produce a highly responsive equine performer, inappropriate modification can make horses useless or dangerous. Horses that resist by fighting or ignoring pressure cues are often subjected to increased pressure via mechanical restraints and stimulants. However, as we have seen, horses rapidly habituate to aversive stimuli, so reaching for more severe bits is ill-advised and may lead to further desensitisation.

The inherent requirements of some equestrian sports to present horses in an 'outline' and make them work 'on the bit' can prompt trainers to use stronger bits as their first approach to achieving what is known as direct (or vertical) flexion. In contrast, educated ethical trainers recognise that where aversive stimuli fail to elicit the desired response and begin to cause behavioural conflict, the application of more force should be avoided. Rather than applying a more

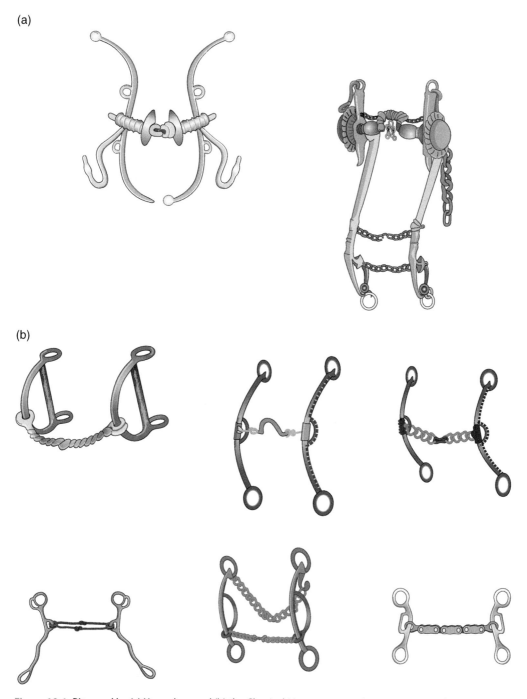

Figure 10.4 Bits used by (a) Xenophon and (b) the Classical Masters were at least as severe as the most severe modern designs (c).

severe bit, they aim to sensitise the horse to light pressures and to shape qualities such as a rounded outline as part of the training of *stop* and *go* responses.

When horses open their mouths to evade the bit, one approach by riders and trainers is to use a noseband that keeps the mouth tightly closed. This has been shown not to

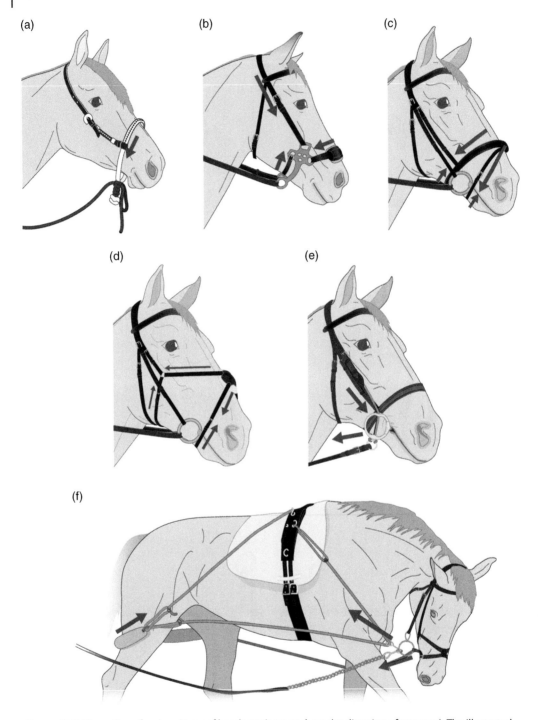

Figure 10.5 The action of various items of headgear (arrows show the direction of pressure). The illustrated items are: (a) Bosal; (b) Hackamore; (c) Flash noseband; (d) Figure-of-eight noseband; (e) Gag; (f) Pessoa.

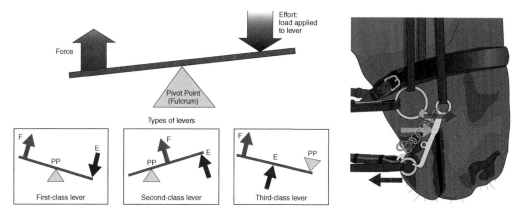

Figure 10.6 The classification of levers depends on the position of the pivot point (PP) or fulcrum and the direction of effort (E) and force (F). The curb bit and chain act as a lever that compresses the tongue and mandible, thus magnifying the horse's pain with little extra effort by the rider. In contrast, curb bits used without chain or chin-strap have no pivot point; therefore, in such cases, forces are not magnified but delayed by the shanks.

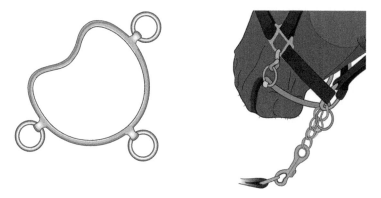

Figure 10.7 A rearing-bit with an inverted port bit presses the tongue onto the bars of the mouth.

elicit relaxation of the jaw but to act as an additional stressor (Fenner *et al.*, 2016). Other devices, such as tongue-ties, restrict normal movements of the tongue (e.g. during swallowing), and prevent the horse from finding comfort. As equestrian sports became more popular and competitive in the 1970s, dropped nosebands gave way to Hanoverian, crossover and grackle nosebands. Then, in the 1980s, 'crank' nosebands emerged. These have an added feature: they can be tightened much further than regular nosebands by a lever action. This highly aversive action seems to sensitise the horse's mouth, making the horse much more responsive to rein pressure and, to some, this gives

the appearance of the horse becoming more 'submissive'.

Cheek pieces may prevent the bit from being pulled through the horse's mouth and equally may make turning pressures on the lateral aspect of the horse's lips clearer to the horse. Rearing-bits (also known as chifney or stallion bits) also have this feature but are generally thinner and have no joint, so they have a more severe action than riding bits such as a regular snaffle. The action of a rearing-bit presses the tongue against the bars and, not uncommonly, may cut the tongue itself (Figure 10.7). Most rearing-bits have an inverted port in the middle and this is their most controversial feature as it drives the tongue into the cavity where it cannot fit and thus severely onto the bars of the mouth. Rearing-bits without a tongue port work on the bars of the mouth rather than the tongue itself. Used correctly, they help to control particularly reactive animals, such as naïve youngsters and fractious stallions that may readily toss their heads and stand up on their hindlegs. Again, the emphasis should be on using light pressure (so that the least amount of pressure creates the maximum effect) and, of course, the pressure must be released promptly after every correct or near-correct response. These bits must never be used in attempts to punish a horse (e.g. by reefing on a lead rope).

Reins

The weight of the reins contributes to the neutral tension of contact. It has been suggested that reins long enough for long-reining may habituate horses to bit pressure, simply because they are heavier than the reins used during riding (Warren-Smith *et al.*, 2007b). Equally, because of the distance the rider is from the horse, long-reins reduce the rider's ability to 'feel' the horse's mouth. The reins may also act as a discriminative stimulus, so the feel of them against the neck can pre-empt turning. When turning, the outside rein can be drawn medially against and across the horse's neck to help train the neck to remain straight during turning. When it comes to turning, different disciplines apply pressure differently to the bit. In some sports, horses are trained to turn by such a neck-reining technique where the outside rein presses against and over the neck.

The reins used in reining competition are necessarily heavy so that they hang away from the horse's neck when not applying pressure to it. Long riding reins hang redundantly from the withers and are sometimes used to trigger forward motion by striking them across the horse's shoulder. Using the reins in this way (where one side is struck more than the other, often as a function of the handedness of the rider) can train a horse to travel in other than a straight line.

The breadth of the bit that has contact with the mouth (or another part of the head) and the action of any levers will also affect the way rein tension is translated to the horse. However, it should be noted that thicker bits are not always more comfortable for a horse. Some horses have rather narrow buccal cavities, and very thick bits may prevent the horse from completely closing its mouth. Bitless bridles are not necessarily a panacea for horses, since they rely on negative reinforcement (and therefore the horse's motivation to remove the pressure) as much as any bitted bridle and may sometimes lack the ability to deliver the clear lateral pressure needed for turns, tending instead to tighten on the horse's head before effecting a turn. However, they do avoid oral conflicts (Scofield and Randle, 2013). It is, therefore, important that when equitation scientists report studies of rein tension, they must specify the dimension and design of the gear used.

Side-Reins, Martingales and Tie-Downs

Side-reins (Figure 10.8), martingales and tie-downs that apply pressure to the nasal planum via the noseband (in the case of the standing martingale and tie-downs) or the mouth via the reins (in the case of the running martingale or draw-reins), prevent evasive raising of the head (Table 10.2). The rider can use the lever action of the running martingale to pull the head lower. Critics rightly point out that these gadgets force the horse into an outline rather than train self-carriage through lightness. Rather, when the head is forced downwards, the muscles of the neck and topline are not 'suspending' the head and neck but, instead, the horse is attempting to raise its head against aversive pressure. We know this because as soon as we release the reins on a horse, with a device such as a martingale on, it raises its head immediately. Gadgets, such as side-reins that fix the head position, deny the horse's need to move its head forwards and backwards in the walk and the canter, which consequently become stilted.

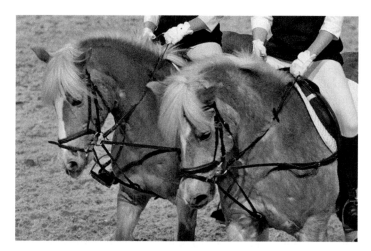

Figure 10.8 Side-reins and draw-reins are used to coerce the horse into adopting a rounder outline, compromising the *stop/slow* response. (Photo courtesy of Minna Tallberg.)

Table 10.2 The sites in which various devices are attached. The severity of action (implied by the degree of shading) would depend on various factors such as the tightness of nosebands, the length of straps and the inclusion of elastic.

	Ventral girth	Lateral surcingle	Bit	Noseband (upper)	Noseband (lower)	Reins	Browband/ crown piece	Gaskin
Side-reins[a]								
Draw-reins[a]								
Standing martingale								
Running martingale								
Chambon[b]								
Market Harborough[c]								
Pessoa[d]								
Elastic rein inserts[e]								
Dropped noseband								
Hanoverian noseband (including grackle, figure-of-eight, crossover)								
Crank noseband					*			

a Used by trainers who prioritise outline before lightness and rhythm. At best, these devices use negative reinforcement to arch and shorten the neck and give the impression of correct training, but they force the wrong muscles to carry the neck, which usually results in a contracted neck.

b Uses negative reinforcement to train the horse to lower its head, thus reducing hollowness or hyper-reactivity and facilitating rounder topline. Possibly replicates postural calmness (see discussion in Warren-Smith *et al.*, 2007b).

c Uses force to obtain head-carriage for trainers who struggle to obtain lightness and roundness with dorsal muscle groups.

d Causes intermittent pressure on the horse's mouth, from its hindleg action, to force it into a rounder outline.

e Used for beginner riders with the intention to moderate unintentional cues and peak pressures (e.g. Heleski *et al.*, 2009). However, cue clarity may also be blurred by the elastic insert, possibly teaching riders to apply stronger pressures than appropriate with regular reins.

* May include secondary lower strap.

The position of the horse's head and neck is pivotal in balance and so the effect of the standing martingale on locomotion should not be underestimated. Standing martingales should never be used for jumping, but running martingales may be justified in the case of racehorses that toss their heads vigorously when literally fighting for their heads and may, in the process, hit their jockeys in the face.

The straps between the rings and girth on a running martingale and the noseband and girth on a standing martingale can be tightened to the extent that the horse is forced to carry its head in a low position, receiving negative reinforcement by lowering its head. These devices defeat any attempt to achieve self-carriage and, because the horse rapidly adopts a new posture that riders become accustomed to, the devices continue to be used. If this device is to be used at all, the length of the straps of a running martingale should be adjusted so that they engage only when the poll is extended vertically.

Standing (fixed) or running martingales should not be confused with Irish martingales that simply join the reins under the horse's neck to reduce the chance of the reins falling over the neck and being trodden on.

Dentition and Mouth Pain

The horse's comfort, especially when ridden, can be profoundly affected by its dentition. Put simply, horses have not evolved to accommodate a bit (of whatever volume) in the mouth, so the intra-oral presence of the bit requires the tongue to move into a more-or-less abnormal position. This, and the need in some disciplines to maintain contact, can reduce the horse's own ability to keep its cheek and tongue away from a sharp element of its dental arcade. The result is resistance (Chapter 13, Stress and Fear Responses) and a narrowing of the margin that represents neutral contact. Essentially, the horse becomes more difficult to maintain in speed, line and posture.

Mouth pain may also be associated with heavy-handed riding or inappropriate gear. For example, some jointed bits can cause pinching between the second premolar and the labial commissures. Wolf teeth, especially those with loose roots and cusps that are directed towards the seat of the bit, may make the horse reluctant to accept the bit and may trigger it to reef the reins out of the rider's hands. This can rapidly escalate into head-tossing (Figure 10.9) (see Chapter 14, Ethical Equitation and Chapter 13, Stress and Fear Responses). The reinforcing nature of this activity seems obvious and is likely to be most profound if the rider usually yields. In the event of a horse fighting the bit, some veterinarians and equine dentists are prepared to remove an appreciable portion of the second premolar to create a 'bit seat' or 'cheek seat', which is supposed to improve comfort in this part of the mouth (Wilewski and Rubin, 1999). While one study reported

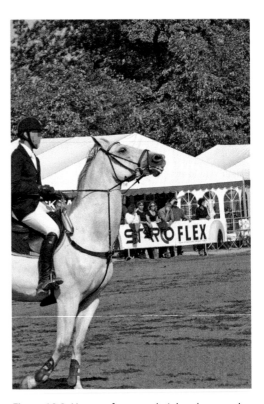

Figure 10.9 Horses often toss their heads upwards when trying to resolve inescapable mouth pain. (Photo courtesy of Julie Taylor.)

improved athletic performance in most horses after the creation of bit seats (Wilewski and Rubin, 1999), an abiding question is whether a simple change of riding technique or bit (e.g. to an unjointed design) would have been equally effective.

Whips and Spurs

If a horse fails to show sufficient forward movement or impulsion, trainers direct their attention to the sides where they can increase the pressure by using whips and spurs and more effectively send the horse forward (or, simply, away from the rider's leg). Although, for some, these stimulants are distasteful, they are not necessarily contra-indicated. They can be introduced so that they can be used minimally and with accuracy to ensure consistency and be employed transiently to fortify the rider's leg signals. That said, whips fortify only if the horse has a clear learned response to the whip, so it is very useful to train the whip/*go* response without leg first.

Apparatus Used in Enhancing Performance

Equipment Used to Increase Range of Limb Movement

In some equestrian disciplines, especially gaited horse classes and dressage, extravagant movements are desired and a high range of limb motion is rewarded by judges. Not surprisingly, trainers have come up with methods and apparatus that potentially speed-up training a horse to lift its legs up to their maximum range of motion. Such devices include weighted boots, action chains, rollers and shackles. While equipment such as weighted boots and action chains allow the rider to influence the horse's movements passively, either by physically training the horse via the added weight or by psychologically inducing the horse to lift its legs higher due to noise or sensory experiences from the equipment, shackles can also be used by the trainer to actively modify the horse's movements by pulling strings attached to the horse's fetlocks. The use of such methods to artificially alter horses' natural movements is highly controversial, particularly if, with the use of shackles, the trainer's timing is incorrect and there is a high potential to disturb the horse's rhythm of movement or to induce physical harm (also see Chapter 12, Unorthodox Methods).

Equipment Used to Enhance Airway-Functioning

Tongue-ties are commonly used in horse-racing to prevent dorsal displacement of the soft palate, although prevention could only be shown in two out of six affected horses, and performance parameters remained unchanged in all horses affected with dorsal displacement of the soft palate (Franklin *et al.*, 2002). With healthy, standing horses, one study reported increased airway dimensions (Chalmers *et al.*, 2013), but positive effects on performance remain to be proved, and so far, other studies have failed to show these effects (Cornelisse *et al.*, 2001a,b). The popularity of tongue-ties, despite limited effects on airway functioning and performance, may therefore be rooted in their additional effect of effectively preventing the horse from getting the tongue over the bit, an action that might serve to defy the trainer's control. The use of tongue-ties is controversial and is forbidden in many disciplines, such as dressage. In certain countries it is forbidden altogether, and in others for racing during winter (to prevent frostbite on horses' tongues). Nasal strips were originally used in racehorses to increase airway dimensions by preventing nasal collapse during inspiration. There is some evidence that this measure does indeed decrease respiratory effort (Holcombe *et al.*, 2002) and the likelihood of exercise-induced pulmonary haemorrhage (reviewed by Hinchcliff *et al.*, 2015). While there is a small chance that nasal strips are harmful to horses, it is the potential effects on performance that led some countries, such as Australia, to ban the use of nasal strips in horse-racing.

Apparatus Used in Restraint

The Practice and Principles of Physical Restraint

Among veterinary professionals, physical restraint of horses (e.g. with twitches or hobbles) during painful procedures is often possible, but rarely preferable to chemical restraint. This is legitimate, if the alternative is a brutal struggle or an opportunity for the horse to learn dangerous evasions. Fundamentally, force can escalate the aversiveness of the procedure and is ultimately likely to compromise the horse–human interaction and make the horse less compliant for future procedures. Numerous handling problems are the legacy of previous mistakes in timing and consistency. Others can have proximate causes in physical pathologies, so trainers should always consider seeking veterinary advice before embarking on any course of behaviour modification. For example, a horse that is reluctant to *step backwards* must be checked for back pain (referred or otherwise) or for specific problems such as wobbler syndrome (Moore *et al.*, 1994).

Once a flight response starts, most naïve horses, when restrained by the head, will continue to struggle until the pressure of restraint is released. This explains why horses should be tied up with a securely fitted head-collar and lead-rope and never by the reins of a bridle or a lead attached to the bit. The rope can be tied with a quick release knot to a length of baling twine, which is attached to a solid object. Baling twine will usually break before a sturdy rope and headcollar. However, there is a paradox here, because a quick escape is reinforcing for the horse, so future struggles become more likely. A preferred approach is to train the horse to *go forward* from light lead-rope tension, and to stand calmly. When first left by the handler, some foundation trainers tie the lead-rope to a car inner tube firmly attached to a secure point on a safe ground surface. If the horse moves, the inner tube reacts like a strong hand. Some commercially available elastic inserts for lead-ropes cannot be recommended as they are often not strong enough, turning into a highly dangerous slingshot if they break under tension.

Even if they are secured by so-called quick-release knots, attempting to release panic-stricken horses can be very dangerous, especially when more than one horse is tied up and motivated by socially facilitated hysteria. It is worth noting also that quick-release knots do not untie readily once they are under pressure, although many horses quickly learn how to untie themselves. Also, with much of the commercially available equipment, parts of headcollar or lead-rope clip will readily break during a horse's violent struggles before the knot can be untied. In these cases, there may be bits of metal from the broken piece of equipment catapulted at high speeds to the surroundings, posing a high risk of injury to both horse and/or trainer. Tying horses at nose height maxim-ises normal head movement within the limits set by the length of rope, which should be short enough to prevent the horse putting its leg over the rope and long enough to allow the horse to turn its head to examine objects that would otherwise be in its blind spot. Horses will work to remove themselves from the threat of discomfort. The danger of horses fighting against physical restraint by blindly paddling their limbs in pursuit of freedom means that hobbles and ropes as means of restraint should be avoided wher-ever possible. Rope-burns and even fractures can result from roping, strapping and hob-bling techniques, even under conditions of best practice.

Roping techniques used to pacify horses during aversive interventions are described exhaustively elsewhere (e.g. Waring, 2003; Fraser, 1992; Rose and Hodgson, 1993). Generally, these have been superseded by chemical agents, since there is no justification for allowing horses to fight against physical restraint when there is no evidence that they can predict that the episode will end. If, dur-ing a handling procedure, a horse is not likely to learn good associations with personnel, then we should avoid it learning anything. The use of over-shadowing techniques to reduce fearful responses to interventions such as farriery, clipping and injections is yet to be empirically explored, but holds tremendous promise in the hands of skilled practitioners (McLean, 2008; McLean and Christensen, 2017).

Horses show an early-morning (i.e. around sunrise) peak in their plasma beta-endorphin concentrations (Hamra *et al.*, 1993) and so are likely to be the least sensitive to noxious stimuli early in the day. As a result, it has been suggested that this may be the preferred time to undertake elective aversive procedures. The natural inclination of horses to flee from threats makes them difficult to deal with in the open and even attempts to corner them in a field or yard for interventions are ill-judged if a stable with a non-slip surface is available. Before any invasive handling or veterinary procedure, anything that may get in the way during a struggle or a forced retreat by the handler, most notably water buckets and wheelbarrows, should be removed from the stable.

When handling fractious and naïve horses, it may be helpful to use calm horses as 'tutors' because of the social-facilitation effect (Christensen *et al.*, 2008a). In cattle, the reverse has been demonstrated, and it has been shown that alarm substances in the urine of stressed conspecifics increase reactivity to aversive events (Boissy, 1998). It would be interesting to learn whether any equivalent messaging occurs among horses. Such substances may linger in transport areas, such as holding pens and trailers, or even in areas used for aversive procedures, such as veterinary interventions.

Physical restraint should not be used in ways that directly compromise horse welfare. Tying horses up for aversive procedures is inadvisable, since their tendency to fight against such restraint precipitates attempts to flee and so increases fear and the likelihood of damage to equipment or, worse still, injury to themselves or to personnel. Restraining horses effectively with a halter has more to do with timing than force, and appropriate behaviour must be negatively reinforced with the release of pressure and

then positively by stroking the animal in anatomical areas previously or intrinsically associated with stress reduction, including the neck and withers. Fear reactions generally manifest as locomotory responses, so gaining control over the horse's legs is very useful. Overshadowing techniques that centre on gaining stimulus control of the horse's legs are important here (Chapter 6, Associative Learning (Aversive stimuli)).

Cupping a hand over a horse's eye on the side on which it is being treated is often helpful for needle-shy horses. The same principle seems to apply when blinkers, shades (pacifiers) or sheep-skin nosebands are used on racehorses. The idea is to reduce the number of fear-eliciting stimuli the horse must cope with. This can have the effect of moderating arousal levels and maintaining the horse's flight response under the control of the trainer rather than the environment. In a similar way, covering a horse's eyes in a fire may allow you to lead it out of a burning stable – it seems that 'out of sight' means 'out of mind'. Originally, pacifiers were made of fly-mesh and were primarily used to stop dust and sand getting in a horse's eyes during track-work. However, trainers soon noticed a serendipitous feature when horses wore these screens: they were much quieter and less reactive to environmental stimuli. It may be that, to an animal that is unable to extrapolate, the fly-mesh cross-hatching radically turned down the volume on visual signals that had reliably triggered hyper-reactivity in the past.

When increased restraint is required, it sometimes takes the form of hobbles, a tail-rope or service hobbles, but these dubious techniques should be used only as emergency measures rather than routine approaches. Distracting the animal with the use of a twitch or rope-gag may occasionally prove useful when dealing with the hindquarters of a fearful horse, but again, overshadowing via the bit is preferable (McLean, 2008). At least in the short term, the distraction caused by the twitch or rope-gag is chiefly pain, even though it may be rapidly modified by endorphins (Lagerweij *et al.*, 1984).

Head Restraints

Headcollars were designed to be placed on the horse from the near (left) side. They should be tight enough to prevent horses from removing them or getting their hoofs caught in them (e.g. while scratching the head with a hindhoof), low enough to assist in control of the head's direction, and high enough to avoid fracturing the nasal bone or cartilage. The noseband should be loose enough to allow the horse to open its mouth and chew. Halters designed to tighten around the head if the horse resists work well when used with the correct technique of negative reinforcement within the pressure/release framework, but the horse should not be tethered by one. The Dually^{TM} halter and stallion chains use a similar principle, tightening and applying pressure around the nose if the horse struggles. Stallion chains can be confusing to the horse, because the eccentric chain pressure tends to result in neck shortening rather than slowing the legs.

Although horses generally lead better from the left side, this is simply a convention in most countries (an exception being Iceland, for example, where horses are traditionally mounted and thus handled from the right side). However, it fails to recognise that there are left- and right-preferent horses (McGreevy and Rogers, 2005). Horses with a motor preference that manifests as left- or right-hoofedness are likely to be more under the influence of one brain hemisphere than the other. Although clear evidence for relationships between sensory and motor bias is currently lacking (Kuhnke and König von Borstel, 2016a,b), this may translate to sensory dominance of one side over the other. So when leading horses from their offside, as is the convention, the influence of the right visual field may be compromised more than the left. Leading a horse sometimes from either left or right side may reveal which side suits that horse better.

The latest generation of halters (such as the Parelli halter and the Dually^{TM} halter) are strong; they tend to exert more pressure than regular headcollars, because they are either made with thinner material or they tighten under pressure. Horses are best controlled if the trainer is standing midway between the horse's head and shoulder. With this approach, accelerating and decelerating signals can easily be issued via the lead-rope. In addition, a flighty horse can be controlled in an open space, as its momentum can be deviated by a sharp tug on the lead-rope. However, when doing so, the horse's hindquarters will tend to swing out away from the trainer, so there is a possibility of colliding with objects to the side.

Although one study concluded that there was no evidence of heart-rate moderation resulting from head lowering (Warren-Smith *et al.*, 2007a), physiological evidence (e.g. from baroreceptors) and practitioners indicate that simply lowering the head may have a pacifying effect on horses (McLean and McLean, 2008). The horse can be trained to lower its head if light downward tension is applied on the lead-rope and the pressure is released as soon as the head comes down.

Where the head goes the body will generally follow, so keeping the head still in cross-ties can be an effective means of reducing lateral movements of the body during everyday procedures such as grooming. The need for quick-release mechanisms applies. Horses should be restrained in cross-ties only via a sturdy headcollar. It is not safe to attach horses to cross-ties, or a single tether, in a rope halter because of the risk of fracturing mandibles during a hyper-reactive response.

War-Bridle (or Rope-Gag)

The war-bridle is an old method that requires no more than a length of rope. It consists of a rope tied in a bowline knot loosely around the horse's neck and then brought forward and wrapped around the horse's nose and mandible and back through the neck loop. When the trainer exerts pressure on the rope, the effect is to compress the mandible (rather like the action of the Dually^{TM} halter). This is renowned for having a profound aversive effect, resulting, with correct application of negative reinforcement, in effective control in many circumstances.

A cord passed under the upper lip and over the poll before being threaded through a loop at the side of the face to form a running noose acts like a twitch when pulled tight. Variations on this theme appear in the literature, and even though they are vehicles for escalated force, they are sometimes advocated for problems in the ridden horse. A piece of rubber tubing slipped over the portion of the rope that presses on the under-part of the lip reduces the risk of injury without appearing to reduce the effectiveness of the device. Inherent dangers with this sort of severe equipment are many and varied. Equitation scientists generally advise against their use and advocate for better timing and consistency in training with regular equipment rather than a continued reliance on more severe equipment.

The 'buck-stop' is a modification of the war-bridle that punishes bucking by causing pain under the upper lip. It does nothing to treat the cause of bucking, which may be directly related to a painful pathology or may be a result of dysfunctions of the *go* and *stop* signals (Chapter 13, Stress and Fear Responses).

Twitches

A twitch is used to apply a constriction to the upper lip of the horse in a bid to restrain it (Figure 10.10). It is simple, effective, easy to apply, and comparatively safe for both horse and operator. For brief, mildly painful procedures, a twitch may help to immobilise the horse, but this is certainly not so in all cases. Some experienced horses see the twitch coming and begin to flee immediately, a response that seems to confirm that pain is involved. Twitches come in a variety of forms, from a simple loop of rope attached to a bull's nose ring, through to a pair of metal pliers called the humane twitch (which in the hands of a novice may cause less tissue damage than a homemade twitch). The narrower the element in touch with the horse, the greater is the pain and likelihood of permanent damage. Twitches with soft, thick rope and plastic handles are generally the safest. When applying a twitch, snare as much of the upper lip as possible to increase the effectiveness of the device and reduce the chance of it slipping. The constriction should be loosened every 15 minutes or so to maintain cellular

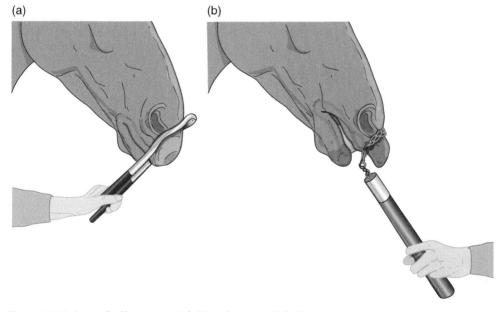

(a) (b)

Figure 10.10 A so-called humane twitch (a) and a rope twitch (b).

perfusion distal to it. In any case, this is advisable since, in many cases, the effectiveness of the twitch tends to wane after this period, possibly because of neurotransmitter depletion at the level of synapses in the opioid pathways. In addition, there are reports of horses suddenly striking with their forelegs during twitching.

Current veterinary thinking suggests that twitching a horse's lip should be undertaken only when chemical restraint is not available (McGreevy, 2004). Twitching should be regarded as a last resort of restraint justified only as a means by which to inject a psychotropic drug. Broadly speaking, the effects of a nose twitch can often be achieved by 'twitching' a fold of skin on the side of the neck (Figure 10.11). Using this technique, trainers can often restrain fearful horses well enough to administer an injectable form of restraint. It may occasionally be helpful to use a skin-fold twitch on a ridden horse (e.g. when the trainer anticipates the appearance of a fear-eliciting stimulus).

In very difficult horses, the ear is sometimes grasped to briefly control the horse while a twitch is put on the upper lip. However, this technique should be avoided, since it is far more likely to create head-shyness in the long term than compliance in the short term. Twitching the ear is not appropriate, since it leads to increased stress responses and may make the animal head-shy (Flakoll, 2016), scar the skin or paralyse the ear. The nose-twitch is believed to work through the mediation of beta-endorphins, but there is also the potential that it works because it involves pain (Webster, 1994). Correct application for an appropriate duration appears to be paramount for the effects of analgesia and calming to happen. While two recent studies reported a decrease in heart rate and changes in heart-rate variability parameters that are indicative of reduced stress when the twitch was applied compared to control a situation without use of a twitch (Ali *et al.*, 2015; Flakoll, 2016), other studies report a transient increase in horses' heart rates when twitched (Morris, 1988) before returning to baseline values. This return to baseline is quicker in crib-biters than in normal horses (Minero *et al.*, 1999), although it is unclear why. Crib-biters are also reported to be less reactive to being twitched than non-crib-biters, and are more likely to remain calm (Minero *et al.*, 1999). These findings may reflect altered dopamine activity in the brains of crib-biters and its consequences for pleasure and rewards.

Forelimb Restraint

Roping techniques are mentioned in this book only for use in emergencies that arise in

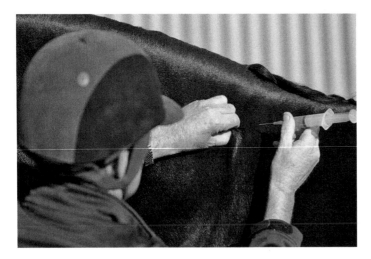

Figure 10.11 Using a skin-fold twitch while giving an injection.

the absence of more appropriate applications of learning theory or veterinary support. Potentially fractious horses can be restrained and their ability to kick decreased by restraining one of the forelimbs. A forelimb can be flexed so that the hoof reaches the level of the elbow and then is held there by a handler. Flexing the leg reduces the power of that leg so the horse is less able to strike. When holding the forefoot of a horse in this way, handlers must grip the hoof only lightly to avoid training the horse to lean. At the same time, avoid giving the horse an opportunity to snatch the foot away, which often happens before a horse kicks out at personnel. However, even when observing these safety measures, some horses are balanced and mobile enough to kick with the diagonal hindleg or to rear. That said, experience suggests that good handling and concurrent overshadowing can overcome many fearful responses that a horse might learn to offer farriers and veterinarians (McLean, 2008).

A 'knee strap' placed around the forearm and the pastern can be used to hold the leg off the ground, but the hazardous responses it can evoke (especially in naïve horses) should not be overlooked. Difficult-to-shoe horses are sometimes restrained in this way, anecdotal evidence suggesting that they learn to maintain leg flexion as a result. A soft surface underfoot is a prerequisite for this approach, because many horses fall before learning that immobility is the correct response when normal locomotory responses are compromised in this way. Generally, however, chemical restraint and, in the longer term, behavioural therapy are the preferred options.

Hindlimb Restraint

Hindlimb hobbles are often used on mares during mating or pregnancy testing. Each hindlimb is attached to a collar around the horse's neck so that the horse can move the legs forwards but not backwards. The straps around the pasterns should be made of a soft but strong material, such as leather, that is unlikely to burn the horse's skin.

The collar must be wide enough to prevent undue pressure being concentrated on a small region of the neck. Farriers and foundation trainers sometimes train a horse to hold and maintain a hindleg by a modification of the breeding hobbles. A strap is placed around the horse's hind pastern and a rope attached to the strap. The rope is then run through a padded collar placed around the horse's neck. The rope may be run back through the strap (if the horse's leg can be approached), and then pressure on the pulley system lifts the hindleg off the ground. For horses in a situation where the hindlegs cannot be handled (i.e. in the absence of veterinary support), a slip loop is sometimes made in the end of the rope and placed on the ground. The horse is then walked over the rope so that the targeted hindhoof is located within the loop. The rope is then pulled so the loop tightens around the pastern. Once the rope is through the collar, it is shortened until the horse's leg is at the required position. To avoid rope burns, only soft ropes should be used. The rope is then secured so that the handler can approach and handle the hindlimb safely. Because it is akin to one method of casting a horse, it is not surprising that, when undergoing this method, many unhandled horses throw themselves on the ground. For this reason, the procedure should take place only in a safe enclosure with a soft landing (e.g. a round-pen floored with deep sand). The extent to which the horse also undergoes learned helplessness in this situation is worth considering. In general, it is better to apply learning theory than brute force, not least because the horse has more brute force at its disposal. The preferred approach to hindleg sensitivity, for example, is to habituate the horse by hosing it with water. The aim here is to keep hosing until there is no more kicking. This procedure can be expedited with timely overshadowing (as discussed in Chapter 7, Applying Learning Theory).

Hobbles

Serving hobbles are designed to limit a mare's ability to kick a stallion during mating.

Various patterns of serving hobbles have been described elsewhere in horse-management literature. All limit the mobility of the hindlegs by roping them to a band around the horse's neck, and most are fitted with some form of quick-release device. Because they occasionally cause horses to fall (usually while struggling), they should be used only in combination with deep, soft bedding materials. Sidelines follow similar principles, but the ipsilateral limbs are secured. In lunged horses, the bit is even sometimes connected to the hindlegs above the hocks, so the movement of the legs causes pain on the mouth, resulting in retreating from bit pressure (e.g. the Pessoa training apparatus).

Hobbling the two forelegs together at the level of the carpal joints (knees) or the metacarpophalangeal joints (fetlocks) or the first phalanges (pasterns) (e.g. with so-called dinner hobbles), is sometimes used as a means of retarding a horse's progress when leaving it untethered (Figure 10.12). It is also used for horses that habitually strike or kick during travelling. However, these

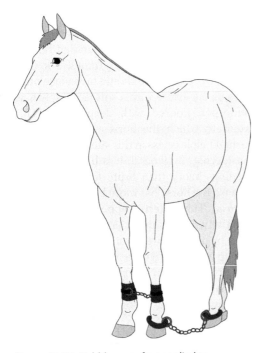

Figure 10.12 Hobbles are often applied to immobilise horses and limit the expression of a flight response.

problems are typically manifestations of in-hand problems with *go* and *stop*. When first applied, hobbles prompt most horses to fight against the restraint. They should not be used by novice trainers and, initially, they must be used in conjunction with soft but not slippery surfaces (in case of falling).

Full-Body Restraint

Lunge-lines restrict a horse's movement within a certain radius and therefore qualify as a form of restraint. Although lungeing is considered a safe way of allowing horses to show post-inhibitory locomotory responses after periods of confinement, it may also allow them to practise inappropriate flight responses. There are strong arguments against training horses to avoid and run from person-nel, which is essentially what many horses learn to do when they show hyper-reactivity (as characterised by a hollow outline) on the lunge. This can lead them to establish aversive associations with the trainer. If lungeing is embraced as a training or exercise practice, it is important that personnel use downward transitions to train horses to maintain their speed and to change the direction of lungeing frequently to avoid unbalanced wear-and-tear and laterally biased training.

Reports on Welsh ponies (Debbie Goodwin, personal communication, 2006) and the Blackfoot Native American remounts (Ewers, 1955) being run into boggy ground as a preliminary step in the breaking process may sound inhumane. After all, the subjects cannot escape and can easily be flooded with aversive stimuli because the boggy ground acts as a form of restraint. However, in a sim-ilar vein, Grandin (2007) has reported on the use of pressure all over the body and legs of unhandled horses as a means of restraining them for habituation and gentling. In this method, pressure is applied using wheat that is poured over and around the horse as it stands in a holding box at the end of a corral chute through which its head and neck emerge. The calmative effect of this restraint is reported to last only 20 minutes, although it is not clear why. However, it has been shown that preventing mobility by restraint can cause habituation to aversive stimuli (Baum, 1970). Further investigation of the role of overshadowing in this and other methods of achieving full-body restraint is needed. There is a clear link between the prevention of locomotory responses and the development of habituation to aversive stimuli. This would help to explain the mechanisms that underpin hobbling techniques in the early training of dairy cattle, horses and elephants.

Pharmaceuticals and Nutriceuticals

Chemical agents that modify the behaviour of horses must not be used without veterinary advice. The risk of falling and loss of coordination should never be underestimated, since it can lead to the horse scrambling and suffering severe injuries.

Tryptophan

Serotonin (5-HT) (or its precursor, 5-hydroxytryptophan (5-HTP) may induce sleep and, importantly, may reduce anxiety. It is produced chiefly by neurons in the rostral pons and midbrain. It is synthesised from the amino acid tryptophan, so oral supplementation with tryptophan may increase serotonin concentrations in the brain (Hahn, 2004). Dietary tryptophan has been used to mildly 'sedate' horses, but this is a topic of some debate since tryptophan in low doses (relative to recommendations for commercial products) has also been shown to stimulate horses (Bagshaw *et al.*, 1994). The 5-HT system is the mediator of learned and sustained fear responses, and decreased 5-HT concentrations have been associated with violent psychopathological behaviour in humans (Lee and Coccaro, 2001). However, there are no scientific publications that support the efficiency of tryptophan for reduction of fearfulness in horses. Accordingly, the present experimental evidence concludes that we should not rely on an acute dose of tryptophan to calm horses (Grimmett and Sillence, 2005; Malmkvist and Christensen, 2007; Liss and Wolframm, 2011; Noble *et al.*, 2016).

Better understanding of the causes of fear and improvement of training methods are more reliable in terms of reduction of fearfulness in horses (Malmkvist and Christensen, 2007).

Reserpine

Reserpine is a product of the root of *Rauwolfia serpentine*, an Indian climbing shrub. It depletes amine concentrations in the brain, including serotonin, noradrenaline and dopamine. Noradrenaline is an excitatory neurohormone in the brain, so its depletion explains the calming or tranquillising effect of reserpine in the horse (Tobin, 1978). Its calming properties have been exploited for management and training purposes. The lasting nature of the drug (up to 10 days) accounts for its appeal to those seeking to modulate equine flight responses, especially during traditional foundation training. There is considerable variability in the pharmacokinetics of reserpine in horses, with reports of adverse reactions (especially among stallions), including erratic behaviour. It has lost favour among veterinarians because of its role in anaesthesia deaths because of hypotension

Take-Home Messages

- Pressure is a function of force applied to a given surface area and is ubiquitous in horse-training. Force applied to a small area can result in very high pressure.
- Tack is designed to either disperse pressure (e.g. in the case of the saddle) or direct pressure (e.g. in the case of head restraint).
- In tack designed to direct pressure, the narrower the interface with the horse, the more severe the apparatus and the greater is the need for excellent timing in pressure-release.
- Safety considerations are paramount when restraining horses.
- Good technique is more sustainable than instruments or equipment that allows trainers to apply more force.

Ethical Considerations

- Devices that generate endorphins and ultimately restrain horses may do so through the intermediacy of pain and, therefore, may be less ethical than pharmacological restraint or behaviour therapy.
- Technological advances may facilitate restraint without due regard for welfare.

Areas for Further Research

- Animal welfare science must address the possibility of learned helplessness resulting from radical restraining techniques.
- The emergence of polymers and so-called smart materials may yet enhance the effectiveness of traditional items of saddlery.
- The development of materials that will be placed in the mouths of horses merits particularly close scrutiny.

11

Biomechanics

Introduction

This chapter is not intended as a definitive work on equine biomechanics – this subject is more thoroughly treated in appropriate texts (e.g. Back and Clayton, 2001). Rather, this chapter will describe the limb movements in sufficient detail to explain the nature of the locomotory requirements that the trainer and rider's signals are intended to control during equitation. As discussed in Chapter 8, Training, the rider's cues should target the onset of the swing phase of a discrete biomechanical action, such as retraction, protraction, adduction or abduction, and therefore a working knowledge of equine biomechanics is advantageous for optimal training.

Locomotion

While kinematic features of equine locomotion have been extensively studied (especially forward locomotion), very few data are available on the neural basis of movement in horses, so much of what we know about locomotion stems from laboratory studies of rats and cats. However, there are good grounds on which to extrapolate these data to horses (Gramsbergen, 2001).

Neuromuscular coordination of locomotion is complex yet predictable. Just as an orchestra's strength is the result of individual contributions by the musicians, the horse's mobility can be traced to individual components. The locomotory responses that allow horses to go forwards, backwards, faster, slower, sideways, and to turn result from individual muscles. They comprise the basic responses that riders endeavour to place under the control of their signals, a process known as *stimulus control*, (Chapter 7, Applying Learning Theory). These locomotory responses can be broken down into four basic ways of moving that can be thought of as building blocks for all movements in-hand and under-saddle in all equestrian disciplines (Figure 11.1):

1) Acceleration;
2) Deceleration (including reverse);
3) Turning with the forelimbs; and
4) Turning with the hindlimbs.

When we consider the possible directions the horse's limbs can take to allow the four basic responses listed above, it follows that different muscles or muscle groups account for each one. Biomechanics identifies the four main ways in which limbs can move that result in locomotion (Back, 2001) (Figure 11.2):

1) Protraction (moving the leg forward);
2) Retraction (moving the leg backwards);
3) Abduction (moving the limb away from the medial plane); and
4) Adduction (moving the limb towards the medial plane).

Protraction and retraction account for acceleration and deceleration, while abduction

Equitation Science, Second Edition. Paul McGreevy, Janne Winther Christensen, Uta König von Borstel and Andrew McLean.
© 2018 John Wiley & Sons Ltd. Published 2018 by John Wiley & Sons Ltd.
Companion website: www.wiley.com/go/mcgreevy/equitation

(a)

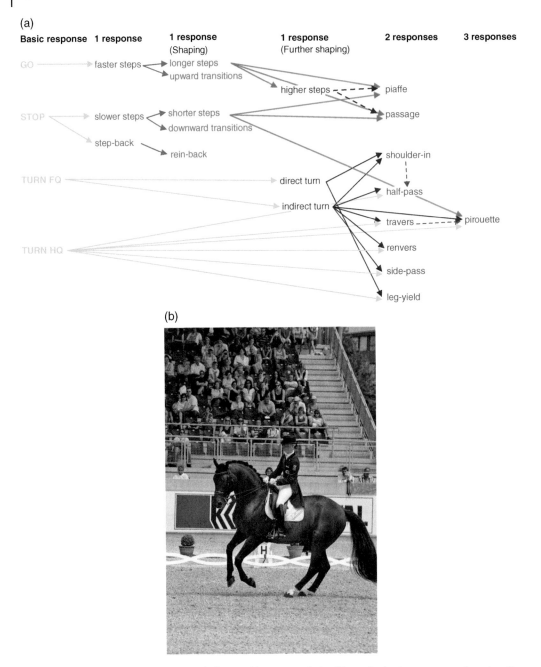

Figure 11.1 (a) All movements required of trained horses are derived from the basic responses of acceleration, deceleration, turning the forequarters (FQ) and turning the hindquarters (HQ). Dotted arrows refer to shaped preparatory movements that usually precede elicitation of the targeted movements. (b) In dressage, the canter pirouette represents a movement that consists of a cascade of the largest number of single responses: shortened canter, turn of the forelegs and turn of the hindlegs. (Photo courtesy of *The Horse Magazine*.)

and adduction produce changes of direction and lateral movements (McLean and McLean, 2008). The relative amounts of these four limb movements at any moment provide the precise direction of travel. All movements therefore can be described as having specific amounts of retraction, protraction, abduction and adduction, depending

(a)

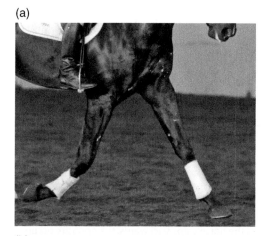

(b)

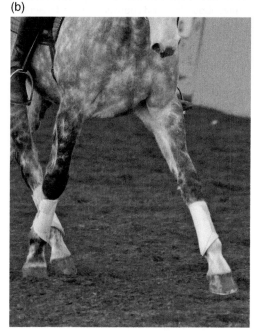

Figure 11.2 (a) Training the horse to go forwards or backwards is a matter of reinforcing the biomechanical responses of protraction and retraction of the limbs. (b) Training the horse to turn the forelimbs, hindlimbs or both requires reinforcement of abduction and adduction of the limbs.

on the direction of the limb in the stance phase, as compared with the swing phase (Figure 11.3).

The Stance Phase and the Swing Phase

When the limb is in contact with the ground, it is said to be in the *stance phase*. This phase

begins at impact and ends at lift-off (Clayton, 1989) and refers to any moment of ground contact that occurs during locomotion (Figure 11.3). The stance phase supplies the power for locomotion, which results from the horse exerting forces against the ground produced by the action of the muscles. Generally, the angle of the limb to the ground in the stance phase is an indicator of the direction in which the hoof is pushing against the ground. Friction between the hoof and the ground allows locomotion to happen. Gaits are characterised by repetitive cycles of limb movements known as strides (Clayton, 1989). In biomechanics, the event demarcating the start and end of successive strides is the moment of impact of a hindlimb on the ground.

The *swing phase* defines the period when the leg is not in contact with the ground (Figure 11.3). While the swing phase supplies no power to the horse's locomotion, it nonetheless has an important effect on locomotion in that its velocity and magnitude can vary so that the power of the subsequent stance phase is altered. Additionally, in all gaits, the swing phase is not only concurrent with the stance phase of the contralateral limb, its velocity is proportional to the power that the contralateral limb exerts in its stance phase. Thus, the velocity and magnitude of the swing phase reflect changes in impact velocity and power of the contralateral limb in the stance phase (unless the horse is lame). The larger swing phase of the leading forelimb at canter reflects the greater power of the non-leading forelimb in effecting acceleration and turns towards the direction of the leading leg. For trainers, identifying the swing phase is important for efficient and ethical training, because this phase of the limbs provides the optimal moment to make changes in speed or direction. During the swing phase, the limb is free of external mechanical limitations and the neural motor circuitry is free to adjust the limb kinematics and dynamics. That said, in the stance phase, strong mechanical proprioceptive constraints predominate (Maes and Abourachid, 2013). This biomechanical information suggests

(a) (b) (c)

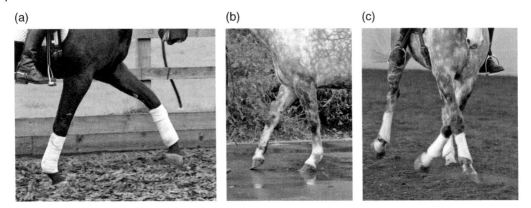

Figure 11.3 (a) When the horse goes forwards, protraction of the limbs occurs in the swing phase, while retraction of the limbs occurs in the stance phase. (b) When the horse steps backwards, the opposite occurs. (c) On the other hand, going sideways is conferred by consecutive abductions and adductions of the forelimbs and hindlimbs in swing and stance phases.

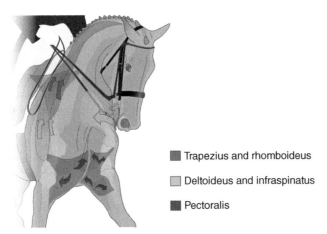

■ Trapezius and rhomboideus

☐ Deltoideus and infraspinatus

■ Pectoralis

Figure 11.4 Locomotion requires certain muscles to move the limbs and other associated muscles to stabilise them.

that the optimal moment to stimulate movement in a limb is at the onset of the swing phase and it is likely that this window of opportunity diminishes towards the end of the swing phase. This may explain why trainers as early as Grisone (1550) believed that the walk is the preferred gait for education. The walk provides the optimal training gait, because the swing phase can be more accurately targeted. Many current trainers continue to emphasise the value of training basic responses at walk.

Stabilising Muscles

Some muscles that contract for specific movements are *mostly* responsible for that movement, with other muscles playing a lesser role. If you think of protraction as the opposite to retraction and abduction as the opposite to adduction, it is easy to understand that during stance-phase retraction, the protractive muscles are not flaccid but are active to some extent in that they stabilise the limbs (Figure 11.4). During stance-phase protraction, the retraction muscles stabilise the limb. The same stabilising effect occurs during abduction and adduction. Without the antagonist muscles, the limbs would be unstable and uncontrollable.

The Mechanics of Locomotion

Going forwards, backwards, changing direction and going sideways are a result of what the limbs are really doing when they move and subsequently make ground contact. Horses are considered very cost-efficient movers (Minetti *et al.*, 1999). In each gait, horses at liberty move at a preferred speed that correlates with the minimum cost of transport (i.e. energy spent per unit body mass and distance moved) for that gait (Hoyt and Taylor, 1981; Wickler *et al.*, 2001; Griffin *et al.*, 2004), with walking being the overall most economical gait in horses (Reilly *et al.*, 2007). Also, even though being unguligrade (walking on hooves) is generally considered to be an adaptation for speed (Walker and Liem, 1994), Reilly *et al.* (2007) suggest that it seems to have evolved in horses to make walking more cost-efficient rather than making running gaits cheaper, as unguligrade limbs serve as supreme pendulums. Furthermore, gait transitions in horses at liberty seem to occur at a speed that maximises metabolic economy, presumably triggered by a system of biomechanical and metabolic factors (Wickler *et al.*, 2003; Griffin *et al.*, 2004). In the absence of human interference,

when carrying increased weight, inter-gait transitions occur at progressively lower speeds (Farley and Taylor, 1991).

Forward and Reverse

Going forward implies retraction in the stance phase and protraction in the swing phase. When going forward, retraction has already begun before the limb makes ground contact (Back and Clayton, 2001; Pilliner *et al.*, 2002). This allows some limb velocity to be generated before ground contact to minimise loss of power when ground contact is first made. On the other hand, reversing means that the protracting limb is in the stance phase while the retracting limb is in the swing phase.

It is likely that, while slowing down, horses may decelerate relatively passively, in that their momentum simply peters out with each stride. Alternatively, the horse may slow using the energy of *active protraction in the stance phase* (Figure 11.5). Such active transitions

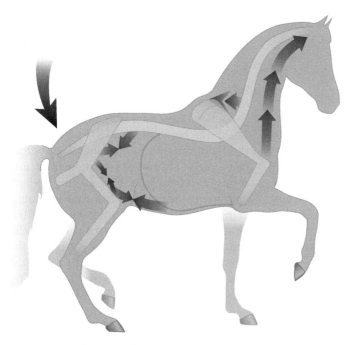

Figure 11.5 The lowering of the croup that is the hallmark of collection is first seen in the stop response when the hindlegs increase their role in deceleration. The muscle groups used are the sub-spinal, sub-lumbar, abdominals and others, such as the *iliacus* and the *psoas*. In addition, the raised head in collection raises the foreleg through the connection of the *brachiocephalic* muscle to the humerus of the foreleg.

may occur with abrupt deceleration (e.g. sliding stops), which are necessary in sports such as polo, campdrafting, cutting, and mounted games. The biomechanics of reversing and actively slowing are little studied. In dressage, transitions are typically required in a smooth rhythm within three beats of the relevant gait (McGreevy and McLean, 2007). Argue and Clayton (1993a,b) describe transitions in dressage as either Type 1, where there are no intermediate steps in between, say, walk and trot, or Type 2, where there may be some intermediate steps, such as a shorter broken trot step. They found that in walk and trot transitions, Type 1 transitions characterised the more highly trained dressage horse, whereas Type 2 transitions between trot and canter showed no association with level of training. More research must be undertaken here, where the transitions are signalled by the rider at precisely the same moment. For example, if the rider were to initiate the transitions when the outside foreleg began the stance or swing phase, it is likely that the number of footfalls could be measured from the beginning to the completion of the transitions. This would allow a standardised measurement of the transition from initiation to completion for research purposes.

Changing Direction: *Turns of the Forelegs*

Turning the forelegs allows changing direction and moving on curved lines, including circles. Alterations in direction generally result from recurring sequences of abduction/adduction or adduction/abduction of the forelegs. At any moment during a turn of the forelegs, one of the pair that is abducting or adducting will be in the swing phase while the other is in the stance phase.

However, there may be associated differential alterations in acceleration and deceleration that may also facilitate turning. Horses may lean in when turning and this may be especially apparent in the faster gaits, such as canter and gallop. When horses turn by leaning in, the actions of the legs involve acceleration rather than significant amounts of abduction and adduction. In sports that require turns at high speeds, such as campdrafting, polo, and all racing codes and games, leaning in may be the predominant form of turns, instead of, or including, large degrees of abduction and adduction of the forelimbs (and hindlimbs).

Training a horse for the sport of dressage requires an upright horse (on the vertical plane) at all times, and leaning in (i.e. the opposite of uprightness) is avoided; each hoof should make contact with the ground squarely. The cavalry history of this sport meant that armoured soldiers required horses to stay vertical and carry as much weight as possible on the hindquarters, so dressage training requires that turns begin with abduction before adduction so that the execution of movements, such as half-pass and pirouette, begin appropriately. For example, during a correct turn to the right, the first step is an abduction of the right forelimb in the swing phase with a simultaneous abduction in the stance phase of the left forelimb (this limb drives the turn). The next step involves the right forelimb adducting in the stance phase while the left forelimb adducts in the swing phase (Figure 11.6). In dressage, the discrete biomechanics of the turn of the forelegs require the use of the reins for optimal achievement of stimulus control.

In the forequarters of the horse, powerful abduction muscles facilitate fast turns at speed; the horse drives itself in a turn from the large muscles of the outside shoulder (the *trapezius*, *rhomboideus*, *deltoid* and *infraspinatus* muscles) by abducting the limb opposite to the direction of the turn. Reining, campdrafting and polo horses owe their abilities to turn suddenly to the powerful abduction muscles, which explain the heavily built shoulders that characterise the best of these equine athletes. This greater power of abduction in the horse's forelimbs contrasts with primates (including humans), who required greater adductive power for arboreal locomotion. Unlike humans, horses do not have clavicles (collarbones) for attachment of the adductors. The horse does not require a collarbone as its limbs move predominantly fore and aft. In equids, the clavicle is represented by a tendon within the *brachiocephalic* muscle.

On a curved line or a circle greater than 6 m in diameter, what is known to dressage trainers as 'bend' occurs when the hindlegs fall into the line of the foretracks (Figure 11.7). On circles smaller than 6 m, it is difficult for the hindlegs to step into the foretracks owing to the poor ability of the horse to bend its thoracic and lumbar vertebrae. Of course, commensurate with the tightness of the turn, there is generally a symphony of protraction/retraction blended with abduction/adduction.

Changing Direction: *Turns of the Hindlegs*

The horse is also able to change direction by *turning the hindlegs*. When hindlegs and forelegs turn simultaneously, turns are more rapid because the degree of direction change is increased. These dual turning abilities are adaptive for a prey animal during escape procedures. Such turns characterise sports that require rapid alterations of direction, such as reining, campdrafting and polo. However, in dressage, simultaneously opposing turns of the forelimbs and hindlimbs are not

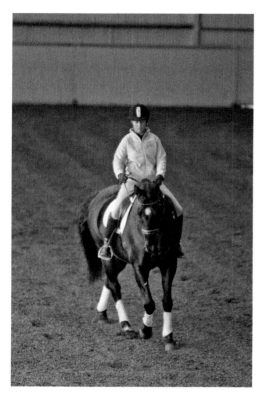

Figure 11.6 *Turning the forelegs* involves consecutive abductions and adductions. Smooth turns are a result of a consistent tempo and stride length during these biomechanical actions.

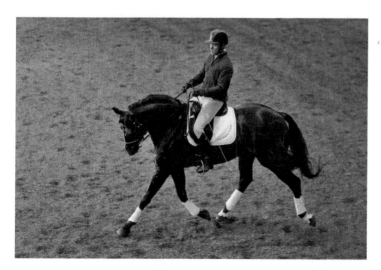

Figure 11.7 In the sport of dressage, horses are required to step into their foretrack line with their hindhooves on all curved lines greater than 6 m in diameter. This means that the vertebral column of the horse should show some flexion, which is known in dressage nomenclature as 'bend'.

prescribed, because of the requirement to maintain a significant proportion of weight directly on the hindquarters, a central precept of the sport.

For correct *turns of the hindquarters* in dressage, adduction of hindlimbs must come before abduction. The first step of a hindlimb turn begins with a simultaneous adduction of both hindlimbs, one during the swing phase and the other during the stance phase. Adduction of the hindlimbs is then followed by abduction, and so on (Figure 11.8). In other words, the hindlegs cross and then open. Note that *turns of the hindlimbs* differ from those of the forelimbs in that forelimb turns involve abduction first, whereas hindlimb turns involve adduction first. Again, the direction is a result of whether the adductions and abductions are in the swing phase or in the stance phase. For example, stepping sideways with the hindlimbs to the left involves a simultaneous adduction in the swing phase of the right hindlimb with an adduction in the stance phase of the left hindlimb, followed by abduction.

Changing Line: *Sideways*

When forelimbs and hindlimbs turn in the same direction and to the same extent, the horse goes sideways (i.e. it changes line but does not change direction). Because going sideways results from turns of both fore and hindlegs, it has the combined biomechanical characteristics of those turns. Therefore, the individual turns of the forelimbs and hindlimbs are generally trained first.

In reining, pleasure and trail classes, going sideways is called a side-pass, while in dressage training it is known as leg-yield. Sideways movements, such as leg-yield, that involve some forward movement as well as

(a)   (b)

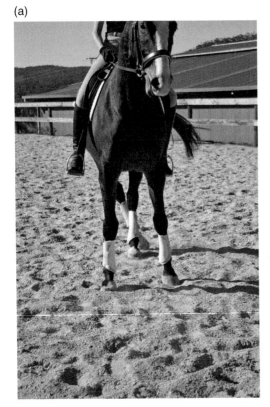 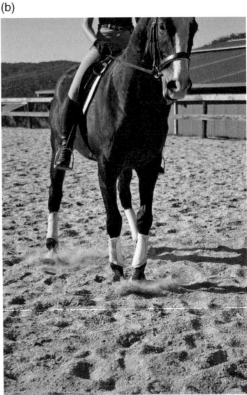

Figure 11.8 Turning with the hindlegs or going sideways involves consecutive adductions (a) and abductions (b). (Photos courtesy of Amelia Martin.)

going sideways, require a blend of abduction, adduction, retraction and protraction – the relative amounts of each depend on the steepness of the sideways movement. Early dressage training of leg-yield requires that the tracks from each hoofprint follow a 22-degree diagonal line (Figure 11.9). (A 22-degree line is represented by the KXM, HXF diagonal lines of the standard 60 m × 20 m dressage arena.) In more advanced training, the angle of lateral movements becomes steeper.

Consider a leg-yield to the left at walk. Because the walk begins with a foreleg, the first step of a left leg-yield will be by the abduction of the left foreleg in the swing phase and the simultaneous abduction of the right forelimb in the stance phase. Immediately following the abduction of the left forelimb, adduction during the swing phase of the right hindlimb occurs as well as the simultaneous adduction in the stance phase of the left hindlimb.

Transitions

The horse can make significant speed alterations by changing from one gait to another through walk, trot, canter and gallop. These alterations are termed *inter-gait transitions* (McGreevy and McLean, 2007). The horse is also able to effect speed changes within the gait, either by altering the speed of the legs or, alternatively, by lengthening or shortening the stride. These are termed *intra-gait transitions* (McGreevy and McLean, 2007). Riders and trainers generally and collectively group these transitions as either *upward* or *downward* transitions.

(a)

(b)

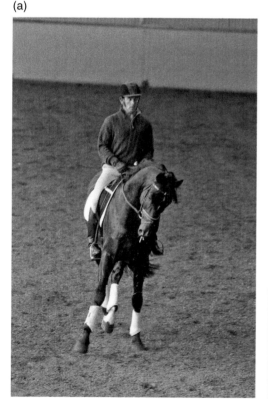
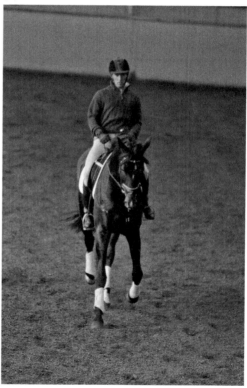

Figure 11.9 As with all training, it is much more efficient to shape and consolidate the required behaviour gradually. Therefore, when the horse is learning to leg-yield, simply going sideways (a) is rewarded at first, regardless of whether the horse is straight in its vertebral column or not. Straightening (b) is dealt with later. (Photos courtesy of Amelia Martin.)

The Gaits

The purpose of the gaits is to provide speed within the parameters of energy efficiency. A gait can be defined as 'a complex and strictly coordinated, rhythmic and automatic movement of the limbs and the entire body length of the animal, which results in the production of progressive movements' (Barrey, 2001). Gaits can be classified according to symmetry. Walking and trotting are symmetrical gaits, where left and right footfalls are evenly spaced in time. In contrast, canter and gallop are asymmetrical gaits, where the right and left limbs move in a dissimilar way. Gaits can also be defined by the presence or absence of a suspension phase (Barrey, 2001). Suspension is the period when all four limbs are in the swing phase (Clayton, 1989). Walking gaits have no suspension phase.

Gaits are commonly described as 2-beat (trot, pace), 3-beat (canter) or 4-beat (walk, ambling gaits and gallop), which corresponds with the number of footfalls or beats that can be heard within each stride. Most riding horses have three natural gaits, although in Anglophone countries, there is additionally a distinction made between canter and gallop, as an increase in speed leads to a progressive shift from the three-beat rhythm in canter to a four-beat rhythm that is considered to be a separate gait, the gallop (Figure 11.10):

- **Walk** (a four-beat gait);
- **Trot** (a two-beat gait);
- **Canter** (a three-beat gait); and
- **Gallop** (a four-beat gait).

Some breeds, known as gaited breeds, are genetically predisposed to exhibit other gaits, such as pacing (an alternating bilateral

(a)

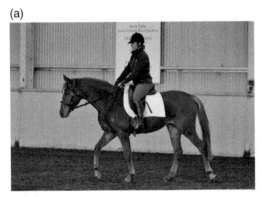

(b)

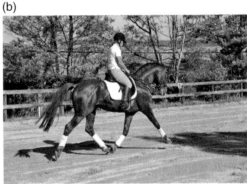

(c)

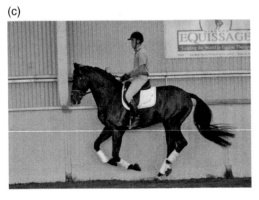

(d)

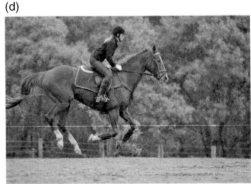

Figure 11.10 Each of the four gaits, (a) walk; (b) trot; (c) canter and (d) gallop, has different beat and suspension characteristics, although the shift from a canter to a gallop may be a gradual one, leaving it open to debate whether these two should be considered as two distinct gaits or just an alteration of rhythm within one gait. (Photos courtesy of Amelia Martin.)

two-beat gait shown by some harness-racing horses and some Icelandic horses) and/or ambling gaits, such as tölting (in Icelandic horses, a rapid alternating unidiagonal four-beat gait similar to the walk), and racking (similar to tölting and found in some breeds in the Americas). While most horses with a genetic predisposition to these extra gaits readily show the gaits at liberty, some may require extensive training to be able to exhibit the gait under a rider. Also, unlike with the walk and trot, gaited horses are frequently able to gradually shift the rhythm of the ambling gait towards the rhythm of either trot or canter, which places special demands on the trainer, if the desired goal is to achieve distinct gaits.

Walk

The walk is an alternating transverse four-beat gait. When the horse is standing relatively squarely, the first leg to leave the ground is a foreleg. Beginning with the left foreleg, the sequence of steps is LF, RH, RF and LH (Figure 11.11). In the walk, each limb typically strikes the ground at a rate ranging from 50 to 60 beats per minute (Clayton, 1995). In synchrony with the walk, the horse's neck extends and contracts. For this reason, the rider's hands follow this movement and should also move forward and back, otherwise, the walk becomes stilted. In a stilted walk, the flexions of the limb joints are differentially altered. This effect may be particularly visible in dressage horses that have been bred and are trained to show a large degree of overtrack (i.e. in a free walk, the horse's hindhoofs step several hoof-lengths in front of the track of the corresponding front limb). Only a diligently forward-moving horse with a relaxed back can produce these movements, which is why such a walk is highly valued in dressage. However, it is questionable whether such an extreme overtrack is adaptive under more natural living conditions, as it appears to be safer for a horse to step with its hindhoofs exactly into the tracks of the forehoofs. With a longer walk, such as in a free or extended walk, the

rider's hands should show the largest magnitude of movement. Nevertheless, measurements of rein tension during riding show characteristic, gait-specific, periodic peaks (e.g. Kuhnke *et al.*, 2010), indicating that riders typically do not completely follow the horse's movement and thus do not maintain an equal contact as would be ideal for the preferred clarity of signals.

Trot

The trot is a symmetrical, diagonal two-beat gait in which the limbs form diagonal pairs. There is a period of suspension between each diagonal pair of limbs. The sequence of footfalls is RH + LF and LH + RF. In some specific postures and circumstances, the diagonal pairings are slightly asynchronous, which is known as diagonal advanced placement (DAP) and is discussed later. At trot, each pair of limbs typically strikes the ground at a rate ranging from 70 to 80 beats per minute (Clayton, 1994a). In the trot, the neck does not extend or contract during locomotion as it does in the walk and canter.

Canter

The canter is an alternating uni- or bi-diagonal three-beat gait with a period of suspension after the third beat. The footfalls of the canter, with the right foreleg leading, are RF, LH and RH + LF. As in the trot, there may also be some DAP of the single diagonal pair of limbs under certain conditions. In canter speeds required for dressage, the limbs or the pair of limbs strike the ground at rates ranging from 70 to 110 beats per minute (Clayton, 1994b). The canter is thus the most variable gait in speed.

The canter is an asymmetrical gait, because the three beats comprise a leading hindleg, then a diagonal pair (foreleg + hindleg), followed by the leading foreleg and terminating with a moment of suspension. When horses at liberty turn in the canter (or gallop), they generally prefer to lead with the inside foreleg. The non-leading foreleg has a shorter swing phase than the leading foreleg and this

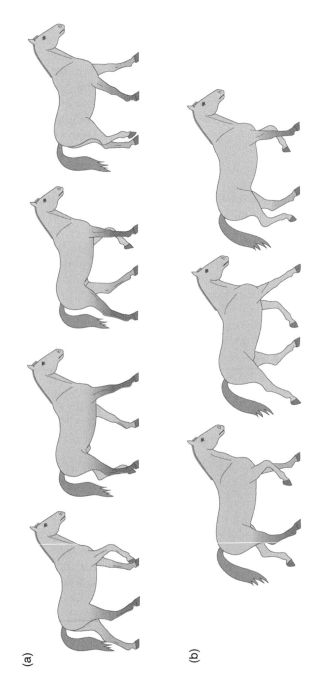

Figure 11.11 The cycle of limb movements at walk (a), trot (b), canter (c), transverse gallop (d), tölt (e) and pace (f). Colour coding shows right (red) and left (blue) weight-bearing limbs.

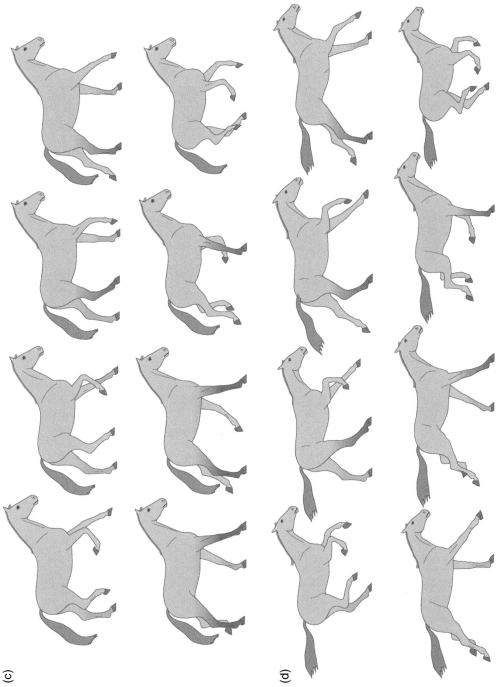

(c)

(d)

Figure 11.11 (Cont'd)

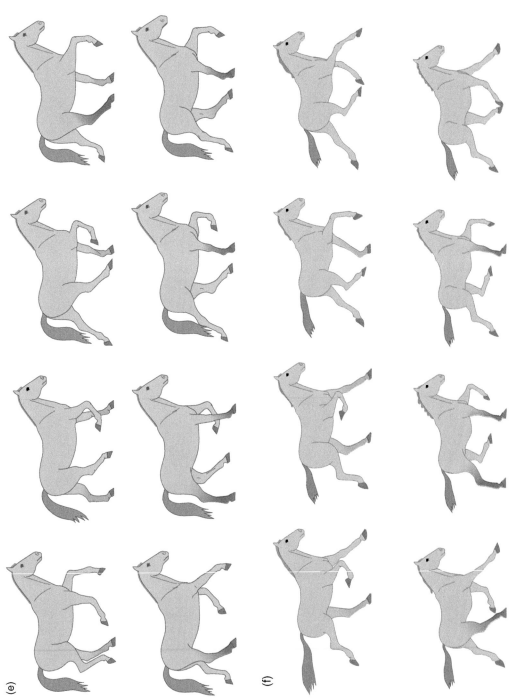

(e)

(f)

Figure 11.11 (Cont'd)

asymmetry probably confers different stance phase characteristics on the forelegs. It is likely that this arrangement facilitates efficient turning, since counter-canter (cantering on a circle with a leading *outside* leg) is difficult for most horses. Counter-canter is more difficult to achieve under-saddle than 'true canter', because during counter-canter the leading foreleg now takes the role of abduction in the stance phase.

In the changes of various gaits into the canter, the initial limb to begin the canter differs. Decarpentry (1949), with the benefit of moving film, was the first to describe this. For example, he found that when the horse makes the transition from trot to canter, the first limb to begin the canter is the leading forelimb. However, when the horse makes the change from one leading leg to the other in the canter (a flying change), the first limb to begin the new canter is the outside hind. This has implications for the signals used in training and retraining. For example, to execute a flying change, any signal should target the new outside hindleg immediately following the suspension phase.

Gallop

The gallop is a four-beat gait derived from the preceding gait, the canter. It is similar to the canter except that the speed is greater and the diagonal pair of legs is separated. Speed is the product of the dual components of stride frequency (SF) and stride length (SL) and can be estimated as follows: Speed = SF × SL (Barrey, 2001). Stride length increases linearly with the speed of the gait, while stride frequency increases non-linearly (Leach and Cymbaluk, 1986).

The sequence of limbs in the gallop is generally transverse (Figure 11.12); however, in fatigued horses or where the forelimbs change before the hindlegs, rotary gallops may be seen (Barrey, 2001). In both rotary and transverse gallops, the hindlegs follow each other sequentially; in a transverse gallop, the third limb placement following the preceding hindleg is the opposite foreleg, followed by the final foreleg. Thus, the first foreleg is contralateral to the preceding hindleg. A typical transverse gallop sequence with the right foreleg leading is LH, RH, LF and RF. A transverse gallop on the left lead is RH, LH, RF and LF. A rotary gallop, on the other hand, follows a rotary sequence of footfalls and can be clockwise or counterclockwise depending on the leading leg. A rotary gallop with a leading right foreleg has a clockwise sequence of RH, LH, LF and RF, while a rotary gallop with a leading left foreleg is counterclockwise, LH, RH, RF and LF.

Pace

The pace is a two-beat gait that bears similarities to the trot, except that the unilateral rather than diagonal pairs of legs are moved almost simultaneously (Figure 11.11). As with the trot, there is a suspension phase between the stance phases of each pair of legs. There are only a few breeds of horses capable of producing a racing pace, such as some harness-racing horses and Icelandic horses. Recent research revealed that it is a mutation in a single gene that predisposes a horse to show this additional gait (Andersson *et al.*, 2012).

One study suggests that the mutation apparently first occurred in the UK, from where horses were brought to Iceland (Wutke *et al.*, 2016) and other parts of the world. Today, the 'gait-keeper' mutation is present in various breeds all over the world, with 68 of 141 investigated breeds possessing this mutation (Promovera *et al.*, 2014). Harness-race horses that are homozygous for this mutation earn more prize-money over their lifetimes (Andersson *et al.*, 2012), compared to horses heterozygous for this mutation. These findings, along with the fact that the mutated allele is fixed in both American Standardbred pacers and trotters (Andersson *et al.*, 2012), suggest that the mutation makes horses capable of maintaining a symmetrical gait at a high speed rather than switching to a gallop (Promovera *et al.*, 2014), which is generally the preferred gait for high speeds in horses lacking this mutation.

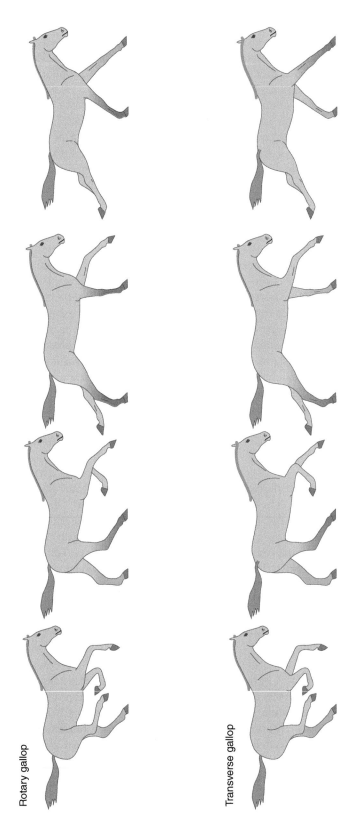

Rotary gallop

Transverse gallop

Figure 11.12 Horses may make a transition from a transverse to a rotary gallop during fatigue or when lead changes are initiated by the forelimbs. The footfall sequences of a rotary gallop are similar to those of a disunited canter.

In its desired form, the pace is ridden or driven at racing speeds, although a similar pattern of footfall, with a reduced suspension phase, or none, may occur as a result of tension and inappropriate interference by the rider with the horse's movements, especially during the walk. Unlike the racing pace, this form of pace is highly undesirable, because originates from in tension rather than being a naturally present movement pattern. With Icelandic horses, the transition to the pace is commonly ridden from a gallop, as it is difficult, with most horses, to achieve a correct transition from other gaits. In contrast, with harness-racing horses, the transition is instead made from a walk because the gallop is generally discouraged in harness-racing horses as it leads to elimination if shown during a race.

Ambling Gaits (Tölt, Rack, Running Walk, Paso, Marcha, Fox Trot, Stepping Pace, Single Foot, etc.)

Ambling gaits are four-beat gaits that show marked, breed-specific differences in rhythm, including regular 4-beat-rhythms as well as lateral and diagonal ambling. Ambling gaits can vary in speed, but are typically faster than a walk and slower than a gallop. The ability to perform an ambling gait seems to be linked to the same genetic mutation that is responsible for the ability to pace, although in contrast to the pace (e.g. typical of an Icelandic horse), a single variant of the mutation is sufficient for a horse to be able to perform an ambling gait. A large number of breeds, such as the Icelandic horse (Figure 11.13), Paso Fino, Peruvian Paso, Mangalarga Marchador, Rocky Mountain Horse, American Saddlebred, Tennessee Walking Horse, Missouri Fox Trotter and the Marwari, possess the ability to perform ambling gaits. Probably due to difficulties that gaited horses have with showing a clear gallop, Przewalski horses along with most sporthorse breeds rarely show any form of ambling gaits (Andersson *et al.*, 2012). In contrast to the non-gaited breeds that typically show distinct rhythms of the gaits walk or trot, many gaited horses are capable of

rather gradually shifting the rhythm of one gait towards the rhythm of another, so that differences between individual gaits may become blurred. A horse's and rider's individual weight distribution and balance also play a role in the rhythm offered by a horse, and shifting the horse's balance by placing the rider's weight differently on the horse's back or by adding weighted shoes or boots, may induce a horse to maintain a more desired rhythm. Future research in this area will be valuable to trainers of gaited horses seeking to gain a better understanding of how different factors influence the horse's movement characteristics.

Jumping

Jumping obstacles occurs mostly at the canter and gallop, although riding at the trot is important to establish self-carriage and good technique. Clayton (1989) describes three functional phases of the jumping effort: the approach phase; the jump phase (including take-off, jump suspension and landing subsets); and the move-off phase (Figure 11.14). She proposed that the approach strides themselves can be labelled so that approach stride 2 precedes approach stride 1, and so on. Similarly, the move-off strides can be labelled as move-off stride 1, 2, and so forth. This approach allows for a systematic analysis of jumping kinematics. For example, labelling each stride allows description of the characteristics of a precise stride.

Barrey (2001) described the footfalls of the jumping effort as the trailing hindleg and leading hindleg at take-off, the airborne phase, followed by the trailing foreleg, then leading foreleg in the landing phase. At take-off, the canter or gallop mechanics are altered so that the hindlegs are more synchronised than before to allow more power in the take-off (Barrey, 2001). The airborne phase is a long dissociation of the diagonal during which a lead change can take place. Many jump trainers, as well as dressage trainers, use this phase in training flying changes. Indeed, some trainers use a pole on the ground to increase the period of suspension

(a)

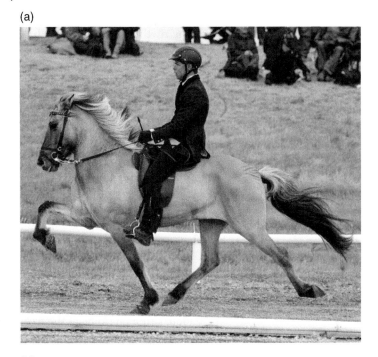

(b)

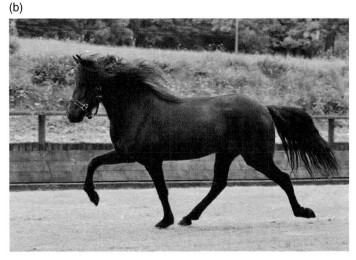

Figure 11.13 Icelandic horses showing the typical one-leg (a) and two-leg (b) support phase of a tölt under a rider (a) and at pasture (b). (Photos courtesy of Igelsburg Verlag.)

and so increase the likelihood that a flying change will occur when the trailing hindleg is stimulated by the rider's new outside leg or whip-tap to initiate a new canter stride. The trailing hindleg is the first leg to begin the new canter stride (Back and Clayton, 2001).

The correct posture of the horse during the jumping effort should be parabolic (Figure 11.15) so that the topline is involved in the jumping arc. A good jumper raises both knees evenly, and evenly flexes both knee joints of the front legs. A lowered foreleg is thought to be associated with errors such as unevenness in rein contact. The hindlegs should tuck up high and, at the peak of jumping elevation, the horse may kick out with both hindlegs. Mistakes with the hindlegs are thought to be associated

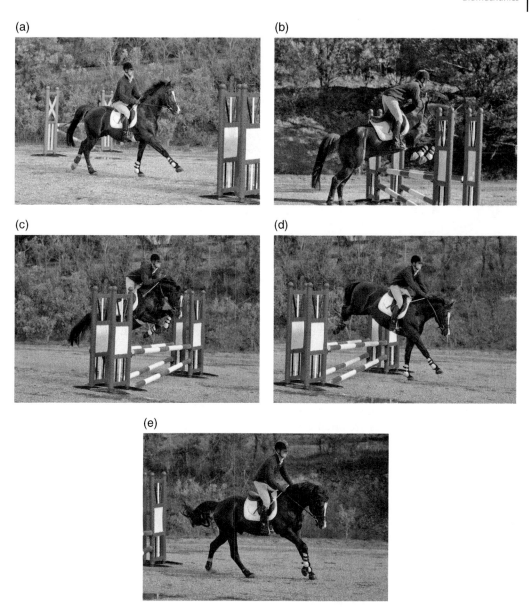

Figure 11.14 The three phases of jumping: (a) the approach phase; the jump phase (including (b) take-off, (c) jump suspension, (d) landing subsets); and (e) the move-off phase.

with the rider's seat and posture, such as sitting up too early.

The Central Pattern Generator

When a foal is born, the gaits are already present. The diagonal pairs are also in place in the trot and canter. The diagonal connections of the horse's legs apply further, so that in all gaits, there is more-or-less diagonal duplication. For example, in the four-beat walk, a longer stride of the right hindleg is associated with a longer stride in the left foreleg, and so on. Similarly, during turns, when the right foreleg abducts, the contralateral hindleg tends to adduct. Thus, a sharp left turn of the forelegs results in a sharp right turn of the hindlegs. Though undesirable in dressage for reasons mentioned earlier,

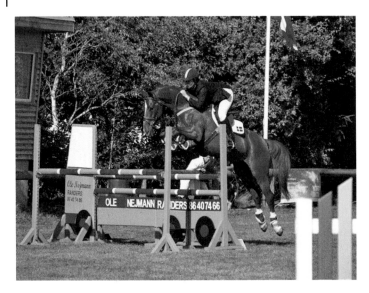

Figure 11.15 Show-jumping trainers aim to train horses to take off close to the obstacle and thus to make the shape of the jumping effort parabolic, rather than longer and flatter. This shape (also known as a bascule) requires the horse to arch its neck and flex its back and allows it to jump as athletically as possible. (Photo courtesy of Susan Kjaergard.)

this diagonal synchrony is clearly adaptive for wild equids under predatory pressure in that it confers faster changes of direction. Trainers, coaches and riders are often aware of this diagonal mirroring effect: in a trained horse, a certain threshold of tension on a rein will turn the forelegs one way and hindlegs the other.

The diagonal connectedness, contralateral synchrony and maintenance of gait rely on a type of neural circuitry, called a neural oscillator, which coordinates limb movements. These neural oscillators are also known as central pattern generators (CPGs) (Gramsbergen, 2001) (Figure 11.16) and, to some extent, they are independent from the brain. It has long been known that when the spinal cord is severed, alternating trunk and limb movements can still occur. Gramsbergen (2001) reports that, while locomotion is initiated in the mesencephalic brain stem, fibres project to the CPGs located in the spinal cord itself. He surmises that CPGs are among the first neural circuits to develop in neuro-ontogeny and tend to remain largely unaltered throughout life.

The existence of CPGs implies that movements in the forelimbs are more-or-less reflected in the hindlimbs. Furthermore, the

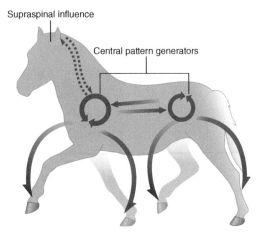

Figure 11.16 The central pattern generators (CPGs) are directly responsible for the precise synchronisation of the limbs in each gait. For example, in the trot they coordinate the alternating sequence of diagonal couplets.

forelimbs may have greater significance in locomotion than is currently believed by modern horse-trainers, in that the CPG of the forelimbs directs the hindlimbs. For example, studies in altricial neonates, such as rats, suggest that forelimb locomotion precedes hindlimb locomotion (Gramsbergen, 2001), which is known as the cephalocaudal gradient. This may have implications in quadrupedal ungulates, such as horses, in the neural connections and sequences of the various gaits. For example, many dressage trainers attempt to maintain the hindquarters behind the forelegs to achieve straightness (hindhooves into foretracks), instead of the approach of more enlightened trainers who recognise that gaining precise stimulus control of the forelegs in deceleration and turns automatically results in straightness (Kyrklund, 1998; McGreevy and McLean, 2007; McLean and McLean, 2008). In addition, the complex circuitry of the CPGs also extends to coordinating both forelegs and both hindlegs in terms of velocity, and therefore power, of the swing in synchrony with the stance. Thus, a fast swing phase in the right forelimb converts to a more powerful stance phase in the left forelimb.

The Vertebral Column

The amount of mobility of the horse's vertebral column is a significant issue for equitation. The cervical vertebrae of the horse's neck are very mobile laterally and dorsoventrally. It is well known in the discipline of dressage that problems of balance arise when the horse's neck is carried to one side. Because the head and neck make up around 10% of the horse's total bodyweight, a neck bent and carried to one side adds extra weight to that foreleg, adding to its adductive power in the stance phase and causing falling-in or falling-out. For this reason, neck straightness is a high goal in dressage and many trainers adhere to the maxim that the neck should not express more bend than the rest of the horse's vertebral column.

The thoracic and lumbar vertebrae of the horse is much less flexible than generally believed (Jeffcott and Dalin, 1980). While objective studies on the degree to which a horse is capable of bending are lacking, Faber *et al.* (1999; 2000; 2001a,b) studied the dorsoventral bending, lateral bending and axial rotation characteristics of the equine spine at walk, trot and canter (Figure 11.17). They reported

Maximal ranges of motion

Vertebral Movement	Walk	Trot	Canter
Dorsoventral + / −	7°	5°	16°
Lateral + / −	5.5°	3.5°	5°
Axial + / −	13°	3°	8°

Figure 11.17 Dorsoventral flexion/extension, lateral bending and axial rotation are characteristics of the equine thoracolumbar column in walk, trot and canter (Faber *et al.*, 2001a,b).

that lateral bending of the thoracolumbar vertebral column occurred only to a small degree and that the amount varied with the gait. Dorsoventral movement was greatest in the canter, while lateral bending was greatest in the walk. The greatest amount of axial rotation was found to occur at walk. In studies of canter conducted on a treadmill, they reported that bending occurs chiefly in two places: T10 and L1 (with less consequential movement at S3). While dressage prescribes that horses should evenly bend the vertebral column laterally when ridden on curved lines, we should be mindful of the variable bending capabilities of different sections of the vertebral column (Figure 11.18).

Roundness

Roundness refers to the arched head, neck and apparent dorsoventrally rounded body posture acquired by the horse in correct dressage training. It is characterised by self-carriage where the horse has learned to persist in his speed, directional line, and head, neck and body posture without support from the rider. However, roundness is frequently a forced response where the rider increases tension on the reins until the horse shortens its neck, or uses concurrent rein tension and

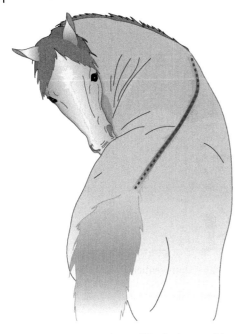

Figure 11.18 Horses have difficulty in scratching their rumps with their teeth owing to the limitations of lateral bending of the thoracic and lumbar vertebrae compared with the cervical vertebrae.

leg pressures to 'drive the horse onto the bit' (Chapter 12, Unorthodox Techniques). Although this is contrary to the tenets of classical and ethical dressage, it provides the illusion of roundness and collection and is known as false collection. However, dressage experts, can readily perceive the incorrect outline, where the neck is shortened and the loins are hollow. The result is that the rider's tight control on the reins to maintain this posture and the incorrect neck and back muscles involved prevent correct development of the topline. There are significant welfare issues surrounding such training, which manifest in a raft of problems ranging from tension and conflict behaviours to wastage.

In correct training, the horse's head should be suspended from his withers in self-carriage and the weight in the rider's hands should be the weight of the reins and a light connection to the lips and tongue of the horse. Such lightness is the putative goal of Baroque training styles and modern ethical training. It is imperative that, from the horse's

viewpoint, pain is escapable and controllable, so lightness, of course, is important for the horse at every stage of training, and those methodologies that embrace correct round-ness training and constant self-carriage are more correctly aligned with the correct application of learning theory than coercive methods.

Collection

The horse at liberty carries most of its weight on the forelegs, so untrained horses carry themselves on the forehand in an apparent downhill way of going. Collection implies an uphill way of going (Clayton, 2004). It is characterised by a highly arched neck where the poll is the highest point and the topline physique of the horse is highly developed. The collected horse has learned to lower its hindquarters using a combination of muscles, including the abdominal and sub-lumbar muscles, which increases the engagement of the hindquarters (Clayton, 2004). The development of collection redresses the previously mentioned downhill situation, where the hindquarters now step in advance of a line dropped from the stifle (Pilliner *et al.*, 2002) and lower. However, measurements in high-level dressage horses showed that under a rider at either a walk (von Peinen *et al.*, 2009) or a collected trot (Weishaupt *et al.*, 2009), nearly 60% of the weight is still carried by the forelimbs. Changing from the collected trot to passage (i.e. inducing a yet higher level of collection) led to a shift of about 5% of the weight to the hindlegs (Weishaupt *et al.*, 2009).

A collected posture is said to put the horse in a stronger position to engage its hindlegs while carrying a rider (Figure 11.19), and the resulting shift in the horse's centre of mass may make the rider's weight cues more effective, allowing the rider to further reduce the intensity of the cues. It is also commonly thought that a more collected way of moving is, due to the reduced forces acting through the forelimbs, healthier for the horse. Notably, however, horses used for dressage are at greater risk of suffering from problems of the

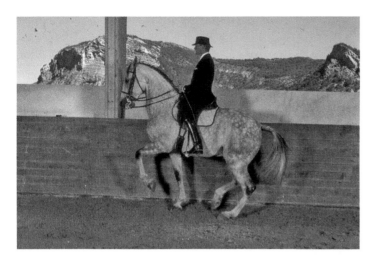

Figure 11.19 Collection involves a shift of weight from the horse's forehand to its hindquarters. This shift is a function of altered stride kinematics and joint flexion of the hindlegs, flexion of the horse's lumbar vertebrae and raising the head and neck. This posture is a prerequisite for all higher dressage movements. (Photo courtesy of Cadmos Verlag and Philippe Karl.)

locomotory system, compared to horses used for other disciplines, such as show-jumping or hacking (König von Borstel *et al.*, 2016a), which typically place less emphasis on collection. It would be interesting to investigate whether these differences are, for example, a result of the higher range of limb motion typically shown by selectively bred dressage horses and higher wear-and-tear resulting from these movements, or if unskilled riders using incorrect techniques when attempting to achieve the postures and movements desired in dressage also contribute to these figures.

While it has generally been supposed that collection is mainly a product of the hindquarters being lowered, Clayton (2004) points out the greater significance of the sling muscles (*serratus ventralis*, *pectorals* and *subclavius*) of the horse's forequarters and the muscles in the upper part of the forelimbs. Tension in these muscles raises the forequarters, increasing the uphill posture of collection.

The relevant hindleg muscles are also developed by the extra weight carried by the hindlegs and the more anterior steps. The net torque of the hamstrings arises from three major attachment sites: the caudal aspect of the hip (extensor torque), stifle (flexor torque) and hock (extensor torque), so variations in thrust probably arise from variations in the contributions of different components of the hamstrings (Clayton, 2007, personal communication). In addition, the sub-spinal and sub-lumbar muscles, the *psoas* and the *iliacus*, are also likely to make a large contribution to collection. This may be one reason that collection must be trained gradually: the symphony of muscles used in its expression differs from typical propulsion and must, therefore, be gradually strengthened.

As collection develops, a quality known as cadence also appears. The concept of cadence is derived from music, where it identifies a rhythmical motion accentuated by a pause. The period of suspension is at its greatest during the progressive development of collection leading ultimately to passage and piaffe. This suspension makes for a clear pause of the horse's legs in the swing phase, which is known as *cadence* (Figure 11.20). The current debate surrounding the dressage training style called hyperflexion (where the horse is induced to hyperflex the cervical vertebrae to the point where its nose almost touches its chest) includes some criticism of the less fluid cadence of horses trained in this way (Chapter 12, Unorthodox Techniques). Classical dressage purists claim that it is an artefact of tension.

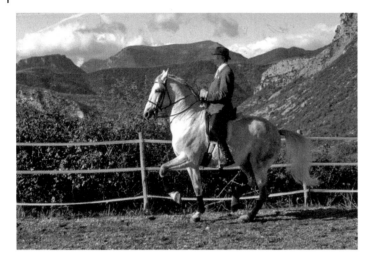

Figure 11.20 Cadence is the term ascribed to the accentuated suspension phase in the collected trot and its derivations (piaffe, passage). (Photo courtesy of Cadmos Verlag and Philippe Karl.)

Muscular Development Effects of Horse Sports

Collection is a result of the physical development of particular muscles, including the dorsal (topline) muscles; it is *not* a quality that can be quickly produced by forcing a particular neck outline. Because of the weight of the horse's forequarters, including the head and neck, significant muscular effort is required to support them. The nuchal ligament and the muscles at the base of the neck, such as the *trapezius*, are attached to the muscles of the back (*latissimus dorsi*). The withers act as a fulcrum. When the horse moves, there is increased tension on the back as well as the topline of the neck and this tension is exacerbated during transitions. During downward transitions, the effects of deceleration and gravity on the horse's descending head and neck place excessive pressure on the muscles of the back. With repetitions, these transitions strengthen and have an anabolic (muscle-building) effect on the topline muscles of the back. On the other hand, with inertia during upward transitions, the back muscles exert extra pressure on the associated neck muscles, which contributes to their development also.

As velocity increases, the effects of transitions are greater in the development of the topline. Indeed, with every doubling of speed, the tension on the topline and limbs quadruples. This is expressed by $E = {}^1/_2\, mv^2$, where the energy involved (E) is equal to half the mass (m) multiplied by the velocity (v) squared. This equation has profound effects for the dressage horse in terms of muscular tension and subsequent development. Because the increase in muscular effort has an anabolic effect, the anabolic requirements for the increased physical development of the dressage horse are proportional to the various speed loads it has been subjected to during training. Thus, it is the transitions at higher speeds (e.g. collected canter to extended canter and *vice versa*) that have the most anabolic effects compared with transitions at walk or trot. For these reasons, the development of the collected physique is a gradual process, beginning with increments in impulsion. The risks of conflict behaviours and subsequent wastage are high if the young horse is forced to adopt such an outline in its early development.

As the correctly trained dressage horse develops, the limb muscles for collection increase in tone and this is likely to have an effect of bringing the hindhooves closer to the forehooves, where the horse now shows the more collected posture described as 'sitting'. On the other hand, horses that are used in horse trials, racing, polo, games and reining, predominantly rely on their hamstrings for speed, and these horses tend to show the stance known as 'camped out', where the hindhooves during immobility stand farther from the forehooves. The shoulder muscles of the correctly trained reining horse also reveal considerable mass and tone.

Diagonal Advanced Placement (DAP)

The term 'diagonal advanced placement' (DAP) is used to describe the interval between the diagonally paired foreleg and hindleg making contact with the ground. It has a positive value if the hindleg meets the ground before the foreleg, and negative if vice versa (Figure 11.21). A DAP value of zero tells us that the diagonal pair contacts the ground simultaneously. A positive DAP arises when horses move with an elevated forehand and this is said to indicate good balance (Holmström *et al.*, 1995). In passage, diagonal pairs move with two well-defined suspensions in every stride, and large positive

DAPs have been recorded. The DAP tends to take on the largest positive values in the most successful contemporary dressage horses.

Interestingly, data from the Seoul Olympics showed that 15% of the extended trot strides analysed had a negative DAP (Deuel and Park, 1990). In the same event, the DAP for piaffe in several horses was negative (Argue, 1994; Holmström *et al.*, 1994), but the highest placed horses had a positive DAP (Clayton, 1997). The existence of DAP has been central to arguments in the current hyperflexion debate. Sometimes it has been implied that any DAP, positive or negative, signifies incorrect training and lack of self-carriage. Preliminary results (unpublished data from Nierobisch, 2016) suggest that there is no direct correlation between the degree of dissociation of front- and hindlimbs in the swing phase and the angle of the horse's noseline, but the angle of the noseline *per se* may not be a good measure of correctness of training (Weishaupt *et al.*, 2016). Unfortunately, in the data collected so far, there has been no quantitative rein tensiometry to test the veracity of the claims one way or the other. There is scope for more research on this topic.

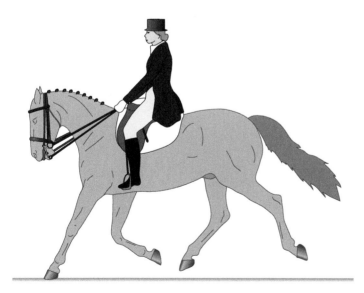

Figure 11.21 Negative DAP occurs when the foreleg begins its stance phase before its diagonal hindlimb. Positive DAP is when the opposite situation occurs: the hindlimb begins its stance phase before the forelimb.

Take-Home Messages

- The horse has four locomotory responses (acceleration, deceleration, turning with the forelimbs and turning with the hindlimbs) that are the basis for all movements in-hand and under-saddle.
- Achieving stimulus control of the forelegs in deceleration and turns automatically results in straightness. This directly contradicts the widely held but erroneous belief that straightness is a result of the hindhooves tracking into the foretracks.
- The thoracic and lumbar spine of the horse are much less flexible than is generally believed.
- In optimal training, the horse should be in self-carriage, and the weight in the rider's hands should be no more than the weight of the reins plus a light connection to the horse's lips and tongue.

Ethical Considerations

- Incorrect training methods that promote concurrent rein tension and leg pressures being used to 'drive the horse onto the bit' result in false collection and compromise the welfare of the ridden horse. Such reduction in welfare may manifest as conflict behaviours and ultimately lead to wastage.

Areas for Further Research

- Characterisation of the transitions between gaits and how these are affected when the rider initiates the cue for a transition.
- Investigation into the relationship between stress levels and cadence, or lack thereof, especially with regard to the reduced cadence that accompanies hyperflexion of the neck.
- Measurement of the relationship between DAP and training methods.

12

Unorthodox Techniques

Introduction

This chapter examines some potential sources of compromised welfare in ridden and non-ridden horses. The practices involved are unusual or radical, and some of the interventions we cover are popular but not orthodox.

Of the practices discussed here, the most confusing to horses are those that apply contradictory pressures (e.g. that send the horse forward while simultaneously halting it). Even without using mechanical devices, riders can coerce their horses to assume certain gaits and postural responses. In equestrian parlance, the horse is said to show lateral flexion, vertical flexion and longitudinal flexion (Figure 12.1), noting that the term 'longitudinal flexion' may confuse some veterinary readers, since it describes what they would call extension. Some of the ways in which these types of flexion can be achieved can compromise horse welfare. This chapter is intended to demonstrate how, although such techniques may bring some short-term benefits to the rider, they are likely to have deleterious long-term side-effects (and also short- and medium-term) for the horse.

Simultaneous, Contradictory Pressure

Perhaps the most insidious and widespread of all unorthodox techniques is the concurrent stimulation of two opposing operantly conditioned signals, such as reins (the *stop* response) and legs (the *go* response). This concurrent signalling places the horse in a biomechanically impossible situation, because the muscles it uses for *go* forward and *stop* are antagonistic so, again, the result is a detraining effect. Detraining is not just a matter of losing the 'brakes' or 'accelerator', the subsequent confusion can induce conflict behaviours in horses. Like all animals, horses seek to avoid pain. When they are prevented from doing so (e.g. when trapped between reins and legs), they become hyper-reactive, using *active* coping mechanisms. They are actively trying to escape, but escape is thwarted. Hyper-reactive escape behaviour switches to other active coping strategies such as hyper-reactive predator-removal behaviours (e.g. bucking, rearing and shying). In a milder form, hyper-reactive responses as a sequel to thwarted escape behaviour may manifest as more exaggerated movements, such as a higher amplitude of leg motion in the trot, which may be perceived as more expressive movements by a lay audience. Perhaps because of the audience's reactions, such movements produced by contradictory pressure are sometimes rewarded by judges. Clearly, there is a need to distinguish between expressive movements that are the result of the horse's natural range of movement plus proper training and development of a horse's self-carrying ability, and those that are the result of attempts to cope with contradictory pressure. Active coping mechanisms share similar characteristics and brain pathways as

Equitation Science, Second Edition. Paul McGreevy, Janne Winther Christensen, Uta König von Borstel and Andrew McLean.
© 2018 John Wiley & Sons Ltd. Published 2018 by John Wiley & Sons Ltd.
Companion website: www.wiley.com/go/mcgreevy/equitation

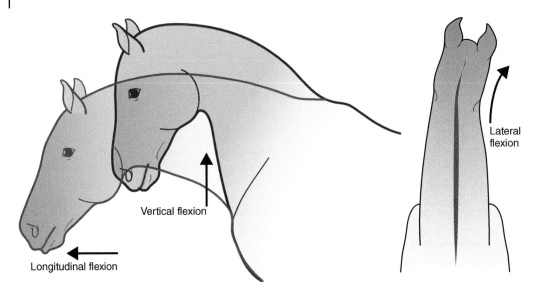

Figure 12.1 Longitudinal (neck extension), vertical (poll raised) and lateral flexion as used in equestrian (rather than veterinary) parlance.

cutaneous pain: in rats, they include hyper-reactivity, increased vigilance, raised heart rate and raised blood pressure (Keay and Bandler, 2008).

If the pain persists over a sufficiently long period, and the horse cannot resolve it, hyper-reactive behaviour can progress to passive coping behaviours, where the horse is now hypo-reactive and seemingly gives up. Its bucking and shying may diminish, but the horse is heading towards learned helplessness, where it is, on the surface at least, careless about pain. Internally, the horse may show all the physiological signs of chronic stress. Passive coping states such as learned helplessness show similar characteristics and brain pathways as deep visceral pain: hypo-reactivity, apathy, decreased vigilance, lowered heart rate and lowered blood pressure (Keay and Bandler, 2008).

Inducing Confusion by Using One Signal for More than One Response

When young horses undergo foundation training, they learn that increased tension on a single rein is the signal for *turning* the forequarters by a process of abduction of the forelegs (in equestrian parlance, this rein signal is known as the direct *turn* signal or opening rein). It is an important early response, because during challenging moments the reins, among an array of other classically conditioned signals such as seat or postural signals, provide the deepest signals that can induce the *turn*. So, maintaining the integrity of the basic operantly conditioned response is important for safety. However, it is now common for many trainers and coaches to use the single rein not for its original locomotory response, but simply to bend the horse's neck in an exaggerated fashion as a way of stopping the horse instead of using or re-training the operantly conditioned foundation response of equal tension on both reins. Forcing the horse to bend its neck from rein tension blurs the distinction between cues for an effective change of direction and simply bending the neck. This is because the signal is the same or similar while the response is different, with the result that the turn is detrained. The same can be said of using both reins to achieve the 'on the bit' head and neck posture at the expense of slowing.

Forcing the 'On the Bit' Head and Neck Position

In many horse sports, head and neck posture resulting from the relative positioning of the cervical vertebrae and the atlanto-occipital joint is given high priority and is typically manipulated via rein tension (Figure 12.2). It is common to see the horse's neck either extremely flexed (c) or extended (d) in a wide range of activities, including (but not limited to) cross country, dressage, driving, reining and show-jumping. Although over-bending does occur in nature, it lasts for only brief periods. Sustained over-bending, however, is becoming increasingly common for the ridden horse. A so-called broken neck (Figure 12.3) is not a reference to a fractured vertebral column but a description of how horses with their necks flexed artificially by force appear to show the greatest amount of flexion at the junction of cervical vertebrae 4 and 5. An abrupt change in the longitudinal flexion can

be seen in the crest of horses undergoing this intervention.

A horse is said to be over-bent when it carries (or is forced to carry) its nasal plane behind the vertical. At this point, minimal further flexion is possible. If the horse has been forced to show this flexion by rein tension or resistance in the rider's hands when it attempts to extend its neck, it can do nothing more to get relief from the pressure in its mouth. This leads to deficits in training (i.e. the quality of the *slow/stop/step-back* responses declines) and subsequent conflict behaviours result from the confusion. This technique may be carried out because riders are unaware of the correct neck outline that is required by the sport of dressage (nasal plane at or just in front of the vertical line). The correct posture is an emergent property of the correct shaping of both the operant rein tension and leg pressure responses. Instead, many contemporary riders use increasingly strong rein tension until the horse brings its mouth towards the rider's hands and thus

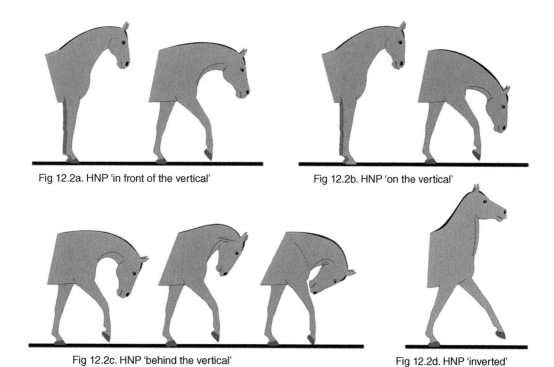

Fig 12.2a. HNP 'in front of the vertical'

Fig 12.2b. HNP 'on the vertical'

Fig 12.2c. HNP 'behind the vertical'

Fig 12.2d. HNP 'inverted'

Figure 12.2 (a), (b), (c) and (d) Head and neck postures (HNP) with different dorso-ventral flexions. (Illustrations by Cristina Wilkins, courtesy of ISES.)

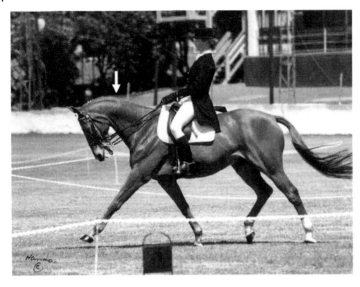

Figure 12.3 A horse with a so-called broken neck (arrow indicates the abrupt change in the positions of cervical vertebrae 4 and 5 relative to one another). (Photo courtesy of Sandy Hannan.)

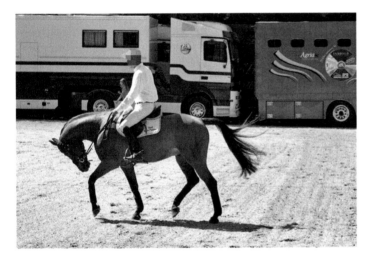

Figure 12.4 An example of a horse being hyperflexed under-saddle. (Photo courtesy of Julie Taylor/EponaTV.)

shortens its neck in an attempt to relieve bit pressure. This neck-shortening is believed by many to be an acceptable practice to achieve the required head and neck outline.

Hyperflexion (Rollkur)

Rollkur or, as it is known by the Fédération Equestre Internationale (FEI, 2006), hyperflexion, describes the technique where the horse's neck is dorsoventrally hyperflexed by bit pressure to the point where the horse's chin may even touch its pectoral region (Figure 12.4). Proponents of this method claim that they shape this response gradually and that the horse is ridden in this frame for only short periods. They attest to biomechanical benefits of this outline in inducing greater flexion of the hock joints. However, many observers have described long durations, and question how this technique might achieve greater flexion of the hock joints.

The veterinary committee of the FEI has stated that hyperflexion of the neck is a degree of longitudinal flexion of the mid-region of the neck that cannot be self-maintained by the horse for a prolonged time without welfare implications. Furthermore, it has stated that hyperflexion as a training tool must be used correctly, as the technique can be an abuse when attempted by an inexperienced/ unskilled rider/trainer. However, to date, there is limited evidence that a horse's or rider's training and skill levels have any significant effect on observed welfare implications of this technique. Instead, signs of reduced welfare are observed regardless of performance levels (König von Borstel *et al.*, 2015).

Hyperflexion is believed to decrease stride length and increase elevation of the hindlimbs, while also increasing the dorsoventral oscillation of the lumbar vertebrae (van Weeren *et al.*, 2006). Certainly, its current prevalence among elite dressage competitors strongly suggests that it lends some competitive advantage in that its use must help to produce a performance the judges wish to see. But, significantly, it is a practice that would detract considerably from scores if it were used in competition itself. Instead, it appears as part of the warm-up routine at many elite events. A literature review and meta-analysis revealed a number of gymnastic effects of this practice (König von Borstel *et al.*, 2015). Of the 55 reviewed studies, 35 investigated aspects related to gymnastics. Approximately one-quarter (26%) of these studies concluded that training in hyperflexed head and neck postures has beneficial effects on gymnastic attributes, while another 23% concluded that it has detrimental effects on gymnastic attributes. The results within the remaining studies were inconclusive. The gymnastic attributes that have been investigated relate to changes in breathing, the workload of specific muscles, overall workload, kinematics: performance marks and so-called submission.

As far as breathing is concerned, several studies showed evidence of airway obstruction during hyperflexion (van Erck-Westergren, 2011; Go *et al.*, 2014 a,b,c; Zebisch *et al.*, 2014b), leading, for example, to increased inspiratory pressure but not to arterial hypoxemia (Sleutjens *et al.*, 2012). The workload

in muscles most notably affects those of the so-called topline. The brachiocephalicus is more active, while the trapezius, splenius and rectus are less active in a hyperflexed head and neck posture, indicating that horses' neck muscles are being trained in an undesirable way for riding (i.e. strengthening the ventral, commonly known as underline, rather than dorsal, commonly known as topline) neck muscles (Kienapfel and Preuschoft, 2014; Kienapfel, 2015). Observed changes in overall workload are based on measurements of lactate concentration and heart rate, and some studies suggest that overall workload is increased by a hyperflexed head and neck posture (Sloet van Oldruitenborgh-Oosterbaan *et al.*, 2006; Wijnberg *et al.*, 2010).

Meanwhile, the reported kinematic changes related to increased back motility (Rhodin *et al.*, 2005; Gomez Alvarez *et al.*, 2006; Kattelans, 2012) and limb motility (Rhodin *et al.*, 2009; Kattelans, 2012), while step length decreased (Weishaupt *et al.*, 2006; Waldern *et al.*, 2009; Ludewig *et al.*, 2013) and stride duration increased (Weishaupt *et al.*, 2006). While some of these effects are considered desirable in the interest of more expressive movements, they may also put the horse at a higher risk of injury (Rhodin *et al.*, 2009). Also, with most studies, significant differences were limited to specific situations (e.g. one but not the other gaits, Weishaupt *et al.*, 2006), and other studies failed to find significant changes in these parameters when investigating horses with a rider rather than without one (Rhodin *et al.*, 2009).

Performance marks and evidence of so-called submission depend somewhat on the level of competition. Marks were either lower, no different or higher, when horses were ridden or warmed-up in hyperflexed head and neck postures (Kienapfel *et al.*, 2014; Lashley *et al.*, 2014). Rideability in young horses was judged to be superior when horses were ridden with the horse's cranio-facial profile behind the vertical (König von Borstel *et al.*, 2011a), potentially because these horses were considered to be more submissive.

While overall the gymnastic benefits remain rather obscure, a review of the welfare implications of this practice reveals a much clearer picture. Of the reviewed studies (König von Borstel *et al.*, 2015), 42 evaluated impacts on welfare, and 88% of these studies concluded that hyperflexed head and neck postures negatively affect equine welfare. Results of the remaining studies were inconclusive, with only one study (van Breda, 2006) suggesting welfare advantages of training horses in hyperflexion.

In particular, hyperflexed head and neck postures have been shown to cause upper airway obstruction (van Erck-Westergren, 2011; Sleutjens *et al.*, 2012; Zebisch *et al.*, 2014b). Airway obstruction is a serious welfare concern, as it leads to shortness of breath, which is known to be highly aversive to animals due to the associated respiratory effort as well as the distinct sensations of air hunger and chest tightness (Beausoleil and Mellor, 2014).

There are also pathological changes in the structures of the neck – flexion of the neck leads to changes in neck length (Kienapfel and Preuschoft, 2011) and intersegmental angles of cervical and thoracic vertebrae (Clayton *et al.*, 2010; Fjordbakk *et al.*, 2013). Pronounced flexion leads to an increase in intervertebral foramina dimensions which, according to Sleutjens *et al.* (2010), potentially leads to interference with nerve function. Furthermore, flexion leads to an increase in lamella sheet width, resulting in increased tension in elastic structures (Nestadt and Davies, 2014), such as the nuchal ligament origin (Elgersma *et al.*, 2010). According to Weiler (2002), this increased tension results in insertion desmopathies, which can be observed in dressage horses that have been trained in flexed and hyperflexed head and neck postures.

In addition, there is evidence of impaired vision (Harman *et al.*, 1999; McGreevy *et al.*, 2010). Inability to see the ground towards which the horse is moving may lead to anxiety (von Borstel *et al.*, 2009) and/or attempts to achieve frontal vision by turning the eyeball (Bartos *et al.*, 2008; von Borstel *et al.*, 2009). However, the horse's ability to do so has only been demonstrated with flexion that results

in a vertical cranio-facial profile (Bartos *et al.*, 2008), but it is not clear if horses can further turn their eyeballs to obtain frontal vision with more flexed head and neck postures.

Finally, there is evidence of stress and anxiety due to physiological compromise and rider intervention necessary to achieve the hyperflexed head and neck posture (von Borstel *et al.*, 2009, Christensen *et al.*, 2014) and due to confusion caused by conflicting signals and inability to escape pressure (McLean and McGreevy, 2010a). These negative effects are expressed through behaviours indicative of conflict (Caanitz, 1996; von Borstel *et al.*, 2009; Kienapfel, 2011; Ludewig *et al.*, 2013; Hall *et al.*, 2014; Kienapfel *et al.*, 2014; Zebisch *et al.*, 2014a), avoidance behaviour/responses (von Borstel *et al.*, 2009), enhanced/stronger fear reactions (indicative of heightened states of anxiety, von Borstel *et al.*, 2009) and reluctance to move forward (Gomez Alvarez *et al.*, 2006; von Borstel *et al.*, 2009). As a result of this reluctance to move forward, more rider interventions are necessary (von Borstel *et al.*, 2009; Christensen *et al.*, 2014; Smiet *et al.*, 2014) which, in turn, further increase discomfort as evident from increased levels of behaviour indicative of conflict. Depending on the study design, changes in physiological stress parameters, such as cortisol concentrations (Christensen *et al.*, 2014; Zebisch *et al.*, 2014a), eye temperature (Hall *et al.*, 2014), heart rate (Sloet van Oldruitenborgh-Oosterbaan *et al.*, 2006; von Borstel *et al.*, 2009) and heart-rate variability (Smiet *et al.*, 2014), also indicate elevated stress during hyperflexion.

A meta-analysis (König von Borstel *et al.*, 2015) of these studies revealed that welfare concerns were detected regardless of the duration the posture is applied, the method used to achieve the posture, the horse's level of dressage training, the horse's prior experience with hyperflexion, and the horse's breed (a factor closely related to head-neck conformation). So, this cross-study comparison suggests that the posture compromises equine welfare even if the horses are accustomed to it and its application, and even when they are exposed to it for only a short period.

Contraction

An illusion of collection can be created simply by shortening the neck (Figure 12.5). Horses trained to do this are likely to offer this response when they are subjected to pressure from the bit. The problem is that the same or dangerously similar pressure from the bit should be *slowing* the horse (a basic operant response typically trained during foundation training). The result can be a horse that has habituated to rein signals (i.e. a horse with a desensitised mouth) that on some occasions may be a bolter. False collection is said to occur when there is no significant change in elevation of the withers relative to the hindquarters.

Rapping

Rapping (Chapter 9, Horses in Sport and Work) is the technique of hitting a horse's hindlegs as they pass over a rail during a jump (Figure 12.6). The dorsally directed strike, often achieved by raising a whip or cane at the height of the horse's trajectory, punishes it for jumping adequately and thus trains it to overcompensate when sizing-up fences. This is believed to make the horse more cautious when jumping and reduces

the risk of it hitting a fence when pushed in competition (e.g. when forced to flatten its trajectory while jumping against the clock). The main argument against rapping is that it punishes horses for making a correct judgment of the height of a fence. It is forbidden both at events and during training, but the ban is extremely difficult to enforce during training. While it is appropriate that the FEI takes a dim view of this practice, many observers feel that practices known to accompany dressage training (such as forcing the mouth shut with crank nosebands) are even more of a priority, because they are arguably harsher and certainly more relentless.

Gingering

Gingering is the use of irritants (traditionally, peeled ginger) *per rectum* with the aim of causing rectal discomfort. It is a practice known to occur in the show-ring, especially where high postural tonus (e.g. a raised tail carriage) is considered desirable. For this reason, it is more likely to be found in shows for Arabians than for other breeds. Considered a breach of the rules under most codes of showing, it is difficult to detect once the agent itself has been passed by defaecation. Inarguably, any manipulations

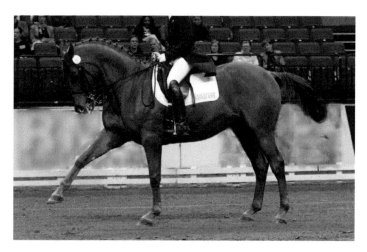

Figure 12.5 When strong rein tensions are used to produce a collected outline, false collection typically occurs with concomitant hyper-reactive associations and increasing levels of conflict behaviour. (Photo courtesy of Minna Tallberg.)

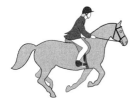

Figure 12.6 An illustration of the so-called 'rapping' technique, banned by the Fédération Equestre Internationale. It involves hitting the horse's hindlegs as it jumps a fence to make it allow greater clearance than each obstacle would seem to require.

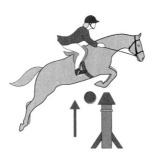

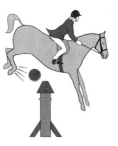

of the horse's tail carriage or conformation (including, of course, docking) should be undertaken only when there is a veterinary reason (Lefebvre *et al.*, 2007).

Soring

Damaging the skin of the pasterns with caustic topical applications and then fitting chains or beads so that they lie on the damaged tissue can cause extravagant lifting of the lower limbs and flexion of the fetlocks. This is practised in show classes where high limb action is highly desired (e.g. for Tennessee Walkers), but practices such as this are more likely to be controlled if veterinarians remain aware of them and prioritise the welfare of the animals in their care. Legislation may have outlawed many such interventions, but policing the rules relies on the cooperation of the veterinary profession. Detection depends on being able to correctly age any evidence of scarification on the horse's limbs; old lesions are not likely to cause current behavioural modifications and can easily be blamed on a previous owner, handler or groom.

Weighted Boots and Training Shackles

Some trainers use gear equipped with extra weights to increase the horse's muscular effort for a given movement, with the intention of increasing efficiency or speed of training.

Other manifestations of the same principle involve training horses in extra deep soil, such that the horse must make an increased effort to lift and move its legs. Weighted boots are also used on gaited horses to shift a horse's balance, thereby making it more likely that the horse will adopt a certain gait. While these training methods are not considered natural and fair by some, they do not necessarily deviate from the principles of ethical training, since they simply increase the effort required from the horse for any given movement. However, with added weights to the horses' limbs, there certainly is an increased risk of soft tissue injury, so when using these devices, a horse's levels of fitness and fatigue needs to be carefully monitored. Beyond these items of equipment that act passively on the horse by requiring more muscular effort for the movements, there are also devices designed to actively interfere with a horse's movements (e.g. by manually lifting the legs beyond a range of motion the horse would naturally offer) (Chapter 10, Apparatus). Apart from the risk that the horse may get entangled in these contraptions, there is clearly a risk that incorrect timing of such interventions with the horse's limbs may cause lasting disturbances in rhythm, if not fear and confusion.

Sedation and Nerve Blocks

Where a lack of reactivity in horses is highly prized in the show-ring (e.g. in Western pleasure riding), a raised tail carriage may detract from the horse's score. So, competitors may, surreptitiously, use nerve blocks or even neurectomy to reduce tail movement (Houpt, 2000). The tail may appear to be clamped between the hindlegs or suspiciously inactive, but detection is difficult and depends on the use of electromyography.

There are also numerous reports of competitors using psychopharmaceuticals (notably, sedatives) to make horses more tractable. One of the ironies of this practice is that the recipients of these treatments are often horses that have, just prior to the event,

been overfed with concentrates and so are less likely to be manageable. Over-feeding horses so that they look in top show condition and confining them to contain their energy and reduce the need to groom them merely increases their ebullience.

The practice of manipulating the behaviour of horses with pharmaceuticals (including fluphenazine, acepromazine and zuclophenthixol) is unethical and is rigorously monitored by the FEI. Nevertheless, even in local shows, competitors may be tempted to eliminate undesirable responses, usually ones that make the horse difficult to control. Largely confined to the show-ring, this intervention is also dangerous since it can affect the horse's ability to move safely and so is of great concern when it arises in jumping competitions.

Electric Training Devices (Shock-Collars and Spurs)

Electric shock-collars, which can be triggered remotely to release a discharge, have received considerable attention from animal trainers. Undesirable long- and short-term behavioural changes in dogs, notably those indicating distress (Schilder and van der Borg, 2004), and problems with the use of electric shock-collars in horse-training have been described (McGreevy and Boakes, 2007). Dogs that have received shocks (even remotely triggered shocks) begin to react fearfully towards their owners (who become a predictor of the aversive stimuli).

Electric spurs have been designed to avoid bodily injuries inflicted by conventional spurs. As such, to some observers, they give the impression of somehow being a more animal-welfare friendly training device, compared to conventional spurs. However, it should be kept in mind that, in the absence of classical conditioning to achieve a gradual refinement in cues, electric spurs are likely to be used such that they produce levels of pain comparable to that caused by conventional spurs that deform (and sometimes penetrate) the horse's skin. Clearly, such levels of pain are unacceptable in ethical horse-training, particularly if used with sustained intensity throughout the course of training. Thus, the risk of spurs being used with sustained intensity is considerable, as may be the case with electric spurs, because they do not produce visible lesions.

There appear to be two major problems associated with the use of electrical devices in training horses. First, perhaps due to the nature of an electric shock, which spreads throughout the entire body, animals sometimes appear to have difficulty relating the resulting aversive sensation to their preceding action, and so instead of being related to the animal's own actions, their consequent avoidance learning may be directed to other stimuli, such as the presence of the owner or particular locations. Second, under practical conditions, it is difficult to precisely control the intensity of the electric shock because environmental conditions, such as humidity in the horse's hair-coat, may influence electric conductance and thus the intensity of the shock perceived by the horse.

Electric shock-collars have also been used to punish crib-biting, but horses often moderate their stereotypic behaviour when wearing the collar only to resume it as soon as the collar is removed, sometimes with a transient increase in the response, possibly as the result of a post-inhibitory rebound (McGreevy and Nicol, 1998).

Horse-Walkers

Although a mainstream means of exercising stabled horses, horse-walking machines have come under scrutiny over concern that they are dragging machines that force horses to undertake locomotion. Notably, horse-walkers are commonly designed so that partitions can be electrified to ensure that horses avoid making contact with them. In many countries, national animal-welfare laws do not allow the use of electricity to force animals to move. Nevertheless, electrified walker-designs are persistently offered for sale, suggesting that they are commonly used in practice, at least when introducing naïve horses to horse-walkers. Other designs allow owners to tie-up horses within the walker by their headcollars. The implication that they merely pull horses seems to ignore the reality that these devices also feature rubber boarding that taps the horse's hindquarters should it begin to lag and that many people use walkers without tying the horse's head. Either way, and regardless of walker design, coercion is certainly involved but, paradoxically, the coercive forces may be more consistent than many trainers, and this may explain why horses' stress levels do not differ between the use of walkers with or without electricity (Giese *et al.*, 2014), and why, generally, accidents involving horse-walkers are rare.

The use of walkers (without electrified panels) in foundation training for horses, especially during backing, has been reported (Murphy, 2007). Effectively, it is a form of overshadowing in that the pressure of the headcollar that evokes a leading response is used to overshadow the pressure of the rider on the horse's back. There are concerns about the dangers to both horse and rider should a flight response emerge within this sort of assembly, which is clearly not designed with foundation training in mind.

Water-Deprivation

It is believed by some that depriving horses of water makes them appear more compliant. Certainly, clinical dehydration will compromise the ability of horses to show flight responses, many of which are seen in confused and poorly trained horses and few of which are desirable. Furthermore, as Xenophon (translated by Morgan, 1962) proposed, depriving a horse of water allows a trainer to use water as a reward. For example, this is seen in methods that advocate the imposition of dehydration as a valid step for remediating horses that refuse to be led into a trailer. Horses may have the ability to adapt to considerable periods with little water, but dehydration is highly questionable on ethical grounds and should never be advocated, since it can cause irreversible renal damage.

Conclusion

There are numerous questionable practices in current equitation. It is usually, but not always, easy to see why they might work, but the ethics and sustainability of their use are subject to continuing debate. If learning theory is applied correctly and no overly aversive stimuli are involved, methods that appear, at a first glance, unethical may be more welfare-friendly than many traditional training techniques. On the other hand, widespread training techniques that ignore the principles of learning theory can indeed be deleterious to horse welfare.

Take-Home Messages

- Horses are so behaviourally flexible that they will give the appearance of tolerating relentless pressure.
- Pressure can be used to force a horse to adopt a given posture in a time-frame much shorter than is the case in conventional training. However, in contrast to correctly trained responses, the results are not sustainable and the same amount of pressure must usually be applied each time the horse is required to adopt that posture again.
- If techniques compromise horse welfare and future trainability for short-term gains, they can be considered neither sustainable nor ethical.

Areas for Further Research

- Investigation into learned helplessness as applied to the ridden horse.
- Establishment of the range of rein tensions on a scale from neutral to aversive.

13

Stress and Fear Responses

Introduction

Stress responses have evolved to help animals overcome emergency situations under natural conditions. Thus, stress responses are adaptive when stressors are short-term. However, prolonged stress is costly in terms of energy and maladaptive (i.e. with negative consequences on, for example, health, reproduction, memory and learning). In this chapter, we will look at the concept of stress and two major classes of stressors that relate to horse-training: fear-eliciting stimuli and painful stimuli. Pain is interlinked with fear because once a horse has perceived a painful stimulus, that stimulus and similar stimuli are likely to elicit fear at future encounters.

The concept of stress was developed in the middle of the 20th century by Walter Cannon and Hans Selye, who were both investigating physiological reactions to harmful stimuli. They found that the body's reactions were approximately similar, regardless of the type of aversive stimulation: hunger, thirst, illness, fear, pain or heat. All resulted in relatively non-specific physiological reactions. These results led to the development of the *standard stress model* (Figure 13.1). According to this model, a stressor leads to two main sets of physiological reactions:

1) activation of the sympathetic part of the autonomic nervous system; and
2) activation of the hypothalamic-pituitary-adrenal axis (HPA-axis).

The central nervous system assesses whether a stimulus represents a significant challenge to the animal. If it is perceived as threatening (i.e. a *stressor*), the biological defence consists of a combination of behavioural, autonomic and neuroendocrine *stress reactions*, and the individual is in a *state of stress*. The body's immediate physiological reaction to a stressor is characterised by activation of the sympathetic system, which prepares the body for action. The fight or flight reaction of the sympathetic system is initiated by stimulation of the hypothalamus, which transmits signals via the reticular formation in the brain stem to the spinal cord to cause sympathetic discharge. This immediately results in several physiological changes, which lead to a greater physical and mental ability, so that the animal can perform more strenuous physical activity than would otherwise be possible (Korte, 2001). Sympathetic stimulation increases both the rate and force of the heart's contractions, as well as arterial blood pressure. Blood flow is redirected, with the blood vessels constricting to supply less blood to non-critical areas (e.g. the gut, which inhibits digestion) and more blood is directed to the skeletal muscles and the brain. The transmitter at the neuromuscular junction is noradrenaline, a close relative of adrenaline. These hormones and neurotransmitters prepare the body for bursts of physical exercise, for example, when about to flee from a threat (Sapolsky, 2002; 2004).

Equitation Science, Second Edition. Paul McGreevy, Janne Winther Christensen, Uta König von Borstel and Andrew McLean.
© 2018 John Wiley & Sons Ltd. Published 2018 by John Wiley & Sons Ltd.
Companion website: www.wiley.com/go/mcgreevy/equitation

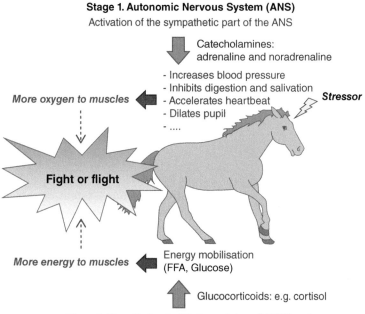

Stage 1. Autonomic Nervous System (ANS)
Activation of the sympathetic part of the ANS

Catecholamines:
adrenaline and noradrenaline

- Increases blood pressure
- Inhibits digestion and salivation
- Accelerates heartbeat
- Dilates pupil
- ....

Stressor

More oxygen to muscles

Fight or flight

More energy to muscles

Energy mobilisation
(FFA, Glucose)

Glucocorticoids: e.g. cortisol

Stage 2. Hypothalamic-Pituitary-Adrenal (HPA)-axis

Figure 13.1 The standard stress model. When the brain perceives a stressor, two main sets of physiological reactions prepare the body for bursts of exercise ('fight or flight') and activate a range of other reactions (e.g. reduced pain perception and immunological responses).

The sympathetic system is counteracted and modulated by the parasympathetic system, where the actions are principally opposite to those of the sympathetic system. The parasympathetic system becomes active when the body is engaged in processes relating to general body maintenance, such as eating and ingesting food. It slows the heart and respiration rates, and stimulates digestion and growth. The normal state of rest is predominantly characterised by parasympathetic activity. In stressful situations, the parasympathetic activity decreases in favour of a higher sympathetic activity, enabling the animal to react appropriately (e.g. with flight).

The second physiological stress reaction is characterised by the release of glucocorticoids (cortisol in horses) from the adrenal cortex. The hypothalamus produces corticotrophin-releasing hormone (CRH) and vasopressin (AVP). These hormones stimulate the pituitary gland to secrete adrenocorticotropic hormone (ACTH), which in turn activates the adrenal cortex to release glucocorticoids. The glycolysis in both liver and muscles increases and

blood glucose concentrations rise, facilitating energy availability over prolonged periods. The reaction of the HPA system takes a few minutes and is somewhat slower than the sympathetic response, which happens in a matter of seconds. Circulating corticosteroids reach a peak some minutes after an acutely stressful event (Korte, 2001; Sapolsky, 2004).

Together, glucocorticoids and the secretions of the sympathetic nervous system (adrenaline and noradrenaline) account for most changes in the body during stress. Other hormones are activated as well. The pituitary secretes prolactin, which plays a role in suppressing reproduction during stress. Both the brain and the pituitary also secrete endogenous morphine-like substances, *endorphins*, which help blunt pain perception (Sapolsky, 2004). Just as some glands are activated in response to stress, other hormonal systems are inhibited. The secretion of various reproductive hormones, such as oestrogen, progesterone and testosterone, is inhibited. Growth hormones are also inhibited, as is the secretion of insulin, which plays a role in energy storage (Sapolsky, 2002; 2004).

Perception of Stressors

Interestingly, the way an individual perceives a stressor is important to the severity of the stress response, so exactly the same external stimulus can induce different levels of stress. This was demonstrated by Jay Weiss in a series of experiments in which he showed that factors such as *predictability, control* and *outlet for frustration* modulates stress reactions (Weiss, 1972). Weiss exposed groups of rats to standardised mild electric shocks, which resulted in an increased rate of stomach ulceration (a typical measure of the severity of stress in rats), compared to rats that were placed in the same apparatus but did not receive any electric shocks (Figure 13.2a). Then Weiss gave one group of rats a warning signal (a beep) before the electric shock. Although these rats received exactly the same number of shocks as the unsignalled group, they developed significantly less

severe gastric ulcers. This difference was suggested to be caused by the *predictability* provided by the warning signal (i.e. if a stressor is predictable, it is perceived as less severe than an unpredictable stressor (Figure 13.2a).

In a follow-up experiment, Weiss gave one group of rats an opportunity to avoid or escape the electric shock by pressing a lever. Another group of rats served as paired controls, receiving the same number of shocks as their partners in the lever group when the rats failed to turn off the electricity. The only difference was that these rats did not have a lever (i.e. they had no *control* of the stressor). The latter developed significantly more severe gastric ulcers (Figure 13.2b).

In similar types of experiments, Weiss demonstrated that if rats are given a bar of wood to gnaw on, they are less likely to get ulcers compared to control rats that receive the same number of electric shocks. This happens because the rats have an opportunity for *outlet for frustration* and the same effects can be achieved if the stressed rat is allowed to eat or drink something, or sprint on a running wheel (Sapolsky, 2004).

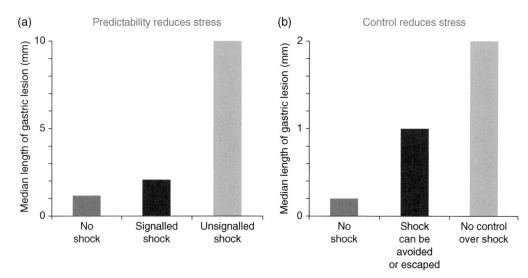

Figure 13.2 (a) Effects of predictability. Rats exposed to unsignalled mild electric shocks develop more severe stress-induced gastric lesions (ulcers) compared to rats that receive no shock and signalled rats that suffer the same number of shocks but receive a warning signal before it. (b) Effects of control. Rats that can show a behavioural response (lever-pressing) to avoid or escape the shock develop less severe ulcers than paired rats that get the same number of shocks but have no control. (Modified from Weiss, 1972.)

Another factor that affects the perception of stressors is *social support*. Humans and non-human animals that have social support from conspecifics during stressful events show reduced stress reactions (Lepore *et al.*, 1993; Gust *et al.*, 1996; Ruis *et al.*, 1999). In practice, this means that horse-trainers and riders have plenty of opportunities to modulate the stress-inducing effect of an aversive stimulus through giving the horse opportunity for *control, predictability, outlet for frustration* and *social support*.

It should also be noted that there is no simple division of stress into categories of 'good' and 'bad' stress (or 'eustress' and 'distress', as suggested by Selye (1979)). Any frequent stressor, including 'good' stressors (such as mating), can have a detrimental effect on an animal's welfare (Ladewig, 2000). Rather, stressors should be viewed as a continuum, from low to severe in intensity, occurring infrequently to frequently, with a short to chronic duration and with different opportunities (e.g. predictability and control) (Figure 13.3). Stress responses are adaptive and help the horse to overcome acute stressors. However, the combination of many/severe/frequent or long-lasting stressors may exceed the horse's capacity to cope, inducing problems that affect its health and learning. It should also be noted that not only external stimuli (e.g. electric shocks) but also lack of

fulfilment of behavioural needs (thwarted motivations) induce stress responses. Thus, a horse kept under appropriate conditions (fulfilment of behavioural and physiological needs) has more resilience towards stress induced by training and competition. Good management and housing can therefore be regarded as fundamental to optimal training.

Consequences of Prolonged or Chronic Stress

The body's stress reactions are ideal to overcome acute stressors, such as an attack from a predator, an aggressive conspecific, or short-term extreme weather conditions. Energy is mobilised and delivered to muscles and the most vital organs, pain perception is blunted and expensive anabolic processes are suppressed until the emergency situation is over. From this perspective, stress reactions are adaptive. On the other hand, we all know that stress can make us ill. This is because the body's stress reactions have evolved to overcome acute, physical stressors. These are the type of stressors that most organisms are exposed to in their natural environment. Stress-induced illness occurs when the body's alarm system is activated too often and/or for too long. If the body is constantly mobilising energy through breakdown of stored

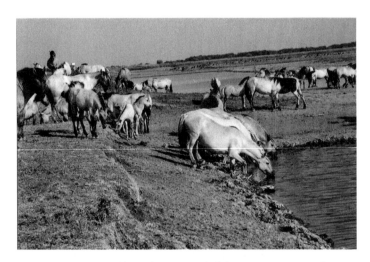

Figure 13.3 Horses at liberty have control of their environment to the extent that they can retreat or attack.

protein, it leads to breakdown of muscles and results in weakness and fatigue. Other negative effects of chronic stress include increased vulnerability to infections and gastric ulcers. In horses, a study involving Danish Warmblood horses used for either dressage or show-jumping reported a high frequency of gastric ulcers (e.g. 55% of 96 horses had glandular ulcers; Malmkvist *et al.* (2012) (Figures 13.4 and 13.5).

Reproduction is also inhibited by chronic stress. Circulating cortisol concentrations have an inhibitory effect on preovulation secretion of luteinising hormone, and thus results in a failure to ovulate (Nangalama and Moberg, 1991). Cortisol is also known to have a modulating effect on the release of other gonadotropins, such as follicle-stimulating hormone. From an evolutionary perspective, it makes good sense that chronic stress, caused by events such as low forage availability or high population density, reduces reproduction and therefore population growth rate.

One of the most complex issues in stress physiology is the interaction between stress and the immune system. It is well-known that glucocorticoids suppress the immune system (Sapolsky, 2002). However, there is actually a transient increase in immune function following a stressor, probably caused by activation of the sympathetic nervous system, and the suppressing effect of glucocorticoids

ensures the return to baseline. It is thus only during profound and long-lasting influence of glucocorticoids that the immune system is suppressed below baseline (Sapolsky, 2002). For example, Blecha (2000) has shown that HPA-axis activity in response to extreme environmental conditions or stressful management practices negatively affects the immune system. In addition, stress hormones affect the brain. Cortisol has a negative feedback on the HPA-axis at different levels, including in the brain. This feedback mechanism ensures that the concentration of plasma cortisol decreases after the acute stressor. Research has shown that long-term stress, via elevated concentrations of cortisol, can have a negative effect on the neuron number and the formation of new cells in the hippocampus with negative consequences for learning and memory (Morris, 2007).

Typical Stressors for Domestic Horses

Domestic horses can experience a wide range of internal and external stressors, including fear-eliciting and painful stimuli, and lack of fulfilment of biological needs, as well as psychological stressors, such as loss of control and predictability. One of the most common stressors in domestic horses

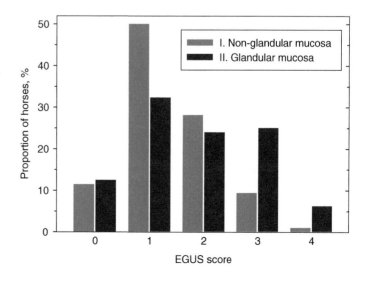

Figure 13.4 Occurrence of lesions in the glandular and non-glandular (squamous) mucosa in Warmblood riding horses (n = 96), according to the Equine Gastric Ulceration Syndrome score (EGUS). Horses with scores 2–4 are considered affected (i.e. 55% had lesions in the glandular mucosa and 41% in the non-glandular mucosa). (Modified from Malmkvist *et al.*, 2012.)

I. Non-glandular (squamous) mucosa

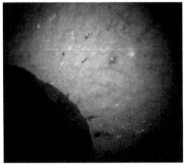

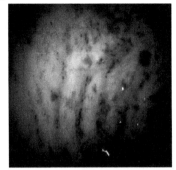

Healthy mucosa (EGUS score 1)

Extensive superficial lesions
(EGUS score 3)

II. Glandular mucosa

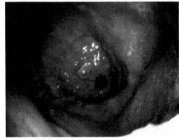

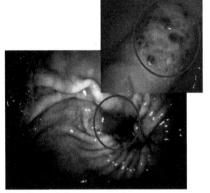

Healthy mucosa

Significant inflammatory changes

Figure 13.5 Examples of healthy and moderately affected mucosa. Lesions in the upper non-glandular mucosa may relate to inappropriate feeding with too little roughage. Lesions in the deeper, glandular part of the stomach have been related to chronic stress. (Photos courtesy of Nanna Luthersson.)

is social stress. Horses are sometimes stabled with limited social contact with other horses and research has shown that singly stabled horses have a strong motivation for social contact (Christensen *et al.*, 2002; Søndergaard *et al.*, 2011). Chronically socially isolated horses even show a depressed cortisol response on a CRF challenge test, suggesting a desensitisation of the HPA-axis (Visser *et al.*, 2008). Thus, keeping horses in social isolation is a severe stressor that will lead to physical and mental damage. Similarly, social instability may act as a stressor that increases aggression (Christensen *et al.*, 2011a). In summer, lack of appropriate shade and insect harassment are also typical stressors for horses (Holcomb *et al.*, 2013; Hartmann *et al.*, 2015).

Another significant class of stressors for domestic horses relate to training: when the training intensity is not adapted to the individual horse, when the rider is too heavy, when equipment is ill-fitting, when goals are unrealistic, leading to harsh training methods, and when trainers and riders are ignorant of correct application of learning principles. All these are examples of training-related stressors that may lead to significant welfare problems. Furthermore, several studies have shown that certain training methods are more stressful than others (e.g. hyper-flexed head and neck positions) (Christensen *et al.*, 2014; Zebisch *et al.*, 2014a). Transport can also be a significant stressor for domestic horses (Schmidt *et al.*, 2010a,b), and even though the horse has been habituated to transport, frequent transport and environmental change when taking part in competitions are additional stressors for competition horses.

Domestic horses may be subject to stressful experiences for various lengths of time. Horse-riding provides a common setting for short- or long-term stress because riders can directly enforce responses and, unlike other animal-training pursuits, can prevent escape by trapping horses between rein and leg pain.

Active behavioural responses are characteristic of acute (short-term) stress. The animal becomes more engaged, vigilant and hyper-reactive when the stressor is escapable. Acute-stress responses may appear disguised when they manifest as redirected aggression, displacement activities (Wiepkema, 1987), or as freezing or quiescence. However, stress typically manifests hyper-reactively as conflict behaviours that range from increased muscle tonus and body tension to aggression, bolting, rearing, bucking, shying, leaping, flipping over, or rushing backwards (McLean and McGreevy, 2004). Conflict behaviours may arise from conflicting motivations, especially when escape/avoidance responses are thwarted. They can be defined as 'a set of responses of varying duration that are usually characterised by hyper-reactivity and arise largely through confusion' (McGreevy *et al.*, 2005).

When stressful situations are regular, conflict behaviours may become ritualised as the effects of prolonged stress accumulate (Ladewig, 2000). Passive emotional coping frequently characterises chronic stress, resulting in disengagement, decreased vigilance, hypo-reactivity and quiescence. The heart rate and blood pressure may be lowered and the horse frequently appears dull. In such situations, trainers may mistakenly believe that the horse is now more accepting of current events, but the quiescence is really a result of inescapable stress and lack of control.

As described above, prolonged exposure to stressors results in physiological degradation (such as immunological disturbances, gastric disorders and damage), and behavioural disturbances (such as development of stereotypies and injurious behaviours, e.g., self-mutilation and increased aggression) (Stolba *et al.*, 1983; Wiepkema, 1987; Moberg and Mench, 2000). Thus, chronic stress has profound negative welfare implications for horses.

The neural basis of chronic stress extends further from the central role of the amygdala. The basal ganglia are implicated not only in stress but also in stereotypic behaviours and alterations in learning. Inside the basal ganglia, the striatum filters and relays information to and from cortical structures and is integral in motivation, action and learning. Chronic stress alters dopaminergic modulation of the striatum in rats, and similar physiological changes appear to occur in the horse (Parker *et al.*, 2008). For example, crib-biting horses have been reported with significantly higher receptor subtypes in regions of the basal ganglia associated with reward (the nucleus accumbens) and significantly lower number of receptors in the basal ganglia region known as the caudatus, the tissue involved in determining action and outcome (Parker *et al.*, 2008). In rats, inactivation of the dorsomedial striatum impairs both reversal learning and strategy switching and is thus implicated in the perseverance of behaviours, including stereotypies (Ragozzino, 2007).

Conflicts in motivation are of great significance in any analysis of horse-training, because of the horse's inability to resolve the stressful situation. Currently, the accurate identification of chronic stress eludes us, and there are no specific tests for it (Ladewig, 2000), so there is a strong need for further research on stress in domestic horses.

Acceptable domestic equine welfare can be defined by the absence of physiological and behavioural disorders (Ladewig, 2003), and through adherence to the Five Freedoms (Farm Animal Welfare Council, UK):

1) Freedom from thirst and hunger;
2) Freedom from discomfort;
3) Freedom from pain, injury and disease;
4) Freedom to express most normal behaviours; and
5) Freedom from fear and distress.

In a training regime where negative reinforcement is predominant and inherent, it follows that its correct use has positive welfare implications. Yet, studies have revealed that many equestrian coaches are not familiar with learning theory. This deficit is at great odds with their responsibility to establish desirable learned responses in animals without causing conflict behaviours (McGreevy, 2007; Warren-Smith and McGreevy, 2008a). Peak equestrian coaching, training and regulatory bodies must legislate for the correct use of learning theory in equestrian activity as a matter of urgency.

Stress and Performance

Stress has major biological consequences for all animals, and stressors can also affect different cognitive processes and thereby learning performance and memory recall in various tasks (Mendl, 1999). Stressors appear to cause shifts, lapses and narrowing of attention and these processes can be adaptive in helping the animal scrutinise a source of danger. Low or moderate concentrations of glucocorticoids (e.g. cortisol) and catecholamines (e.g. adrenaline) can enhance memory formation, while excessively high or prolonged elevations of these hormones lead to memory disruption (McEwen and Saplosky, 1995; Mendl, 1999; Morris, 2007). Yerkes-Dodson's (1908) law neatly illustrates how the association between performance in a cognitive task and the level of stress can be expressed as an inverted U-shaped curve (Figure 13.6). The law also states that the optimal stress or arousal state decreases with increasing task difficulty (Mendl, 1999). Optimal learning, therefore, requires a specific narrow range of stress (e.g. when training a horse to step sideways from the rider's leg pressure, stress levels increase as the horse shows raised muscular tonus levels). When the response becomes habitual to a cue, stress levels decrease to the normal range.

Accordingly, research has shown that fearful horses generally give poorer performances under stressful conditions (Christensen *et al.*,

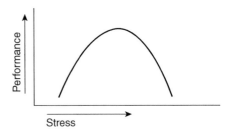

Figure 13.6 Yerkes-Dodson's law describes how stress (arousal) can enhance learning performance to a point and then inhibit it (i.e. at low levels it can be beneficial for learning due to increased attention, but at higher levels it is detrimental).

2012; Valenchon *et al.*, 2013a;b), probably because they do not pay attention to the trainer (i.e. stimuli in the environment outcompetes the trainer for salience) (Christensen *et al.*, 2012). Some scholars have posited that arousal and affective state affect the efficacy of each of the four operant conditioning quadrants (Starling *et al.*, 2013), a suggestion that explains why the best trainers always look for shifts in both these attributes during training. In effect, negative affective states create risk-averse animals and positive affective states create optimistic animals, while high arousal funnels focus and promotes more active behaviours and low arousal more calm behaviours and broader focus. Optimal training therefore predicates that the goals of training are to achieve sufficient calmness in horses and to create training schemas that encourage horses to trial new behaviours. It has already been established (see punishment, chapter 6) that punishment discourages animals from attempting novel responses. The work of Freymond *et al.* (2014) suggests that negative reinforcement, when applied correctly (in terms of minimal and timely removal of pressure) induces positive affective states where, for example the horse may learn that offering responses will result in pressure removal. However, the incorrect use of negative reinforcement is likely to produce risk-averse and highly aroused animals. Despite the unavoidable disconnections in contingencies during shaping and in alterations of schedules of reinforcement, the lower levels of arousal commonly seen in positive rein-forcement scenarios are also likely to produce animals with broader focus and thus the capacity to trial novel behaviours. The para-dox of affective and arousal states on one hand and positive and negative reinforcement characteristics on the other is most satisfac-torily reconciled by combined reinforcement, which offers the greatest promise for future horse training.

Fear Responses

Fear and anxiety places the animal in a *state of stress* which, as described above, can have negative effects on welfare, health and repro-duction (Boissy, 1995). In horses, fear is addi-tionally problematic, because fear reactions can cause serious injury to both horse and human. Indeed, horse-riding accidents are relatively common: the injury rate is one for every 350 hours of contact, which is 20 times greater than motor-cycling (Ceroni, 2007). Surveys have shown that a major part of horse–human accidents occurs when the rider falls off the horse, and many accidents are caused by unexpected fear reactions (Keeling *et al.*, 1999; Thomas *et al.*, 2006).

Fear can be regarded as a 'state of the brain or the neuroendocrine system arising under certain conditions and eventuating in certain forms of behaviour' (Gray, 1987). Stimuli that members of a species will avoid, work to prevent, or flee from, can be categorised as fear-releasing. The central nervous system assesses whether a stimulus or a group of stimuli represents a significant challenge to the animal. This assessment of stimuli may differ between individuals, and the predispo-sition for assessment of stimuli is termed *fearfulness*. Boissy (1995) defined fearfulness as a basic psychological characteristic of the individual that predisposes it to perceive and react in a similar manner to a wide range of potentially frightening events.

Fear-eliciting stimuli are one class of stress-ors that result in the animal being in a state of stress (or more specifically 'a state of fear'), leading to behavioural and physiological

stress reactions to regain homeostasis. According to the standard stress model (Figures 13.1 and 13.7), the main physiological reactions are relatively non-specific to the type of stressor that the individual is exposed to. However, behavioural reactions are more specific to the type of stressor, i.e. whether it is a predator (fight or flight reactions) or extreme cold (increased eating, shelter seeking and minimising heat loss).

Behavioural expressions of fear in animals include active avoidance (flight and hiding), active defence (attack or threat) or movement inhibition (freezing and tonic immobility). Other responses that are considered indica-tors of fear include vigilance, vocalisations (e.g. alarm calls) and production of alarm pheromones (Boissy, 1995). Conflicting motivations, such as motivation to explore and motivation to avoid a potentially aversive stimulus, may also result in displacement activities and frequent alternation of differ-ent types of behaviour (e.g. approach and avoidance). However, since fear does not necessarily lead to an obvious behavioural expression in all cases, and since behavioural reactions are linked to the type of stimulus (e.g. whether it is a visual or an auditory stimulus), both behavioural and physiological measures should be considered when assess-ing the state of fear (Manteca and Deag, 1993; Christensen *et al.*, 2005).

After the acute fear reaction, corticosteroids function to re-establish homeostasis via feed-back mechanisms. The animal must consoli-date its memory of the threat's appearance, location, smell and sound, because such information may predict the occurrence and nature of the next encounter, thereby maximising the likelihood of survival. Thus, corticosteroids act to facilitate behavioural adaptation via their effect on the consolida-tion and potentiation of fear, or the facilita-tion of avoidance extinction (i.e. habituation) (Korte, 2001).

The Adaptive Fear Response

Fear has definite survival value for wild animals. The life expectancy of an animal

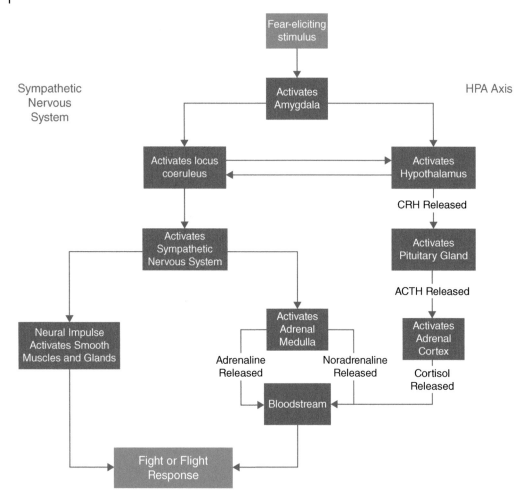

Figure 13.7 The physiological reaction to fear is characterised by activity in the sympathetic nervous system and the HPA-axis, which enable the body to perform more strenuous exercise than would otherwise be possible. (Modified from www.anxietyboss.com.)

obviously increases if it reacts appropriately to avoid sources of danger. In this context, fear-related behaviour and physiological responses are certainly adaptive and the mammalian body has evolved to deal effectively with these acute stressors. However, since fear reactions are costly in terms of energy, excessive fear does not contribute positively to animal fitness. Through the damaging effects of frequently or chronically elevated concentrations of stress hormones, excessive fear can lead to psychopathology and mental suffering, as well as physical damage (Korte, 2001).

Fear has been investigated in many species (reviewed, for example, by Boissy, 1995;

1998; Forkman *et al.*, 2007), and individual responses to fear-inducing events appear to be shaped by interactions between individual tendencies and properties of the stressor and the situation (Boissy, 1998). Despite the importance of fearfulness to both horse welfare and human safety, there has been relatively little research on basic fear responses in horses. Some studies have investigated temperament traits (e.g. Visser *et al.*, 2001; Seaman *et al.*, 2002; Lansade *et al.*, 2007; König von Borstel *et al.*, 2011b), reactivity (e.g. McCann *et al.*, 1988; Lansade *et al.*, 2004; 2005; McCall *et al.*, 2006), or emotionality (e.g. Wolff *et al.*, 1997) in horses, but few have dealt with basic fear reactions, including which types of stimuli and situations are perceived as frightening (Christensen *et al.*, 2005; Lansade *et al.*, 2007). Recent results have demonstrated that ageing affects fear responses: younger horses showed a significantly higher frequency of avoidance but also more exploratory behaviour, while older horses were less behaviourally responsive but showed a shift towards control by the sympathetic nervous system (Baragli *et al.*, 2014). Another study explored the effect of coat colour on fear reactions and reported that the Silver mutation Arg618Cys was associated with increased fear reactions in Icelandic horses (Brunberg *et al.*, 2013).

Given the neophobic nature of horses and the importance and implications of horses' fear reactions for human safety, surprisingly few studies have explored habituation to novel stimuli and the subsequent imperative of developing desensitisation techniques for horses (Christensen *et al.*, 2006; Hartmann *et al.*, 2011; Leiner and Fendt, 2011; Christensen, 2013) (see also Chapter 4, Non-associative Learning).

Dietary Effects on Fear

Some studies have suggested that diet can have a modulatory effect on fearfulness in horses (Nicol *et al.*, 2005, Bulmer *et al.*, 2015). Performance horses are often fed a high-starch diet with restricted roughage and this has been associated with increased occurrence of stereotypic behaviour and health problems (McGreevy *et al.*, 1995a,b; Hothersall and Nicol, 2009; Luthersson *et al.*, 2009; Wickens and Heleski, 2010) (Figure 13.8). Feed with a high starch content results in a higher glycaemic response (increase in blood glucose concentrations, Lacombe *et al.*, 2004), which has been hypothesised to cause high reactivity in horses (Bulmer *et al.*, 2015). Nicol *et al.* (2005) found that, compared with foals fed on starch and sugar diets, foals fed after weaning on fat and fibre diets were more investigative and were more likely to approach unfamiliar people. In addition, they cantered about less, seemed calmer and were less distressed immediately after weaning.

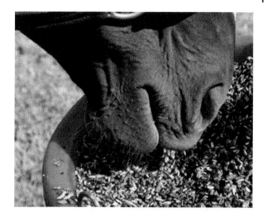

Figure 13.8 Diets with a high starch content are associated with increased stereotypic behaviours and health problems and may also increase reactivity.

Bulmer *et al.* (2015) found that a high-starch diet led to increased heart-rate responses in novel object and handling tests, compared to when the same horses were fed a low-starch and high-fibre diet. Thus, fat- and fibre-based diets may result in calmer patterns of behaviour, whereas there is currently no evidence that dietary supplements, such as tryptophan-containing products, influence equine behaviour (Malmkvist and Christensen, 2007; Noble *et al.*, 2016).

Horse-Specific Fear Reactions

As prey animals, horses are generally more inclined to escape from rather than attack aversive stimuli; aggression is mainly confined to situations where the animal is cornered or trapped or when defending foals from certain predators. Horses generally have a strongly developed flight response and possess morphological characteristics for running away from danger. It is likely that selective breeding over the past few millennia, to facilitate habituation to towing carts and having humans on their backs, has dulled the flight response of horses to some extent. In equestrian circles, it is common to describe some breeds and individual horses as *hot* and some as *cold*, meaning that they are more or less sensitive, and more or less prone to express a flight response when presented with an aversive stimulus. A mixture of hot and cold breeds is known as a Warmblood.

There is a great variation among breeds and individual horses as to their predisposition to express the flight response (Visser *et al.*, 2001; Hausberger *et al.*, 2004; Christensen and Rundgren, 2008; Rørvang *et al.*, 2015a). Murphey *et al.* (1981) showed similar variation in flight response between *Bos indicus* and *Bos taurus* cattle. As also mentioned above, fear responses show a great deal of variation both within individuals and among individuals, depending on the nature and intensity of the perceived stressor; responses can also be modified by age, experience, genetics, physiological state and season (Moberg and Mench, 2000; Hausberger *et al.*, 2004; Brunberg *et al.*, 2013; Baragli *et al.*, 2014).

Because fearful behaviours in horses can have serious implications for safety, relaxation and low levels of fear and stress should be ubiquitous goals in horse-training. Anecdotal experiences have been substantiated by scientific evidence that a rider is able to induce nervousness in a horse, which can potentially lead to dangerous fear reactions (von Borstel *et al.*, 2005; Keeling *et al.*, 2009). The fear response can be the horse-trainer's greatest adversary, inversely correlating with learning and performance (Christensen *et al.*, 2012).

Once the brain has perceived a frightening stimulus, alertness is raised and less-salient stimuli are ignored. That is why a horse in a full-blown flight response can seem senseless, and can gallop into fences and cars or collide with trees and other obstacles.

The jumping response of an intensely fearful horse may be altered to the extent that it scrapes over fences and may drag its legs through the top wires of a fence. A flat hollow jump characterises the flight response and is not uncommonly seen in incorrectly trained eventing horses in horse trials where the performance appears to be semi-controlled bolting (Figure 13.9). It is likely that flight responses are highly implicated in the high levels of rider falls and deaths in that sport. The stronger the flight response, the greater the acceleration tendency and the more the horse is unresponsive to other stimuli, including the rider's signals. Such a horse invariably has what is known as a 'hard (habituated) mouth'. The mouth is really not insensitive, but the flight response outcompetes the rider's signals for salience.

When a horse experiences conflicting motivations, fearful behaviours may be clearly expressed in some cases, but less so in others. For example, a rider on a fearful (or confused) horse may restrain the horse with the reins and the horse's attempts to escape manifest

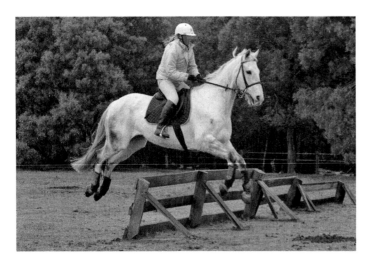

Figure 13.9 The flight response is strongly implicated in horses that jump 'hollow and flat' (i.e. with raised head, extended neck and extended vertebral column).

as hyper-reactive behaviour, such as jogging and increased muscular tonus. On the other hand, a cornered horse at liberty may find escape impossible and may actually approach its 'aggressor'. Such a horse may not outwardly express fear.

One-Trial Learning

While most things we try to train the horse to do require a number of repetitions, the flight response, unfortunately, can be learned in just one experience (Chapter 6, Associative Learning (Aversive stimuli)). It is adaptive for the animal to remember any response that enables it to survive a life-threatening experience. Patterns of escape that result in surviving a predatory attack are instantly recorded for later use (McLean, 2001). Once an animal has acquired a learned fear response, it will rapidly learn to associate any other signal that may predict the original frightening stimulus via classical conditioning, and it will show an avoidance response to this previously neutral stimulus to prevent the original aversive stimulus. The animal may even generalise between such classically conditioned signals, resulting in fear reactions towards a whole class of similar stimuli. In this way, neutral stimuli become powerful triggers of the fear response.

Even if these signals no longer predict the original stimulus, the animal will still react fearfully towards them, because avoidance reactions can be self-reinforcing through the relief they bring. If the reaction eventually wanes, it may spontaneously recur (this is known as spontaneous recovery), or be reinstalled by exposure to another stressor.

For this reason, it has been argued that the emotional memory of fear cannot be erased and that apparently extinguished fear responses should only be considered dormant (Le Doux, 1994). This research has monumental implications for horse-trainers: avoid fearful reactions at all costs (Figure 13.10). If, during human interactions, the horse is showing hyper-reactive behaviours (high head, hollow back, short choppy strides), it may be acquiring associations between fear and humans. Chasing horses can be a recipe for further, and sometimes more severe expressions of the fear response, and for rifts in horse–human bonds. Krueger (2007) found in her experiments on the round-pen technique that 3 of 19 horses in her first set of trials had to be withdrawn on animal-welfare grounds because of 'untypical immense sweating' and the problem that these horses 'did not respond to the experimenter anymore' (however, they did respond in subsequent trials).

(a)

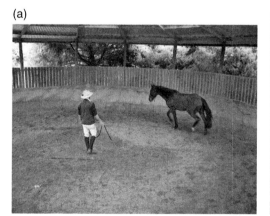

(b)

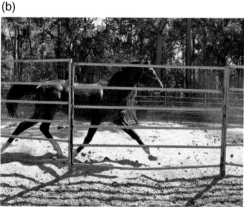

Figure 13.10 (a) Round-pen training should be managed so that there is minimal or no flight response, otherwise it can make indelible associations between fearfulness in the horse and the presence of humans. (b) Flight responses should be avoided at all costs in horse-training. (Photos courtesy of Amanda Warren-Smith and Carol Willcocks.)

As described above, fear can also readily become associated with neutral stimuli and these neutral stimuli then become powerful triggers for the fear response. So, chasing young horses to show off their movement, round-pen techniques, lungeing and long-reining fearful horses are all ill-advised and can have negative welfare implications. There is no ethical justification for inducing fear during training.

Pain

Pain is another stressor for domestic horses that may occur in relation to training. Pain is interlinked with fear, because once a horse has experienced a painful stimulus, it is likely to become fearful of both this and similar stimuli. Also, discomfort and neutral stimuli that the horse associates with the painful stimulus can elicit fear responses. While pain is generally thought of as a sensation, there is justification for it to be described as a state, in that it has more in common with primary reinforcers, such as hunger and thirst, than it has with the senses (Keay and Bandler, 2008). There are qualitative differences in pain of different origins. Cutaneous pain provides a different experience from the deep pain that arises from internal organs or muscles. While skin pain is associated with hyper-reactivity,

hyper-vigilance and rising pulse-rate and blood pressure, deep pain may be associated with quiescence, slowing of the pulse, a fall in blood pressure, sweating and nausea (Keay and Bandler, 2008).

Very few riders indeed would contemplate the notion that riding and handling include regular aversive and even painful events. However, steel bits are placed in the horse's sensitive mouth, and strong, sometimes relentless, pressures may be applied there. The rider may also kick the horse in the thorax constantly, believing that the horse is lazy. The so-called lazy horse, having no means of ameliorating the situation, may then be invaded with spurs or whips instantly and haphazardly. Even a well-trained horse may still have to endure the least obtrusive of pressure from apparatus to induce acceleration or deceleration. In-hand, also, various apparatus may be used to control an animal that is deemed unruly or lazy. The tragedy of such welfare issues is that horsepeople do not willfully mean to injure horses and most would be aghast that such issues can be interpreted in this way.

The pressures applied to horses via the bit, rider's legs, spurs and whips may regularly exceed tolerable levels, or may not be removed appropriately, leading to hyper-reactive behaviours in attempts to escape the stressor (Figure 13.11). The ridden and led horse's

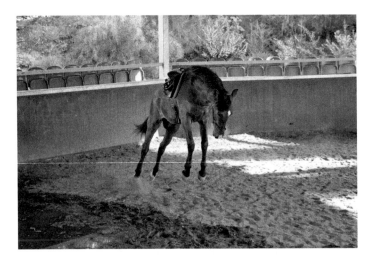

Figure 13.11 Hyper-reactive behaviours (attempts to run away, bucking, bolting, shying and rearing) may relate to fear or pain. (Photo courtesy of Rob Duncan.)

experience of discomfort and pain from incorrectly applied negative reinforcement may constitute the most regularly experienced unpredictable and uncontrollable aversive stimuli, leading to conflict behaviours and other indirect behaviour changes. The term *conflict theory* has been proposed to highlight the significance of the correct use of negative reinforcement and the deleterious effects of getting it wrong (McLean, 2010; McLean and Christensen, 2017). It is most important to acknowledge that negative reinforcement relies on a pressure/pain continuum, so when a horse is reinforced for the wrong response or not reinforced at all, the ongoing exposure to painful stimuli must have a detrimental effect on the horse's mental security. Being unable to predict or control relentlessly strong bit pressure or spur assaults on a regular basis, is likely to amount to a significant deterioration of a horse's mental stability well before the apparent signs of learned helplessness set in.

When they are not trained to respond to the lightest of signals and when they are not consistently in self-carriage, many ridden horses endure discomfort or even pain on a regular basis. They show this in a variety of ways, sometimes as direct responses to the extant aversive stimuli, and at other times as neurotic manifestations of chronic invasions of pain (McLean and McGreevy, 2004; McGreevy and McLean, 2007). Losses of controllability can lead to insecurity which may manifest as neophobia, where the horse may show unusual and sometimes increasing fearful reactions to environmental stimuli. The following section describes some examples of manifestations of fear- and stress-related responses in domestic horses and emphasises not only that the problems may have strong links with dysfunctions in various stimulus–response entities trained by negative reinforcement, but also that the reinstallation of associated responses can provide the key to rehabilitation. While it is important to stress that many of these behaviours may have associated age, breed, sex and genetic predispositions, it is also important to recognise that, by and large, learning and experience confirms or denies these tendencies.

> It is important to note that before undertaking any behaviour modification, such as proposed in this book, a veterinary examination should be used to rule out pain as a cause of unwelcome responses.

Manifestations of Fear and Stress

From the standpoint of behaviour, fear and stress have many guises. Typically, and throughout the centuries, fear and stress responses in horses have been described in anthropomorphic ways (Chapter 3, Anthropomorphism and the Human–Horse Relationship). Usually, these behavioural descriptors categorise them as resistances and evasions and sometimes as vices. Stress-related behaviours that result from training interventions are numerous and diverse. They may show up overtly as a direct result of the horse's interaction with apparatus used in training, handling and riding. Some of these reactions to apparatus are a result of variations in hypersensitivities among individual horses. Some horses show variations in their sensitivity to being touched on the head, body and legs and some are especially reactive to girth pressure.

Head-shyness is a progressive hypersensitivity in the head/ears region, where the horse has learned to rapidly withdraw its head to escape human touch. It is learned by negative reinforcement: the horse learns rapidly that raising its head results in removal of the trainer's hand. Gradual habituation (via systematic desensitisation) can be successful but may be less so if the horse has learned to show escape behaviour. In that case, the next technique may involve overshadowing (outcompeting) the head-shyness with sequences of *step-back* and *forward* until they become more salient than the head contact (McLean, 2008). Horses are quick to develop aversions to unpleasant stimuli. So typically, a horse that is fearful of the human hand has fewer problems with a hand wrapped in a towel. The towel can be rubbed

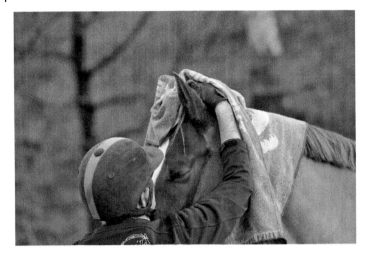

Figure 13.12 Head-shyness may be desensitised by rubbing the horse's head through a towel or other novel or innocuous stimulus, which may be further elaborated by moistening it and then gradually reintroducing human fingers.

around the horse's head and, if necessary, gradually brought closer to the more sensitive areas (Figure 13.12). As the horse habituates to the towel, the fingers can gradually be allowed to protrude from the towel until the horse has lost its hypersensitivity to human touch. The towel may be dampened to add a further variation in tactile stimulus that will assist in habituation.

Similarly, with *bit-shyness*, the avoidance behaviour is reinforced by freedom from contact. This interpretation informs the remedy: systematic desensitisation, perhaps in combination with overshadowing, until the horse habituates to the approach, touch and insertion of fingers and bit into its mouth. Counter-conditioning provides further depth to the remedy in that the approach of the bit or, with head-shyness, touching the head can be trained as a secondary reinforcer that is antecedent to the delivery of food or tactile contact such as wither caressing. Correct skills are necessary in handling horses' heads and especially when inserting things into their mouths. Sometimes horses may raise their heads when the bridle is removed and the bit can become caught for a moment in the diastema of the lower jaw. As the horse raises its head, the mouth pressure may increase and the increasing pain can result in fearfulness of the bit. With bit-shyness, it is

particularly important to ensure that reactions are not caused by pain from, for example, an ill-fitting bit or poor dental care.

Leg-shyness describes the condition where the horse's legs show hypersensitivity to touch. Gradual habituation (via systematic desensitisation) is a typical approach, but the danger of touching the horse's hindlegs cautions trainers to stand in a safe position and to use, say, a long stick with a glove attached to the end that can touch the legs safely and remain in contact until the horse shows a desirable behaviour that can be rewarded (e.g. putting the leg down). The moment of removal is crucial. Another approach is to hose the leg (McLean and McLean, 2008), because the trainer can stand at a safe distance and can gradually vary the intensity of the hose spray so that the habituation process can be more thorough and the horse can remain calmer during this variation. It is usually easier to touch the horse's legs during hosing. Often the horse shows calmer reactions to a person touching dampened hair than dry hair because of context-specific responses (McLean and McLean, 2008). When horses are fearful of aerosols, the same hosing method can be used and, during the hosing, the aerosol can usually be applied with no adverse reaction. The hose spray is then varied and switched off from time to time so that the aerosol and hose are randomly applied and intermingled at first. This is an example of stimulus blending (Chapter 4, Non-associative Learning). It is not surprising that horses develop aversion to sprays, because the hissing sound is probably ethologically relevant as an indicator of events that may be dangerous. It can be appropriate to use counter-conditioning to habituate horses to this sound (i.e. the sound should be immediately followed by food, so that it eventually becomes a predictor of a pleasant event).

Just as horses show large variations in their initial reactions to a rider's leg pressure (Chapter 6, Associative Learning (Aversive stimuli)), they may also show similar variations to pressure on their heads. While some horses may trial *stepping forward* in response to pressure on their halters or bridles, others react strongly by **pulling back from the tether**. If this backwards reaction results in removal of pressure, either by the trainer releasing the pressure or by the tether breaking, the backwards reaction is reinforced. Again, this analysis informs the remedy. The horse should be trained to *lead forward* correctly and it is significant to observe that horses that pull back tend to raise their heads as their first reaction to anterior lead pressure. So repetitions of *lead forward* from pressure are efficacious.

Because horses that resist *leading forward* can easily rear, it is safer to apply the *lead-forward* pressure sideways at about 45 degrees. It is important to set up the training situation so that the horse is more likely to offer a correct response. With some horses, it can be helpful to motivate the horse to *step forward* initially by presenting a food bucket just after the rope signal. A step forward will be reinforced through both the release of the rope pressure and a mouthful of food (combined reinforcement). This is repeated until the horse *leads forward* immediately from a light lead signal and without raising its head. The aim is to get the horse to respond to the rope signal alone. However, many problems are context-specific, so when the horse that has had such effective treatment is tethered,

it may still attempt to pull back. If so, the trainer should initially train the horse to remain immobile next to the post. The horse can then be tethered to a car inner tube attached to a safe strong post. This way, the horse learns that the pressure remains until it steps forward.

Girthing the horse can be another challenging habituation event. Some horses find it highly aversive to have their thoraxes compressed and become **cold-backed (girth-shy, or cinch-bound)**. Through systematic desensitisation, the horse should be initially habituated to an elastic girth (See figure 8.14 in Chapter 8, Training, for a detailed description). It may be necessary to combine the gradual approach with overshadowing by using well-established sequences of *step-back* reactions and then, when calm, sequences of *forward steps* followed by *step-backs* (Figure 13.13).

When horses show problem behaviour with the farrier and are **difficult to shoe**, it is generally associated with fast forward reactions. The worst scenario involves kicking out and this can be interpreted as synonymous with running forwards, because both the kick and running forwards consist of hyper-reactive retractions of the hindleg, the major difference being that one is in the swing phase, the other in the stance phase. Training the horse to remain immobile during any intervention is important. If the horse kicks out when its legs are touched, this can be overshadowed by a single step back applied during the kick. Again, counter conditioning with secondary positive reinforcement can also modify the behaviour very successfully. The behaviour may occur because the horse has not been appropriately handled and habituated as a foal, because it lacks balance, or because it has had a bad experience (in terms of a painful/frightening event, which may also have led to the behaviour being reinforced through release). The reactions may be specific to a particular farrier and, if so, it is necessary to give the horse a number of pleasant experiences with this person, or use a different farrier for a period. Regardless, training should be carried out by the horse's known trainer outside the shoeing situation. If the problem occurs only during shoeing (i.e. the usual trainer can lift the leg and clean the hooves without problems), the trainer should habituate the horse to hammering on the hoof as part of systematic desensitisation, starting at a very low level and only increasing in intensity when the horse reliably fails to react to the previous level. The trainer should pay attention to the horse's behaviour and be careful to reinforce only appropriate behaviour (i.e. termination of hammering when the horse does not move the leg). If the horse has not been properly habituated to lifting its legs and hammering on the hooves by its usual trainer, then obviously, the horse is not ready for shoeing and attempting to shoe such as horse is a welfare and safety problem.

Horses are ethologically compelled to avoid dark, narrow and confined places, so it is not surprising that **loading onto horse floats and trailers** presents considerable difficulty for many horses (Figure 13.14). Those that refuse to load onto trailers often show deficits in their *leading forward* responses (McLean, 2005b), which may either contribute to the loading problem or be exacerbated by it. The first step is to ensure that the horse is not overly frightened of the trailer. If the horse has had a bad experience and is highly aroused, it can be useful to associate the trailer with a positive (rather than aversive) event through classical conditioning. For example, the horse is led to the trailer, the ramp is lowered and a food bucket is presented on the ramp. The next step is to re-train acceleration and deceleration responses in-hand. This should initially be done in the home environment where the horse is calm. When it is then brought to the trailer, it is important to maintain the pressure forward until the horse steps a single *step forward* in the direction of the trailer. This step should be repeated until the horse *steps forward* from a light lead signal. Then the next step is attempted, repeating until the horse *steps forward* from a light signal.

Repetitions continue until the horse steps easily all the way into the trailer without further signalling after the initial signal to *lead forward*. Forward signals may be fortified by tapping the horse on the ribcage with a long-whip in association with the light *lead forward* signal, but the horse should have learned to respond appropriately to whip-tapping in the home environment before this signal is used in the problem situation. The tapping should stop as soon as the horse *steps forward*. Primary and/or secondary positive reinforcement when the horse responds correctly can also be efficient. One study showed that using target training and

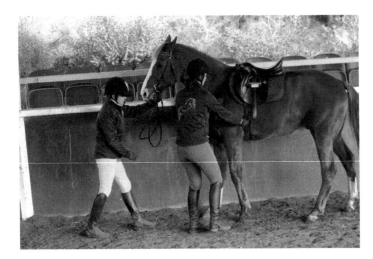

Figure 13.13 The girth-shy response can be successfully overshadowed by simultaneously *stepping* the horse *forward* and *back*. It is useful to initially habituate the horse to an elastic girth (Chapter 8 Training Figure 8.14).

(a)

(b)

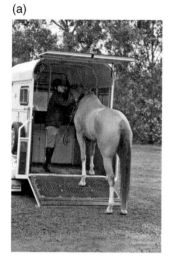
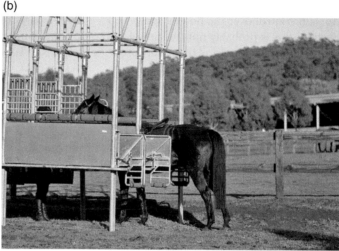

Figure 13.14 Training or re-training the horse to load onto the (a) float/trailer or (b) into racecourse starting gates is a matter of reinforcing the correct response and shaping it so that the smallest correct attempts and all improvements are rewarded. Combined reinforcement (i.e. the use of both positive and negative reinforcers to reward correct behaviour) can be effective.

positive reinforcement to load horses with severe trailer-loading problems was efficient and caused less fear-related behaviour in the horses compared to using only negative reinforcement in the trailer-loading situation (Hendriksen *et al.*, 2011).

Similarly, the horse that **rushes backwards** out of the trailer shows deficits in *leading forward* because, when it rushes backwards, it pulls on the lead-rein held by the trainer in the forward direction. The behaviour may be caused by a bad (painful/frightening) experience in the trailer, so the horse is strongly motivated to get out of the trailer. With some (food-motivated) horses, the solution may simply be to offer highly appreciated food in front of the horse while the ramp and bar are open, so the horse has some motivation to stay inside the trailer. In addition, the horse should be trained to *step forward* from lead pressure, so that it does so immediately and from light signals. When it rushes out of the float, care should be taken not to raise the lead-rein pressure too much for *forward* as the horse may raise its head and connect with the roof of the float, creating more problems. The best solution is to train the horse to *go forward* from whip-taps on the ribcage with the long-whip, and to step forward in

association with light forward lead pressure so that when it rushes out of the float, the trainer can tap the ribcage rhythmically during rushing backwards, ceasing only when the horse *steps forward* again (McLean, 2003).

Problems with starting stalls (starting gates, starting barriers) show up as either refusing to load into the stalls or hyper-reactive behaviours once inside. A number of problems confront the horse when loading into starting stalls, the first being their appearance. They are closed spaces with low overhead frames (except for New Zealand starting gates). In addition, the space is narrow so the horse's body may easily connect with the opened back gates and with the foot platforms. All these are aversive to some horses and as soon as they feel the foot platforms on their sides they may rush out backwards, which only serves to reinforce the aversiveness of the gates. Following consultations by A. McLean, starting gate design in Australia has begun to take these aspects into consideration. Remedying loading problems follows the same principles as described above for loading into trailers/floats. It is important that the horse is trained to stand still (without being held) inside the starting gates through equally thorough training of *stop* and *go* responses.

While the goal of all equestrian disciplines is to gain control over the horse's speed and direction, this is probably not the aim of the horse, so it is not surprising that many problems are associated with speed and direction issues. Furthermore, when riders attenuate the acceleration and deceleration responses by concurrent signalling (simultaneous rein tension and leg pressure), horses may show conflict behaviours that manifest largely as dysfunctions of speed and line.

In many cases the deceleration responses are unintentionally deteriorated, so the conflict behaviours manifest as attempts to escape and run away. *Bolting, rushing, running away, jogging, pulling* and being *above the bit* are all manifestations of poor deceleration responses (Figure 13.15). They are all remedied by re-installing deceleration responses so that the horse can *stop, slow, step-back* and shorten its stride from light

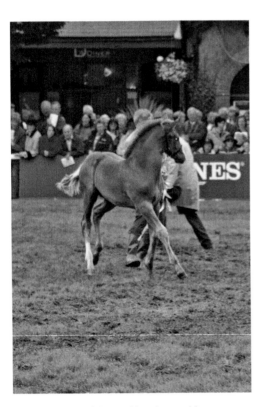

Figure 13.15 Rushing and jogging problems (including bolting) in-hand and under-saddle are largely associated with inadequately trained *stop/slow* responses.

rein signals. This involves returning to the earlier parts of the shaping scale and reinforcing single steps of *stop* or *step-back* responses. For example, the horse is signalled to *step-back* with the reins only for one step of the forelegs and tension is released at the onset of the response. Downward inter-gait and intra-gait transitions are repeated, releasing the rein tension immediately after the transition.

Rushing at jumping obstacles generally begins when the horse either hurts its legs on a pole or the rider pulls it in the mouth over the fence and the pain causes the horse to run away. Soon, the obstacle itself is associated with the pain and it now elicits a running response *towards* the fence. Jumping low cross-rails and gradually training the horse to *stop* from rein tension 6 metres after the cross-rail soon results in the horse losing its acceleration response towards the fence (McLean, 2003). This may need to be repeated at various obstacles. When horses are *above the bit*, the hyper-reactive behaviour and rein heaviness are not always apparent to the rider, but the above-the-bit reaction may be a defensive head-carriage, suggesting painful bit invasions which, in turn, suggest slowing deficits. *Reefing* and *head tossing* are generally also associated with running away behaviours, but they may also be associated with problems in acceleration (McLean and McLean, 2008), so upward inter-gait and intra-gait transitions involving reinforcement of single strides of each gait provide the remedy for these also.

Bucking is a counter-predator behaviour (evolved for feline predators) that presents perhaps the most dangerous and challenging behaviour a horse can offer. Before attempting to train a horse that shows bucking, it is necessary to ensure that the behaviour is not caused by vertebral pain. If pain is not the cause of the behaviour, it may occur either because the horse has not been sufficiently habituated to a rider on its back (i.e. an innate defensive response) or, if the behaviour has escalated after a rider fell off, because the behaviour has been negatively reinforced through the accidental dismount of the rider.

If lack of appropriate habituation is the cause of the behaviour, systematic desensitisation should be applied to gradually habituate the horse to weight and movement on its back, which is, of course, unnatural for horses. While bucking is well-known to be associated with *forward* problems, it is also associated with dysfunctions in *stop* responses (McLean, 2005b). Here, it is important to consider that because bucking involves random acceleration responses or acceleration responses not under stimulus control of the rider (or trainer), and because flight responses can be learned in just a few trials and are difficult to extinguish, the remedy is not to ride *forward* but to *slow* the legs. When horses buck under-saddle, most riders attempt to use the reins, not to *stop* but to maintain balance. The bucking horse does not respond to the slowing effect of the reins but continues to buck, so training effective *stop* and *slowing* responses provides a means of arresting this behaviour. Training horses that buck under-saddle to have better *stop* responses is best undertaken in-hand, focusing on good transitions, such as those from trot to halt in two beats of the forelegs, releasing as soon as the legs are still (McLean and McLean, 2008).

Rearing is another problem characterised by dysfunctions in acceleration, deceleration and *turn* responses. Like bucking, it is often a result of concurrent signalling of both *stop* and *go* signals, or conflicting motivations (e.g. if a rider escalates pressure to an unacceptable level while trying to make a horse approach something it fears). Rearing can also be dangerous for riders, although riding a rear may be less challenging than riding a buck (Figure 13.16). Skilled jumping riders are usually capable of riding rears because of the similarity between rearing and riding tall vertical obstacles. Rearing generally begins with stalling and jibbing, and then progresses to spins and finally rearing emerges. Most horses rear to some extent to the left and the result is further dysfunction in the right *turn* response. Thus, rearing results in deficits of acceleration, deceleration and *turn* responses. Rearing is reinforced by the release of the effort of *going forward*, as well as release of the rider's reins and leg pressures. Rehabilitating a rearing horse is first a matter of identifying the underlying cause of the behaviour and, second, a matter of re-training deceleration, acceleration and *turn* responses and is a job for skilled trainers as it involves removing the reinforcement from the rearing response. Remedying rearing in-hand may involve using a stallion bit, which is vibrated in the opposite direction of rearing during a rear and released as soon as the horse lands.

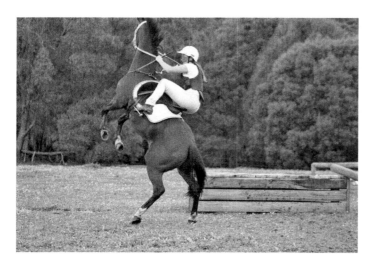

Figure 13.16 Rehabilitating a rearing horse can be very dangerous as the horse can easily be pulled off balance by the rider's efforts to stay aboard.

Freezing is characterised by the horse refusing to move altogether despite strong signalling. When the horse eventually does move, it is likely to be explosive and uncontrollable. This behaviour is most likely to be a 'last-ditch' counter-predator reaction. Because freezing is often followed by a sudden explosive reaction, it can be very dangerous for riders and the horse may lose any sense of self-preservation in its panic. Freezing is typically a conflict behaviour that is a consequence of inconsistent acceleration and deceleration responses and concurrent signalling of *stop* and *go* signals. Because of the degree of dysfunction of pressure-based signals, freezing may have significant links with learned helplessness.

Jibbing, napping, baulking and ***refusing*** may result from frustration or conflict related to deficits in acceleration responses. In general, these behaviours are less dangerous to personnel as they are usually not as hyperreactive as behaviours that involve deceleration. Jibbing and baulking involve random slowing outside the rider's or trainer's stimulus control. The rider or trainer may inadvertently reinforce these behaviours by relenting on the pressures for *forward* at the wrong moment, thus negatively reinforcing these behaviours. Rehabilitating these problems involves re-training the acceleration responses so that these are immediately initiated by the horse from light signals. This involves negatively reinforcing either a single *step forward* or, if that is easily elicited, reinforcing a single stride forward. It may be necessary to increase the motivating level of pressure so the horse is more motivated to move off (e.g. by using whip-taps that increase in frequency). It is important that the whip is not used to deliver sharp punitive pain, but that it instead conforms to the optimal use of negative reinforcement by gradually increasing in speed of whip-taps. Re-training napping also involves re-training acceleration responses, as well as *turns* due to the losses of line. Refusing at jumping obstacles is reinforced by two factors: losses of effort and turning away from the obstacle (Figure 13.17). Thus, successful rehabilitation of refusing at jumps can be obtained by lowering the fence (i.e. using show-jumping obstacles for rehabilitation) and jumping the lowered fence from a standstill or by *stepping back* so that the obstacle does not depart (is not removed)

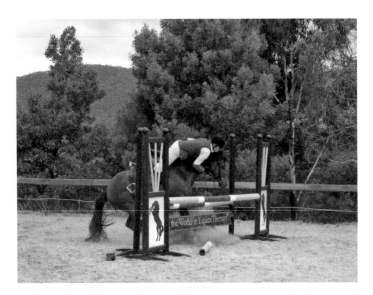

Figure 13.17 Horses can learn to refuse jumping obstacles if riders reward losses of effort and turning away. Once horses have learned to refuse and run out to the side, approaching at greater speeds will generally result in faster swerving.

from the horse's field of vision (McLean and McLean, 2008).

Losses of the designated line intended by a rider manifest as various behaviours, all characterised by greater or lesser amounts of propulsion asymmetry. In these behaviours, the horse drifts sideways with varying degrees of hyper-reactivity. The most hyper-reactive loss of line is seen in *shying*, where the horse suddenly veers sideways. Shying has ethological relevance in escaping predators and is conferred by a rapid abduction in the stance phase of the foreleg proximate to the aversive object, followed usually by an acceleration forward and away from the aversive object. The abduction and subsequent acceleration, like many conflict behaviours, are out of the stimulus control of the rider (or trainer). Remedying shying thus involves regaining stimulus control over the abducting stance-phase foreleg, which means re-training *turn* and *stop* responses. Because the individual reins provide the fundamental signals through negative reinforcement of *turning*, and the two reins provide the means of *stopping*, the reins are instrumental in re-training the *turn*. When the horse shies, the rider should immediately implement a downward transition and then return the forelegs to the designated line. It is often useful in re-training shying to steer the horse's forelegs in a specific line, such as towards the extreme edge of the manège. Typically, shying horses have considerably more difficulty with this exercise than non-shying horses. If the horse shies in response to a particular object, it is also appropriate to habituate the horse to this object (see examples of desensitisation methods in Chapter 4, Non-associative Learning). Research has shown that it may be beneficial to habituate horses to a range of objects simultaneously, thus reducing their general fearfulness towards other objects (Christensen *et al.*, 2011b). *Spinning* is synonymous with shying, except that in spinning the horse continues turning for more than one or two steps. Spinning horses require similar re-training as shying horses, due to the losses of line involved.

Lugging (*hanging*) is where the horse maintains contact on one side of the bit more strongly than on the other, and in doing so it drifts or attempts to drift (Figure 13.18). Sometimes riders hold the reins with stronger contact on one side than on the other, thus preventing the losses of line that normally accompany such inequalities in contact. Lugging is typically seen in racehorses, and this is usually remedied by using a lugging bit – a ring bit that encircles the entire lower

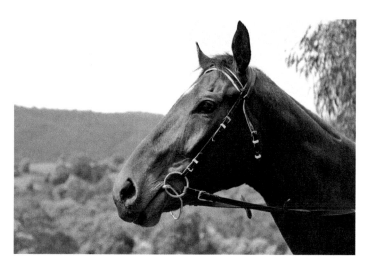

Figure 13.18 Lugging bits are typically used on racehorses to hold them to their designated line and prevent drifting out. This drifting tendency involves losses of speed. A more sensible approach is to train the horse to self-maintain its designated line.

mandible and enables the jockey to pull the horse back on line or hold it on a line. This, however, does not cure the horse. The most effective cure is to re-train the uneven turns associated with lugging. If the horse lugs to the right, then more time is spent on re-training *left turns*, reinforcing single strides of turn until the *left turn* arises from a single light signal. Riding shallow serpentine shapes on the racetrack assists in re-training these turns (McLean and McLean, 2008).

Bridle lameness refers to an apparent lameness as a result of rein contact. Such horses are usually not lame in-hand, but are clearly lame under-saddle. Because it arises from uneven rein contact that is too strong, bridle lameness causes uneven propulsion that becomes habitual under-saddle. Bridle-lame horses require re-training of deceleration and *turn* responses under-saddle where single correct strides are reinforced. *Barging* refers to in-hand problems where horses drift during leading, sometimes stepping on the feet of the trainer (Figure 13.19). These deviations of line also result from uneven propulsion and incorrect leading training where straightness is not reinforced. Downward inter-gait transitions to halt, followed by upward ones where the trainer's hand pushes the horse away from the trainer's body

whenever the horse shows a deviation of line, provide the corrections for this behaviour.

Conflict behaviours resulting from confusions of speed and line signals do not always manifest as alterations of speed or line. Sometimes they may show up as other behaviours. For example, *tension problems involving increased muscle tonus* can be a result of confusions primarily with deceleration responses (Figure 13.20). Whereas confusions with acceleration responses may still result in poor welfare, confusions involving the mouth are generally more serious, most likely because the horse's mouth is so sensitive and not adapted to carrying and being pressured by steel bits. Thus, increased muscle tonus can be indicative of poor deceleration responses, where the horse leans on the bit and slows inconsistently from it. Therefore, the rehabilitation of tense horses may involve reinforcing single strides of downward transitions. Further relaxation is most easily effected by lengthening the stride until the horse stretches its neck forward (longitudinal flexion) and then shortening the stride with the reins so that the horse learns not only to *slow* but also to shorten its stride from light rein signals.

Similarly, *teeth grinding*, *pawing* and excessively *champing the bit* during riding

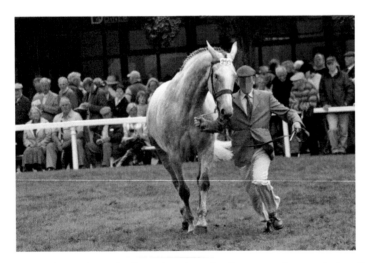

Figure 13.19 Horses that barge into the trainer's space are frequently described as having 'no respect'. However, the simplest explanation shifts the blame from the horse to the trainer; the horse has simply not been trained to maintain its designated line in-hand (i.e. it does not lead straight).

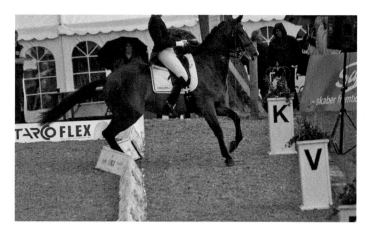

Figure 13.20 A fear response that is thwarted by the reins will lead to increased tension, because when escape is thwarted, anxiety escalates. (Photo courtesy of Julie Taylor/EponaTV.)

may have associations with deficits in deceleration responses, even though they are not necessarily accompanied by obvious accelerations. As with increased muscle tension, these problems can result from inconsistent reinforcement of deceleration responses or concurrent signalling of deceleration and acceleration responses (simultaneous rein and leg pressures). The rehabilitation of these involves the same methodology as above for tension: re-training *stop* responses so that the horse can *stop* and *slow* from light signals, and achieving relaxation in a longer body frame (McLean and McLean, 2008).

Tail-swishing during riding, on the other hand, is typically associated with discomfort in relation to leg, spur or whip use, as well as losses of self-carriage and subsequent dysfunctions in the acceleration responses. When associated with poor acceleration responses, the cause is usually inconsistent negative reinforcement of the acceleration responses, but again, these may also have associations with confusions arising from concurrent signalling of both acceleration and deceleration responses. The remedy for tail-swishing is to re-install acceleration responses so that a single stride is reinforced to arise without resistance and from a light signal, so upward transitions are integral in this process. Sometimes tail-swishing is related only to leg or spur use and may even be a learned response if a previous rider used excessive leg cues. If this is the case, whip-tapping may be used as a supplementary or alternative signal to reinstall the acceleration response to a light leg cue.

Horses may develop ***chronic behaviour disorders*** if their attempts to cope with fearful events regularly fail. These disorders may show up as aggressive or defensive behaviours or as insecurities. Such behaviours may be influenced by testosterone, in that stallions are more inclined to become aggressive than geldings or mares. These behaviours are unique in that they manifest out of the original conflict situation: the horse may simply show aggression whenever it comes into contact with people. Such horses are usually kept in protective custody where they are less exposed to people, which might exacerbate their neuroses.

Biting, kicking, striking and ***threatening*** can become habitual and, furthermore (and quite understandably), can be reinforced by the retreat of people during these attacks (Figure 13.21). Biting during training may also be related to a lack of social contact with other horses outside the training situation, as reported by Søndergaard and Ladewig (2004), where singly-housed horses bit the trainer significantly more often than did group-housed horses. Horses showing severe biting or other undesired human-directed behaviour should be treated with caution and handled only by experienced personnel.

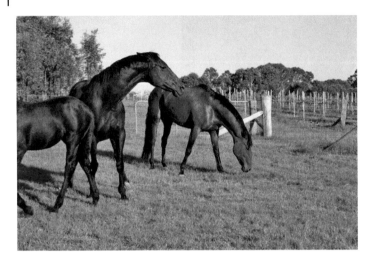

Figure 13.21 Aggression among horses rarely leads to injuries in well-socialised horses, because most agonistic interactions consist of threats without physical contact. Lack of social contact can lead to increased biting during training.

Their rehabilitation may be a lengthy process and requires identification and removal of the underlying cause of the behaviour, as well as thorough in-hand re-training of acceleration and deceleration responses, reinforcing single strides of correct behaviour through the release of pressure until the responses emerge from light signals. It is interesting to note that well-socialised horses rarely injure each other (Christensen *et al.*, 2011a; Hartmann *et al.*, 2012), because most agonistic interactions consist of threats without physical contact (Christensen *et al.*, 2002).

Separation anxiety is common in horses and it is particularly difficult for the young, naïve horse to be left behind in a stable or paddock. Horses have evolved to live in groups and their insecurity when left alone can induce strong stress reactions. If the horse is in a highly aroused state when the other horses return, this may act to reinforce locomotory behaviour. Separating foals from their mothers during weaning is also problematic, yet research on the effects in later life such as increased neophobia is lacking.

If it is necessary to habituate horses to social isolation, it is best done via systematic desensitisation, progressing only when the horse reliably fails to react to the previous level and ensuring that only desired behaviour is reinforced. The horse should initially be trained to leave the other horses, because it is usually less stressful to leave the group than to be left behind. A study found that training a naïve horse to leave the group initially with a companion is not efficient, because these horses showed no evidence of having habituated to social isolation faster than horses trained individually from the start (Hartmann *et al.*, 2011). It is useful to combine the systematic desensitisation procedure with counter-conditioning to make the horse associate isolation with a pleasant stimulus, such as food.

Separation anxiety may also be expressed in horses that are confused and subject to inconsistent reinforcement of responses, because the stress related to this increases the horse's motivation to seek security among other horses. The increased predictability conferred by consistent reinforcement and light, less obtrusive signals may lower the horse's motivation to seek conspecifics. Similarly, horses that show ***horse-shy*** behaviour (being fearful of approaching other horses) may be insufficiently habituated to the unnatural situation of passing close by other (unknown) horses that are trotting or cantering in the other direction, especially in a fenced area where the horse may feel trapped between the wall/fence and the approaching horse. A horse may also become horse-shy if it has prior experience of being attacked or threatened by a passing horse; the latter may not even have been noticed by the rider, as horses can perceive and react to very subtle cues. The rehabilitation of these horses involves systematic desensitisation to initially well-known horses passing closer and closer, and consistent reinforcement of correct responses (McLean and McLean, 2008). When the horse no longer reacts to a well-known horse passing close by, the procedure is repeated with unknown horses.

Take-Home Messages

The following principles apply to horse-training with regard to managing fear:

- Identify the cause of fear and diminish all expressions of the flight response. Habituation to fear-eliciting stimuli can be achieved through various desensitisation methods (as described in Chapter 4, Non-associative Learning).
- When a horse shows fearful behaviours, *slow* the horse's legs with downward transitions.
- Reduce the pressure required to elicit responses trained by negative reinforcement to the least obtrusive cues (light cues).

Ethical Implications

- As a matter of urgency, regulatory bodies for equestrian coaching must legislate for an appropriate use of learning theory in all equestrian coaching activity.
- Fear responses are a major cause of horse–human accidents.
- Excessive fear has negative implications for learning, memory, reproduction and health through the damaging effects of frequently elevated levels of glucocorticoids.
- Fear and pain are interlinked because once a horse has perceived a painful stimulus it will become frightened of this, and similar stimuli, in the future.
- Many ridden and led horses endure pain on a regular basis due to deficits in the tactile signals for *stop*, *go* and *turn*.
- Frequent or chronic stress caused by inappropriate housing, management and training has profound welfare implications for horses.

Areas for Further Research

- An accurate description of behavioural signs of stress in the ridden horse.
- Comparisons of different habituation methods in terms of efficiency and stress imposed on the horse.
- Effects of artificial weaning on horses with respect to neophobia.

14

Ethical Equitation

Introduction

In principle, our use of the horse differs little from our use of other animals for food, fibre, transport, traction, entertainment, and so on (Midgley, 1983; Regan, 1983). However, equitation offers a novel motivation for the use of animals, namely, the drive of some people to use horses in pursuit of a certain psychological satisfaction: 'winning'. The desire to win appears to go beyond the notion of pleasure or even success, because it requires that we outperform other people. Does this make it the ultimate exercise in human pride, vanity and individualism? And if so, does this provide a justifiable motivation for the use of animals, even when pain and suffering may be involved? This line of thinking has prompted cynicism about the use of terms such as the 'equine athlete', as if horses can be willing participants in the heavy slog and self-sacrifice we generally associate with human athletes (Cathy Schuller, personal communication, 2008).

People can be adept at justifying practices they might secretly have misgivings about. Critics may say that until we can prove that horses read scoreboards, there is no evidence at all that they share an interest in winning. They would go on to urge that we dispense with anthropomorphic rhetoric that spuriously suggests such a shared interest in winning, and review some of the common practices that can compromise equine welfare.

Generally, ethical arguments are based on cost/benefit analysis (Jones and McGreevy, 2010). Do the costs for the working horse outweigh the benefits (Table 14.1) for humans or possibly the long-term benefits for the horse as an individual or as a species? After all, training can also assist in enhancing fitness, thereby reducing disease and injury rates, and beyond that, if we were not to use horses for our equestrian purposes, hardly anyone would keep horses and their numbers would be greatly reduced, if not threatened by extinction. If we acknowledge that horses will always be required to work for us, how can we refine their use so that it is morally justified? The debate about what defines ethical horse use and, particularly, ethical equitation, has yet to be heard. A frank appraisal of horse-riding as an ethical pursuit may seem absurd to many riders, but we believe that the issue of ethical equitation is a fascinating and largely unexplored one. Just because we *can* do something to a horse does not make it an ethically sound practice. Horses may appear extremely tolerant, seeming to put up with interventions even when these are broadly aversive. However, this could simply be a manifestation of their outstanding abilities in habituation and associative learning.

If horses were truly able to comprehend their environment, then perhaps they would not be so trainable and rideable and maybe it would be unethical to ride them. After all, if horses *were* capable of reflection, they would

Equitation Science, Second Edition. Paul McGreevy, Janne Winther Christensen,
Uta König von Borstel and Andrew McLean.
© 2018 John Wiley & Sons Ltd. Published 2018 by John Wiley & Sons Ltd.
Companion website: www.wiley.com/go/mcgreevy/equitation

Table 14.1 An example of different aspects of equestrian activities, their associated costs and benefits to both horses and humans and potential measures to optimise cost:benefit ratios.

Aspect	Costs	Benefits for *horses* and/or trainers	Potential measures to optimise cost:benefit ratio
Confinement of horses to husbandry system	Deprivation of freedom to move, forage, associate with desired conspecifics	***Increased quality and length of life*** due to: Safety from predators. Provision of adequate shelter and nutrition. Quick access to other horses	Provision of group housing with sufficient amount and quality of space. Adjusting group composition, if necessary. Careful adjustment of nutrition to each horse's individual nutritional and behavioural requirements
Use of negative reinforcement as main means of training horses	Pressures can cause discomfort, pain or injury. Incorrect use can cause confusion, frustration	Bridles and reins are effective in controlling horses in emergency situations, particularly if horse is well-trained	Correct use of learning principles to refine cues as much as possible. Use of positive rather than negative reinforcement where possible
Use of coercive force to control horse and optimise sport performance	Pain or injury in the horse; possibly also secondary risk of injury when horses are pushed beyond their limits	In some equestrian horse sports, use of coercion may increase odds of winning a given competition/race	Change competition rules so that use of coercion leads to penalties
Inherent risk of accidents due to equestrian activities	Risk of pain and injury	Moderate levels of training ***increase fitness and reduce risk of injury and various diseases***	Finding an optimal level of training intensity to maximise fitness and minimise risk of exercise-related injuries
Survival of the species *Equus*	All of the above	***If horses were not used for work or equestrian purposes, their numbers would be greatly reduced*** as there would be in the modern world limited or no habitat left for horses to survive as a species	All of the above

suffer by comprehending their own enslavement and the ubiquity of pressure during ridden work, of having to jump clearly avoidable obstacles, and of having to carry another being. The horse would be consumed by his longing for freedom to simply be a horse: to eat grass, be with affiliates and be free of human exploitation. That said, there is reason to believe that the correctly and humanely trained horse is not distressed by its interactions with humans. Indeed, ethical training and riding can provide environmental and behavioural enrichment (O'Brien *et al.*, 2008). This is a valid proposition because the horse

has evolved to discriminate and respond to multiple stimuli in a complex landscape covering hundreds of hectares. For the modern horse kept in a comparatively uneventful few square metres, clear, consistent learning outcomes that arise during their interactions with humans most likely fulfil the behavioural need to learn how best to interact with the environment.

This book emphasises the reliance on pressure and release in horse-riding, and how the use of pressure of any sort distinguishes equitation from training in most other species not used for riding or traction.

Given that negative reinforcement is the critical control mechanism, horses cannot be safely ridden without some degree of pressure. Ethical equitation demands that minimal pressure and immediate release is used at all times for both contact (if relevant to the sport) and signalling. If horsemanship relies on consistency (and therefore clarity in training), what are the long-term consequences of inconsistent training techniques? Can poor training affect aspects of the horse's ethogram that do not seem to be directly related to the trained responses? For example, this may explain the anecdotal finding that training flaws confined to human–horse interactions seem to lead to social dysfunctions in horse–horse interactions (McLean, 2005b).

As in other sports, many horse-owners, trainers and riders will arrive at a choice between doing something 'bad' that may increase their chances of winning, or not doing it and relinquishing the possibility of first place. It may be a decision about using a gadget or a drug, withholding food or water, or hurting the horse.

The extent to which sport horses are coerced to perform is often the focus of welfare debates. The roads-and-tracks and steeplechase elements have disappeared from the sport of horse-trials. It is also possible that steeplechasing and the use of the whip in racing may be moderated in response to pressure from outside the racing industry. For example, in Norway, whips have been banned from harness-racing, both during warm-up and races (The Norwegian Harness Racing Association, 2015), and the Norwegian harness-racing and betting industries continue to thrive. The same can be said for Norwegian Thoroughbred racing. The horse-welfare lobby has begun to voice its concerns about other elite equestrian events, too – some people find the dressage movement called piaffe unacceptable.

Equitation science will be able to play a vital role in deciding the outcome of these debates and, particularly in dressage competition, emergent technology will remove subjectivity from judging and will underpin the development of high-welfare dressage. The sport of soccer has set an excellent example of how judges' decisions can be supported by technology (e.g. by introducing goal-line technology to increase objectivity of judges' decisions when keeping scores). Equestrian sports that involve judging decisions might be well advised to learn a lesson from the progressiveness of other sports (König von Borstel and McGreevy, 2014). Science may be able to help us value training of any manoeuvre that is dependent on and achieved through lightness of pressure (i.e. attesting to self-carriage and the horse's self-maintenance of rhythm, straightness and outline) (McGreevy *et al.*, 2005). Imagine dressage scores being awarded for the most humane training techniques. Despite its anthropomorphic connotations, the introduction of the concept of the happy equine athlete by the Fédération Equestre Internationale (FEI) to its rules governing dressage competition can be seen as a step towards better welfare in that sport. Although problematic to judge, the introduction of the happiest horse prize to the Olympics and World Championships for Dressage may yield positive effects.

Whips and Welfare

Across the various sports and equestrian codes, any real consensus on equine welfare indicators is superficial at best. Prime examples of this are regulations governing the use of the whip. Compare these with the FEI's general regulations. The British Horseracing Authority (BHA) has the world's most exhaustive instructions on the use of the whip in racing (BHA, 2009). These stipulate that the whip should be used for 'safety, correction and encouragement only'. The ways in which the whip may and should not be used are described in Table 14.2.

The BHA's disciplinary enquiries usually relate to how the horse ran, for example, a failure to run a horse on its merits; interference with other runners; excessive use of the whip. The first and last of these imply use of

Table 14.2 Verbatim instructions on acceptable and unacceptable use of the whip according to BHA rules.

Acceptable use of the whip	Unacceptable
Showing the whip and giving the horse time to respond before using it	Hitting: • To the extent of injury • With the whip arm above shoulder height • Rapidly, without regard to the horse's stride • With excessive force • With excessive frequency • Without giving the horse time to respond
Using the whip in the backhand* position for a reminder	Hitting horses that are: • Showing no response • Out of contention • Clearly winning • Past the winning post
Having used the whip, giving the horse a chance to respond to it before using it again	Hitting horses anywhere except: • On the quarters (hindquarters) with the whip in either the backhand or forehand position • Down the shoulder with the whip in the backhand position, unless exceptional circumstances prevail
Keeping both hands on the reins when using the whip down the shoulder in the backhand position	
Using the whip in rhythm with the horse's stride and close to its side	
Swinging the whip or actually using it to keep the horse straight	

Adapted with permission from BHA (2008).
* Backhand position means a rotation that is clockwise from the jockey's perspective.

the whip that appears, at first glance, to be contradictory. To be convinced that a jockey has run a horse on its merits ('ridden a horse out'), many punters would need to see him use the whip. So what constitutes excessive use of the whip? This is poorly described, not least because both pressure and frequency must be assessed. Fundamentally, it is difficult to make a visual appraisal of the amount of force being used – although whips with force recorders are being designed and may revolutionise the monitoring of whip use. Rarely, jockeys may be accused of hitting the horse on multiple occasions without giving it time to respond.

This point is critical because jockeys and trainers know that the response of the horse to the whip cannot be assumed. In other words, to some extent the use of the whip, if only as a test of whether the horse has the energy to respond, becomes obligatory. Some horses speed up, others slow down. For example, in a study of Quarterhorses at the gallop, the use of a whip on the shoulder of the leading forelimb, in rhythm with the stride, did not increase speed but reduced stride length and increased stride frequency (Deuel and Lawrence, 1987). To learning theorists, this report might suggest a flawed understanding of negative reinforcement, since the stimulus to run faster was withdrawn following the wrong response (reduction in stride length). An analysis of racetrack patrol videos has shown that 38% of breakdown injuries occur after use of the whip (Ueda *et al.*, 1993). This may reflect the rider's response when a horse begins to pull up with acute lameness.

Racing stewards' judgments commonly focus on frequency of whip use. They base their judgements on whether the number of hits was reasonable and necessary over the distance they were given, taking into account the horse's experience and whether it was continuing to respond. Clearly, this is subjective. It is blurred further by the stewards' need to factor in the degree of force used: 'the more times a horse has been hit, the stricter will be the view taken over the degree of force which is reasonable' (BHA, 2009).

As identified already, these rules are subjective. For instance, the definition of a 'reminder' is questionable (Table 14.2) in terms of learning theory and we might question whether keeping both hands on the reins while using the whip (down the shoulder) constitutes a good riding technique. In current best practice, the whip is swung by the jockey in a clockwise rotation and may not even make contact with the horse; each iteration coincides with suspension of the gallop (Chapter 11, Biomechanics) and any contact coincides with the beginning of the stance phases of each stride.

In performance sports, the whip should be held like a ski pole (Figure 14.1a), not like a

(a)   (b)

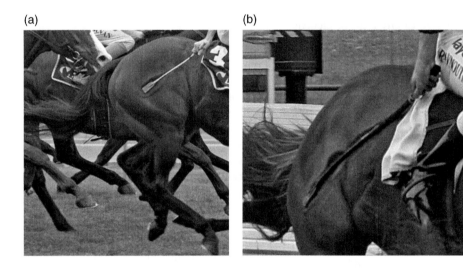

(c)

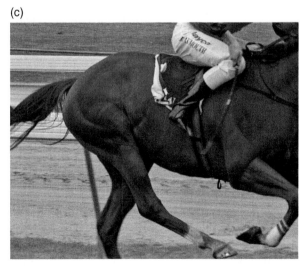

Figure 14.1 The whip can exert different forces on impact, depending on how it is held. Both regular whips (a) and padded whips (b) can leave welt marks (c).

tennis racquet (Figure 14.1b). To align with learning theory, the whip must be applied with very light pressure at first, so it becomes a discriminative signal (Chapter 7, Applying Learning Theory). This can be followed by a contiguous evenly spaced rhythm of increasing or maintained pressure that is removed when the horse offers the correct response. The FEI's General Regulations (2007) stipulate that no person may abuse a horse at *any* time (i.e. not only during an official event). They define abuse as any actions or omissions that cause or are likely to cause pain or unnecessary discomfort. These include:

- whipping or beating a horse excessively;
- subjecting a horse to any kind of electric shock device;
- using spurs excessively or persistently;
- jabbing the horse in the mouth with the bit or any other device;
- competing using an exhausted, lame or injured horse;
- 'rapping' a horse (Chapter 12, Unorthodox Techniques);
- abnormally sensitising or desensitising any part of a horse (Chapter 12, Unorthodox Techniques);
- leaving a horse without adequate food, drink or exercise (interestingly, Xenophon would have been barred, on the strength of his proposal that horses should be kept for periods without food and water so that eventually they associate the human carer with the arrival of these resources); and
- using any device or equipment that causes excessive pain to the horse if it knocks down an obstacle.

How are FEI stewards to decide whether a beating has been excessive? Is it excessive for that horse, its perceived crime or the combination of these because of the horse's 'prior form'? Fundamentally, the term 'excessive' implies that a certain amount of whipping is indeed appropriate or even required. This is of concern since it presumes that an onlooker (in this case, the steward or judge) can calculate a prescribed dose of pain without even having ridden the horse or known its history, let alone the principles of learning theory as

they apply to aversive stimuli in equitation. Fundamentally, it is difficult to make a visual appraisal of the amount of force being used. There are sound arguments for banning the use of the whip altogether in horse-racing. Apart from welfare benefits, this would encourage trainers and jockeys to use more enlightened training methods and, of course, there would still be winners. Perhaps, too, the horses would be easier to re-home at the end of their careers if they were not subject to punishment during their racing careers.

It could be argued that the welfare of the UK racehorse has better safeguards than the horse competing under the protection of the FEI, since at least the ways in which it cannot be whipped are stipulated. The recent ban by the Danish and Swedish Equestrian Federations on the use of whips and spurs in punishment and a complete ban of whips and spurs in Norwegian harness-racing and Thoroughbred racing has raised the possibility of a global move against the use of aversive stimuli for nonperformance.

Recent studies have revealed how difficult it is to justify the whipping of tired horses. For example, one study has shown that increased whip use is most frequent in the final two 200 m sections of races, when horses are fatigued (Evans and McGreevy, 2011). It demonstrated that increased whip use is not associated with sufficient variation in velocity to explain final placings. There is also a report indicating that the carriage (and, by inference, the lateralised use) of the whip, by the left or right hand appears to be primarily determined by handedness of the jockey, not by the direction of the track. This finding challenges the traditional view that the whip needs to be retained for steering purposes (McGreevy and Oddie, 2011). Additionally, there is also evidence that apprentice jockeys whip horses on average more than three times as often as non-apprentice jockeys (McGreevy and Ralston, 2012). These findings, taken together, indicate that the suffering horses endure from whip use has no purpose and is due to tradition rather than reason.

The racing industry relies on the use of the padded whip to reduce pain and on the rules of racing to ensure that whip use is not abusive. However, there is no research to indicate that the padded whip is pain-free, although it is reasonable to assume that, if it were used in the same way and with the same force as a traditional whip, it would have less impact, thereby causing less tissue damage and thus less response with less-intense associated pain in general terms. However, still photographs and high-speed video footage of whip use during Australian flat races indicate that when padded whips are used, both the padded and unpadded sections can make contact with the horse (McGreevy *et al.*, 2013) and that strikes where the unpadded section of the whip makes contact with the horse are more common than when only the padded section makes contact (McGreevy *et al.*, 2013). Additionally, there is evidence that the rules of racing are difficult to police (McGreevy *et al.*, 2013; Hood *et al.*, 2017).

One study has identified whip use as a potential risk factor for horse falls (Pinchbeck *et al.*, 2004) and specifically suggested that there were increased risks of falling from whip use 'immediately before an obstacle is jumped and while a horse is progressing in position during the race. This may be due to increased speed and/or the horse being unbalanced by whip use.' As mentioned above, an analysis of racetrack patrol videos suggested that 38% of breakdown injuries occurred after whip use (Ueda *et al.*, 1993). Possible explanations for this association include that riders respond to horses beginning to pull up with lameness by using the whip, that increased speed from whip use reduces safety or that riders use the whip to avert a potential fall as a breakdown begins (i.e. for genuine safety). These findings may suggest that whip use actually decreases safety, and that whip use for so-called correction may be counter-productive.

The racing industry has failed to counter any of these criticisms, so it seems likely that the use of the whip in racing will eventually disappear. If this happens, whip use in other equestrian codes will next come under close scrutiny, although guidelines on the ethical use of whips could assist in the retention of whips where their use can be minimised. These guidelines require that negative reinforcement should involve the use of minimal force; that aversive stimuli used to provoke a response should be used appropriately and minimally so that habituation and stress are avoided; that appropriate timing and release should be adhered to in all training; and finally, that punishment and fear should be avoided in horse-training.

Restrictive Nosebands

Horses tolerate interventions that most species would not. This does not mean that whatever we *can* do to horses is ethical. One of the leading examples is nosebands, which 30 years ago were largely aesthetic rather than functional. These days, restrictive nosebands on horse bridles are being tightened so much in some equestrian competitions that horses are suffering stress, reduced blood flow in the area and ultimately even deformed nasal bones.

The horse's mouth never evolved to accommodate a bit and there is no convenient space in the buccal cavity waiting to be filled by one. When the tongue is depressed by a bit, it does not fit in the narrow inter-mandibular space, so many bits press the tongue against the bars of the mouth. Fluoroscopic studies show that the bit rests on the tongue, rather than on the bars of the mouth, as was originally believed (Clayton, 2005). The regular snaffle bit is designed to apply pressure broadly across the tongue and, some believe, also the upper palate. Jointed bits tend to form a peak as tension increases in the reins; these are said to have a nutcracker action across the tongue and into the upper palate. Certain types of bits may be associated with a reduction in swallowing frequency (Manfredi *et al.*, 2005) possibly by restricting movements of the tongue that are necessary in deglutition. So, it is easy to see why horses would need to move their tongue and mandible while wearing a regular snaffle bit. When we add the second bit of a double bridle, we must expect more of such movements and when the rider picks up the reins to take up a contact, the need for the horse to make minor adjustments, as it seeks comfort, increases still further.

Excellent equestrian technique relies on steady and sensitive hands that give clear cues and avoid the application of relentless pressure. In dressage, judges reward tactful riding in the scores they assign for so-called submission – a notoriously subjective collection of marks on which judges agree least (Hawson *et al.*, 2010b). Submission scores include lightness of contact through the reins and so they are one of the few ways in which good horse welfare can be celebrated in competition (König von Borstel and McGreevy, 2014). Certainly, there is more poll flexion than there used to be and arguably more conflict at the level of mouth (Lashley *et al.*, 2014).

It is an established principle of ethical equitation that the horse's relaxation must be benchmarked (McGreevy and McLean, 2007; ISES, 2011). This entails training lightness of rein contact by carefully eliminating expressions of mouth discomfort, such as opening, gaping or crossing the jaw. The rules of dressage anticipate that horses will open their mouths unless ridden lightly and dressage stewards used to check that nosebands were not too tight.

When horses open their mouths to evade the bit, one short-term response by riders and trainers is to use a noseband that keeps the mouth tightly closed. Clearly, this does nothing to help the horse relax its jaw and is likely to act as an additional stressor. The same criticism can be levelled at tongue ties, since they restrict normal movement of the tongue, such as during swallowing, and stop the horse finding comfort. As equestrian sports became more popular and competitive in the 1970s, dropped nosebands gave way to Hanoverian, crossover and grackle nosebands. Then in the 1980s, 'crank' nosebands emerged. These have an added feature: they can be tightened much further than regular nosebands by means of a lever action. They are now common in all three of the Olympic equestrian disciplines but arguably dressage which, by definition, should be all about training, is where their use is least acceptable. In a recent statement, the FEI Director of Dressage, Trond Asmyr said, 'The FEI is currently looking into all aspects of nosebands, including possible ways of measuring tightness' and further stated, 'The FEI rules previously included guidelines which stated that it should be possible to put two fingers under the noseband. This was a very imprecise measurement, due to the different finger sizes of the persons who did the checks, and also how they were used. As a result, this sentence was removed.'

Many equestrian manuals and competition rule-books propose that 'two fingers' be used as a spacer to guard against over-tightening, but fail to specify where this gauge should be applied or, indeed, the size of the fingers. A taper gauge has been developed, based on the mean circumference of adult index and middle fingers (9.89 ± 0.21 cm) (McGreevy *et al.*, 2012). This amount of space under the noseband allows horses to express conflict behaviour and so aligns with the principles of ethical equitation. That said, it does not permit horses to perform the full repertoire of behaviours, including yawning (McGreevy *et al.*, 2012). Unfortunately, as the popularity of crank nosebands has increased, stewards have become less likely to check on noseband tightness.

Sadly, the practice of restricting jaw movement has become entrenched, as it prevents the horse from opening its mouth which, in dressage, is regarded as a sign of resistance or lack of compliance and attracts penalties for the rider. So, here is the paradox: rules that penalise evidence of rough riding (e.g. mouth opening) have prompted the development of gadgets that mask such evidence. By their design, these tight nosebands restrict virtually all normal jaw and tongue movements in the horses, primarily for the sake of avoiding penalties in competition. As the tightness of the noseband increases, there seems to be an elevation in horses' sensitivity to the bit, presumably because it becomes more uncomfortable (Randle and McGreevy, 2011). So, riders may also feel that they have more control of the horse when the noseband is tighter, which is why such nosebands appeal not only to dressage riders but to many show-jumpers and eventers and, to some, this gives the appearance of the horse becoming more 'submissive'.

Relentless pressure from nosebands has been likened to pressure from a tourniquet and can reach levels associated in humans with tissue and nerve damage (Casey *et al.*, 2013). Nosebands are padded to avoid cutting the skin, but inside the mouth, they force the cheeks against (naturally) sharp molars and are associated with lacerations and ulcers. Damage to the medial aspect of the buccal mucosa may eventuate when it is pushed against sharp molars, but this should not be remedied solely by rasping the teeth. Removing parts of the horse just because they do not suit the rider's purpose is very difficult to defend.

A study of naïve horses wearing jaw-clamping nosebands has shown that, depending on their tightness, crank nosebands compromise or eliminate several behaviours, including yawning, licking, chewing and swallowing. Unsurprisingly, denying horses oral comfort is associated with physiological distress and a post-inhibitory rebound in the restricted behaviours once the nosebands are removed (Fenner *et al.*, 2016). Consequently, on welfare grounds, the use of nosebands that constrict and have potential to cause injuries should not be permitted in training or competition. Tight nosebands can mask unwanted behaviour in horses, which might be indicative of either pain or deficiencies in training or, indeed, both. Unfortunately, the loosening of nosebands might reveal undesirable responses that could be dangerous to riders and other horse–rider combinations. Riders should therefore rule out any pain-related issues in their horses and ensure that their horses are trained according to principles of learning theory to meet the demands of competition.

Given that over-tightened nosebands put so much pressure on horses' nose and mouth areas that they cause distress and obvious injuries to the horses, equestrian competition organisers are under some obligation to decrease the harmful effects of these detrimental devices. In most equestrian disciplines, stewards check that all equipment used on horses complies with the regulations specified for that discipline. Now that there is a simple standard taper gauge that can be used by stewards at competition to measure the gap under the noseband in a fair and objective way, adding a simple noseband-tightness test would be straightforward for competition organisers.

The widespread appeal of noseband tightening and the problems with checking tightness at competitions was revealed by a recent international study of 750 horses showing that, across a range of equestrian disciplines, 44% of horses had no appreciable space under their nosebands and only 7% passed the traditional test of having sufficient space underneath the nosebands to accommodate two fingers (Doherty *et al.*, 2017). The practice of over-tightening nosebands to avoid penalties in competition covers up poor training at the expense of horse welfare. By instituting rules to ensure that nosebands are not tightly clamping horses' mouths shut, horsesport organisations will alleviate horse suffering and also promote excellent training.

Ethical Considerations and Equitation Science

Equitation science can help to inform the decisions we make as equestrians. For example, there is a need for debate around some of the central tenets of horse-training, such as contact and half-halts, which are too loosely interpreted to be universally understood. These issues are currently the source of too much data-free and, therefore, largely semantic, debate among coaches, confusion among riders and conflict in horses.

Perhaps equitation science will permit the rules of equestrian sport to be revisited in the light of more scientific rigour. For example, the FEI rules stipulate that in passage the toe of the forehoof should be elevated to the middle of the contralateral cannon (whereas the toe of the hindhoof should be raised slightly above the contralateral fetlock joint) (FEI 2008). In the individual medal finals at the Barcelona Olympics, none of the horses performing passage achieved this amount of elevation in the forelimbs (Argue, 1994). It may be that equitation science will help to show why this height is difficult to achieve in contemporary training.

Ethical equitation may help us to answer the question: 'Can happiness ever be measured in an equine athlete?' Can we ever be sure of happiness in a horse beyond satiation or absence of pain? Some might say that happiness is an emergent property of higher mental abilities, while others feel that happiness *in horses* occurs simply when they are in a familiar but fresh pasture, with clement weather, familiar conspecific company, no flies and no evidence of predators. There is a growing body of literature on the conscious life of animals, and this may be relevant when trying to determine what 'matters' to them (e.g. McMillan, 2005).

Ethical equitation could also lead to calls for better matching of horses and humans. For example, should certain humans be allowed to ride horses with which they are poorly matched? Are novice riders a potential threat to the welfare of the horses they learn on? Should sentient beings be exposed to complete novices who are not simply learning to ride but also learning to balance? Perhaps, before allowing them to balance and provide negative reinforcement humanely on a horse, we should teach novice riders (including children) the principles of associative learning and negative reinforcement. With human obesity levels rising in the developed world (Flegal *et al.*, 1998; Ogden *et al.*, 2014), the maximum weight of the rider a horse should be required to carry is another aspect of current debate in ethical equitation. Investigation of horse use in military contexts suggests that horses could carry up to 10% of their bodyweight for extended periods of low-impact work without adverse effects. That said, although regular

(circa 125 kg) or cuirassier (circa 160 kg) military tack and rider weight (Nordendorf and Hekele, 1997) frequently exceeded this threshold and we must remember that typical cavalry horses were not of exceptionally heavy build and thus weighed considerably less than 1000 kg. More recent research has focused on the requirements of typical riding sessions of short duration and medium exercise intensity and has revealed increased signs of muscle fatigue, such as elevated heart rates and increased levels of muscle soreness, when horses carried 25–30% of their bodyweight, compared to 15–20% (Powell *et al.*, 2008). A UK survey suggests that these thresholds are commonly exceeded in the general population of horse–rider pairs (Halliday and Randle, 2013). However, additional factors, such as horses' conformation, also play a role, such that horses with wider loins and thicker cannon bone circumferences seem to show less fatigue when carrying the same weight compared to more lightly built horses (Powell *et al.*, 2008). Rider skill level is also thought to play a role in the emergence of equine fatigue, although one study did not observe differences in equine kinematics, heart-rate recovery times or lactate concentrations when exercise bouts with a 90 kg rider were compared with exercise bouts with 90 kg lead (van Oldruitenborgh-Oosterbaan *et al.*, 1995).

Now is the right moment for the bodies that govern horse sports to identify the types of scientific evidence they require when considering the welfare implications of novel techniques and technological advances. The governing bodies of horse sports should encourage research into the most humane application of pressure and alternative means of communicating with horses and reinforcing them.

Horses that are of no further use have low monetary value and are therefore more likely to be neglected. Thus, we can see a direct relationship between welfare and usefulness and so we should look forward to a time when more emphasis is placed on ensuring that sport horses are under stimulus control and not exposed to motivational conflict and thus remain useful after their competitive careers have ended.

It is even possible to look to a time when competitions that use horses (and therefore aversive stimuli under a negative reinforcement framework) reward welfare above all else. This would be especially important if we ever see the emergence of technological advances (such as rein-tension meters) that facilitate restraint with due regard for welfare. The emphasis on lightness that is receiving increased attention in some sections of the dressage world is likely to prove critical here. At the same time, the rules concerning the mandatory use of the double bridle and spurs in higher levels of dressage will come under closer scrutiny. In some countries, the bodies that administer national dressage competitions have moved to make the use of double bridles optional for competitors. In Australia, for example, snaffle bridles can now be worn at all levels of national competition, but if classes are held under FEI rules, then double bridles are still compulsory for tests above and including Advanced (fifth) level.

Ethical horse-use also demands ethical horse-breeding and this raises some interesting questions. For example, if laterality studies and temperament tests identify foals that are likely to prove difficult to train, how will this affect those foals' commercial value and ultimately their welfare. Will a horse's tolerance of poor riding be a quality that we value and therefore select for? Have we in fact been doing this for some time? Biotechnologies (and ultimately cloning) may allow horses of extraordinary ability or tolerance to become more predictably available, meaning that riders and trainers do not have to modify or moderate their own behaviour as much as they currently do.

However, these debates must be considered in light of the fact that, despite the growth of horse numbers used in sport and leisure, these are easily eclipsed by the number of horses in working contexts. There are an estimated 90 million equids in the developing world (FAO statistical database, 2003). Indeed, more than 95% of all donkeys and mules and 60% of all horses are found in developing countries (Fielding, 1991), the majority being used for work (Figure 14.2). Working and competition horses all thrive on the appropriate application of learning theory, even though the responses expected of them often seem worlds apart. Use of relentless pressure when working with animals and lack of will to refine cues certainly merit close

(a)

(b)

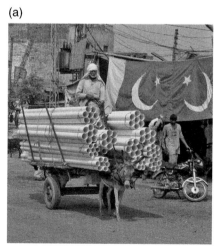 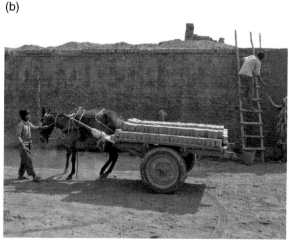

Figure 14.2 In less developed countries, donkeys and mules remain an important source of power. Their health and ability to work can directly affect a family's livelihood. (Photos courtesy of Becky Whay.)

scrutiny from those interested in advancing horse welfare, but overstrain, heat stress, dehydration, malnutrition, and chronic pain due to lack of appropriate medical and hoof care and lesions from ill-fitting equipment play a major role in the welfare of working horses in developing countries (Swann, 2006, Ali *et al.*, 2015) compared to sport horses of the Western world. Just as the military use of horses foreshadowed competitive dressage, perhaps we can look forward to a time when skills refined in competition find a place in working contexts. So, while best practice in training allows riders to get the best out of the horse in competition, the same principles could ensure that the working equid is spared from abuse and the catabolic effects of chronic stress (Moberg and Mench, 2000). The lot of the working horse in the Western context was the primary focus of the first piece of UK anti-cruelty legislation (in 1822) and was highlighted by Sewell (1877), whose popular novel is credited with fuelling the UK animal-welfare movements by making people consider an animal's perspective. It is worth reflecting that, despite the passage of time and the wholesale improvement of awareness, much remains to be done.

Take-Home Messages

- The concept of the happy equine athlete may influence our decisions about how far horses can be pushed to perform for human glory.
- The aim of viewing good horsemanship is undermined when artificial equipment is substituted for or exaggerates genuine riding skills. While such tactics and gadgets may help individual competitors, they may not benefit the sport overall, neither its supporters nor the horses.
- Ethical equitation demands that minimal pressure and immediate release of that pressure are used for both contact (if relevant to the sport) and signalling at all times.
- Whipping horses to ensure that they perform may one day be considered abuse, regardless of the context.
- The welfare of working equids in the developing world in terms of both numbers and severity of welfare issues is arguably a larger problem than the threats to the welfare of sport and leisure horses in the Western world, but this issue is a sensitive one, as the owners' and caretakers' living conditions are often desperate, too.

15

Research Methods in Equitation Science

Introduction

Developing valid and reliable ethograms with a high degree of intra- and inter-observer reliability is fundamental to equitation science. We try to assess the responses of horses in a consistent and standardised way, so that behavioural observations made within training and/or study situations are accurately interpreted. Physiological measures are frequently used, with the proviso that exercise level, fitness and age be taken into consideration when interpreting results. We also collect and record commonly-used physiological measures and provide protocols when these are included. Developing technology allows us to measure interactions between rider and horse more and more easily, for example, with rein-tension gauges and pressure sensors, so we continually make recommendations for current use, noting limitations and future requirements for such equipment used in our studies.

Because we are dealing with both human and animal participants in these studies, animal ethics committees consider the impact on the horses, its mitigation and the justification for any residual stress. We also seek consent from owners, and take care to work within the legal framework of the country in which the research is being conducted. Researchers must consider the suitability of animals being used and whether the work constitutes a legal procedure. Inclusion and exclusion criteria are always defined but

obviously depend very much on the research question. In some countries, even if only the behaviour of the horse is to be assessed, all individuals who are part of an animal experiment must be considered by the animal ethics committee. Habituation to any scientific equipment should be undertaken prior to the study and we must make clear the rights of all human stakeholders to withdraw animals from the study where there are concerns about an animal's response to the equipment.

Before a study begins, if possible and feasible, we suggest that horses in a study have a veterinary examination, preferably by a veterinarian with an interest in horse behaviour. As clinical equine behavioural medicine matures, we are getting better at identifying individuals at high risk of certain disorders and eliminating them from studies of handling, training and riding, because they are likely to skew data if included. For the same reason, we should also try to become more skilled at identifying horses with true learning deficits or that are resistant to extinction, as often seen in stereotypic horses (Parker *et al.*, 2008).

Similarly, in some countries, human research ethics committees focus on how the research may affect riders and other stakeholders, such as the owners of horses used, employers of the riders (where applicable), and owners of venues where the study takes place. All human stakeholders involved must be fully informed of all that is required of them and

Equitation Science, Second Edition. Paul McGreevy, Janne Winther Christensen, Uta König von Borstel and Andrew McLean.
© 2018 John Wiley & Sons Ltd. Published 2018 by John Wiley & Sons Ltd.
Companion website: www.wiley.com/go/mcgreevy/equitation

give their written consent. They retain the right to withdraw themselves and their data from the study at any time (up to the point of submission for publication, at which time, unless researchers have explicit permission, all information is made anonymous). If travel is required, riders should be fully informed well before the study takes place. Fully informed consent must also be obtained where heart rate variability (HRV) measurements are to be taken from human participants, as pathological conditions of the heart may be detected.

When both horse and rider may be required to wear scientific equipment and may be asked to perform particular movements rather than to simply execute normal training routines, accurate science is best achieved by making the measurement situation as 'ecologically valid' as possible. Riders may have further biological information recorded (such as limb lengths, bodyweight), so they need to know before the study that such data will be taken, and what will happen to it (i.e. issues of data confidentiality). Health and safety aspects are a standard requirement for any study and these are usually included as part of approval by an ethical-review process, if such approval is required.

Designing a Study and Reporting Results

Depending on the nature of the study, features such as age, breed and gender may be standardised. When the aim is to evaluate current practices within equestrianism and to gather evidence on which recommendations for future practice can be based, it is important to replicate 'real' situations. Participants are usually recruited from the equestrian industry, but because costs often limit the number of animals used, organising adequate sample sizes for equine research is challenging. When multiple horses and riders are involved, it is even more difficult. Nevertheless, small samples can be useful if all characteristics of the horses and riders involved are recorded fully with an eye on

eventual meta-analyses. Using single or multiple riders both have advantages: a single rider will maximise consistency across horses (but the results of the study may then be attributable to the skills and experience of that individual); with multiple riders, the effects of different horse–human combinations must be considered. However, many editors of peer-reviewed journals would hesitate to accept a study for publication if only one rider were included. Even when testing the effect of two different treatments, any treatment effect may show up only in combination with a certain rider.

Controls included to mitigate potential rider effects will depend on the aim of the individual study and the resources available. A crossover design can be used with small samples to control treatment order effects when multiple treatments are involved. Of course, the order with which treatments are distributed must be balanced. Each treatment can leave a legacy, and although washout periods between treatments help to reduce this effect, they do not guarantee that each horse is at baseline condition at the start of the next treatment in a series. For this reason, order effects should be factored into any regression analysis exploring the effect of a treatment.

Sample Size

Optimal sample size balances statistical power with the practicality and difficulty of accessing a large sample group (Eng, 2003). An appropriate sample size can be calculated using the equation suggested by Eng (2003) of:

$$N = 4a^2 \left(Z_{crit} \right)^2 / D^2$$

where N = sample size; a = assumed standard deviation calculated from previous studies; Z_{crit} = standard normal deviation; and D = confidence interval. Standard deviations of the measures taken should be presented in the results to enable future researchers to calculate the optimal sample size for future studies. With data collection and analyses, planned statistical analysis should be considered during planning and before data collection begins, so that erroneous assumptions are not made. Pilot studies are highly recommended in the early stages of designing a study.

Randomising and Blinding Trials

Variable skill levels and bias in experimenters and other personnel, such as riders and trainers, can affect results. Where interventions take place that are proposed to influence data (e.g. training programs, physiotherapy), it is preferable that as far as possible they should be blinded to personnel until after data collection/analysis is completed. Also, when riders know what is being measured they may, consciously or not, ride differently, so is it imperative that riders are blinded to what is going on. For example, they might not be told when the pressure sensor is wired up to the computer.

An important variable in equitation science studies is the skill level of trainers and riders. Most usable criteria are co-dependent with the horse. The only current usable measure of rider-skill level is the highest competition level at which the rider has ridden. However, this is a crude measure, because skill level may not equate directly to competition level. For this reason, quantifying skill level is an important point for future discussion and some suggestions are included in Table 15.1.

Rider and Environmental Variables

The many variables that affect the behaviour of the horse–human dyad should be clearly described, ideally in a standardised way, in all studies involving ridden-horse behaviour, including sample (horse/pony) characteristics, rider features and environmental factors. Table 15.1 provides a list of variables and a suggested way of reporting them. Although by no means exhaustive, the list includes the main factors to be listed under three headings. Including experimental variable details, in this consistent way, means that it is easier to compare the findings of different studies. Human participant details must be stored securely and should not be attributable to individuals. There is relevant legislation relating to data protection and it is vital that this is adhered to.

If the experiment involves separate treatment groups, these groups should be as balanced as possible in relation to variables such as horse type, horse and rider age and experience. Null findings must also be reported so that studies are not repeated – this sometimes happens when results of completed studies are not published. Null findings also provide information for future studies and give valuable insights into equitation *per se*.

Recording Horse Behaviour

Evaluation and manipulation of the horse's behaviour is fundamental to equitation and equestrian sports (Hall *et al.*, 2013). The horse's behaviour demonstrates the different processes active in its brain and body and, in the ridden horse, this is directly influenced by human action. To report on and discuss equine behaviour we need to clearly define and widely understand an accepted definition of behaviour units. Such a basic ethogram of domestic horse–human interactions is not yet available, but the equid ethogram by McDonnell (2003) is an important standard. An ethogram can be defined as a comprehensive set of descriptions of characteristic behaviour patterns of a species (Lehner, 1996). Most behaviours are described in terms of body movements. Martin and Bateson (1993) recommend that quantitative recording of behaviour be preceded by a period of informal observation, so that we understand and describe both subject and the behaviour of interest. This initial phase of observing and clearly describing behaviour allows relevant research questions for quantitative and experimental research to be formulated.

Table 15.1 Factors to be recorded and suggested mode of recording for each factor: Riding discipline, horse/pony (sample) characteristics, rider features and environmental factors.

Factor	Suggested mode of recording
Riding discipline	For example: English (Dressage/Show-jumping/Eventing/Driving); Western (reining, pleasure, trail, horsemanship, cutting, team-penning); Gaited horse-riding; Baroque riding; working equitation; recreational riding
Horse/Pony	
Age	Years (months)
Gender	Mare/gelding/stallion
	State whether females are, or may be, pregnant or in oestrus
Breed/type	Specific breed or, at minimum, type: Hotblood, Warmblood or Coldblood
	Where crossbreds are being used, state the breeds involved only where there is documented evidence
Past experience	Time span under-saddle, previous training and related discipline, highest competition level
	If applicable, state different use of horse before current use at the time of the experiment (e.g. was it formerly a trotter or a breeding mare?)
Current role	Competitive discipline (if this varies between horses/ponies and/or if they participate in more than one discipline, including level), perceived level of training, non-competitive role
Management style	Type and amount of turnout, as well as companionship of other horses and seasonal variation
	Approximate size and type of turnout in SI units (i.e. pasture/paddock); hours/week of turnout. State whether turn-out is in groups or solitary
	Type of housing: Individual or group housing, size of stall. If individual, description of possibilities for contact with other horses; if group, size of group
Type and amount of feed	Reported in kg/day for roughage, grains and supplements, seasonal or temporal variation
Horse health	Horses should be clinically sound
Familiarity with test-area	Circumstances (e.g. daily riding training) and time-span (e.g. for 5 years)
Rider	
Gender	Male/female
Age	Years
Height/weight	SI units (metres/kilograms)
Riding experience	Time-span (years, months), equestrian qualifications (specify where appropriate), range/discipline(s), competitive level and success (Provincial/local, National, International). Professional role within equestrianism
Familiarity with horse	Time-span and hours/week riding and interacting with horse/pony. Is the horse/pony cared for by the rider? Regularity of contact (daily, more/less frequent?) (e.g. perceived experience in riding). Involvement in training the horse (yes/no/partly)
Environmental factors	
Presence/absence of other horses	Group/individual test. Proximity of other horses/horse-rider combinations
Test area	Indoors/outdoors; riding surface; area; boundary type (open fencing, close-boarded etc.)
Environmental conditions	As appropriate for study: Ambient temperature (degrees Celsius); humidity; wind speed; light conditions
Extraneous variables	Noise, visual stimuli, any other unexpected event (description of event and frequency of occurrence)

The Fédération Equestre Internationale (FEI) currently produces guidelines for assessing certain ridden-horse behaviours in dressage, providing detailed descriptions of movements involved and assessment criteria (FEI, 2012). However, within FEI guidelines only desired behaviours are described in detail and limited reference is made to specific behavioural events. Although it is important to incorporate currently used equestrian behavioural descriptors within experimental studies, we need a more comprehensive ridden-horse ethogram. Most ethograms are not purely descriptive but contain a certain degree of interpretation, so equitation science will help provide evidence on which to base such interpretations and assessment criteria within equestrian sport to arrive at this goal.

In the past, for the sake of adaptation to the individual situation, each paper assessing ridden-horse behaviour essentially contained its own ethogram of ridden-horse behaviour. However, using a common basis would help in comparing different studies, and a list of definitions (McDonnell 2003) (see also Glossary), in addition to descriptors included in the FEI Guidelines (FEI, 2012), provides a valuable starting point for developing a standard ethogram for ridden-horse behaviour.

The first step in studying any species must be a purely descriptive definition of its different behaviours, beginning by describing the movement of body parts alone and in combination with other body parts and leading to an assessment of the whole animal. Objective nomenclature generally demands the use of the Nomina Anatomica Veterinaria (ICVGAN, 2012), with a lay glossary available for use by the wider equestrian community. Lehner (1996) states that since functional descriptions can be confusing and misleading, they should be avoided, except when the function is intuitively obvious or supported by data. This demands that any functional interpretation is always supported by data on the relationship with physiological, social or environmental parameters. A functional ethogram is necessary for many studies, but regular updates are important before undertaking new studies to incorporate the rapidly evolving knowledge of functional interpretation of behaviour units.

Designing an ethogram is about careful observation and description of behaviours. An ethogram is needed for all studies where behaviour is measured. For a reliable and valid ethogram, a minimum requirement for assessment is standardisation of the method – all potential sources of variability must be identified and controlled or at least taken into account and reported. Standardisation also extends to formalising reports of the animal's response (e.g. by using check sheets, videos or voice recordings).

Observers should be trained to score the behaviours in the ethogram reliably and consistently. A fundamental step to ensure the reliability of all assessments in a study is to check the scoring of both inter- and intra-observers. Inter-observer reliability measures the likelihood that different observers will assess the same behaviours on the same occasion in the same manner. Differences between observers may be caused by imprecise definitions in the ethogram that allow individual interpretations. Intra-observer reliability measures the consistency of the scores of a single observer. In theory, the observer's assessment should report the same scores when the animal is observed for a second time under the same conditions (preferably using video images). In all studies with two or more observers, reliability of the observers should be tested in a pilot study and stated. Usually, this is reported using correlation coefficients, Kappa or Kendall. Repeatability, calculated on the basis of variance components from mixed-model analyses, can also be used and has the advantage that the values are corrected for other potentially influencing factors. It is generally accepted that a Kappa or Kendall value of 0.41–0.6 is regarded as average concordance, a value of 0.61–0.80 as substantial and above 0.8 as excellent concordance (Burn *et al.*, 2009).

Another pre-study consideration is how to validate behavioural elements. Validation should demonstrate how each element reflects precisely what it is intended to measure and can be achieved by correlating the results with physiological measures, and other scoring techniques. Since some behaviours occur in different contexts, the validation process can inadvertently complicate some behaviours used as indicators of a single function. Principal Component Analysis can be applied to interpret these functions and study the underlying motivation, although it is chiefly used to reduce the number of variables and explain the biggest part of any reported variation.

Video images are useful for training purposes, especially to test the reliability of observers over time. No study results have yet revealed how many video images are necessary (i.e. the minimum number) to test for reliability or to provide adequate training material. To be most useful, the horse's midline should generally be perpendicular to the lens in video images and cameras should preferably be mounted on a tripod. Colour footage and a minimum of 25 frames per second are preferred. In cases of long-reining or driving, this may require the use of two synchronised cameras. If possible, multiple synchronised cameras can also record behaviour from different angles simultaneously.

Descriptive definitions of behaviours are a starting point for research on proximate and ultimate causes, functional attribution, physiological correlations or ontogeny. A growing array of technical instruments to measure physical and biochemical variables allows detailed quantitative studies on the interpretation of described behaviours. Techniques such as accelerometry, morphometry, kinematics, heart rate, infra-red thermography or assays of hormones, neurotransmitters or other biochemical markers, will help validate and elucidate the functional interpretation of behaviour units. This will lead to an equine ethogram with evidence-based functional definitions. Behaviour patterns should be reported in frequencies (or duration, where appropriate) per hour of riding, or calculated as percentages of total riding time so that studies can be compared easily.

Physiological Measures

To evaluate the (emotional) response of a horse to ridden work, several physiological measures are commonly used, with the proviso that factors such as exercise level, fitness and age are considered when interpreting results. Most importantly, the relationship between physical activity and changes in heart rate (Figure 15.1), HRV and hormonal responses must be accounted for. When monitoring heart rate, only changes over and above those that can be accounted for by physical activity can be attributed to emotional (stress) responses. Studies by Schmidt *et al.* (2010c) and Jansen *et al.* (2009) provide examples of how this measure has been used to monitor emotional responses in ridden horses. Among other measures currently used, based on the physiological response to stress, are changes in HRV, cortisol release and, more recently, changes in surface temperature as measured by infrared

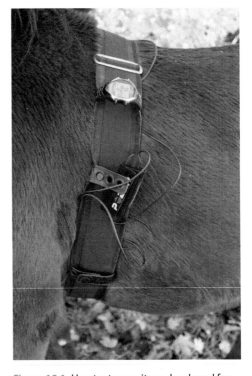

Figure 15.1 Heart rate monitors, developed for endurance training, have been used for studies in equitation science.

thermography (IRT). There is more to discover about the thresholds at which stress, as assessed by the different physiological parameters, becomes negative or even pathological.

Human mental states (e.g. nervousness) are known to have measurable effects on horse heart rate (von Borstel *et al.*, 2005; von Borstel, 2008; Keeling *et al.*, 2009), so all participants and observers should ideally be blinded to treatments. Unless standards for error correction in heart-rate raw data are determined beforehand, the statistician/person dealing with the data should ideally also be blinded to treatments (this will be hard to accomplish, though in the current structure of research, where resources are limited and usually one student conducts the practical aspects of a research project for his/her thesis):

1) *Measuring endpoints.* The Task Force of the European Society of Cardiology (1996) gives some recommendations regarding minimum lengths of measurement periods for different HRV parameters to be valid. These relate to human HRV, but since the underlying physiological mechanisms tend to be similar across species, we can use these values as a good starting point for horses, too. It is important to ensure that endpoints are biologically, clinically and behaviourally meaningful.

   Assessing repeatability of equine cardiac data in various situations is currently topical (König von Borstel *et al.*, 2011b, 2012). High repeatability *per se* neither demonstrate a method's validity nor the value of measuring within a certain time-frame, but low repeatability does demonstrate lack of validity.

   With low-frequency/high-frequency (LF/HF) measurement, where to draw the lines for LF and HF bands has yet to be established. Software such as Kubios for analysis of HRV data uses the human range as the default setting (so many researchers in the equine area probably just used these values), even though they may not be appropriate. For example, Physick-Sheard *et al.* (2000) suggest

frequency bands of (LF) > 0.01–0.07 and (HF) > 0.07–0.5 cycles/beat in horses.

2) *Best current tools for measuring.* The Holter monitor represents the gold standard, producing an electrocardiogram (ECG or EKG) trace continuously for 24 hours or longer, but it can be expensive. It is often also impractical because of its limited mobility. According to validating studies done on humans (e.g. Macfarlane *et al.*, 1989; Thivierge and Leger, 1989; Kingsley *et al.*, 2005; Gamelin *et al.*, 2006), Polar™ equipment is among the most accurate available. However, much has changed in the past 10 years and significant problems with some Polar™ heart-rate monitors have been reported (Górecka-Bruzda *et al.*, 2012; Suwala *et al.*, 2012), so ideally each device should at least be cross-validated against a second machine.

   Machines set up for clinical use may be less suitable for scientific purposes, for example, if the monitor temporarily loses the signal (e.g. when electrodes lose contact), missing data can cause problems with the interpolation of heart-rate data. Drop-out must be carefully checked for because there are serious implications for HRV data analysis. Default settings must be turned off before measurements begin.

3) *Standardising calibration.* The standard way of validating HRV-measurement tools is to compare measurements with ECG-recordings obtained simultaneously. Thivierge and Leger (1989) considered correlation coefficients of 0.85 and higher and standard errors of the estimates and systematic errors of less than 5% of the average ECG values as requirements for a heart-rate monitor to be considered valid.

4) *Relating statistical tests to sample size.* With small sample sizes, HRV data tend to be non-normal, but logarithmic transformation to approximate normality often achieves good results. Thus, parametric statistics, such as ANOVAs, and linear mixed models are fine, the latter being especially good as they can deal with unbalanced data. This is well worth noting because, during HRV measurements,

technical failures frequently result in missing data. Non-parametric statistics, such as Mann-Whitney-U-tests, are also appropriate. Where animals are used as their own controls, methods for paired data or repeated measurements are appropriate.

A major concern is how to deal with outliers, both in the original data and in means and other measurements calculated from them. Some common correction methods include filtering settings provided by the manufacturer's software, or removing individual values outside the physiological range, but there is no consensus on which methods are most appropriate. Since the biologically relevant difference is not known for the different HRV measurements, it is difficult to deduce required sample sizes. We need to reach consensus on how to recognise and deal with artefacts in the raw data. In addition, we should develop protocols on how to handle data and control for multiple comparisons.

The problem of how to control for multiple comparisons is not specific to HRV data. Some argue that it is not necessary at all or at least not under certain circumstances (Rothman, 1990). The best approach would probably be to assess each situation for risks and benefits of type I and type II errors and to decide on how to adjust for multiple comparisons, depending on which type of error would have more severe consequences. In any case, the use or non-use of adjustment methods should be clearly stated and decisions to overlook any adjustment should be justified by the authors. Some researchers routinely use Tukey-adjustments (e.g. König von Borstel *et al.*, 2011b) for multiple comparisons with HR data when each individual comparison is of interest.

Whether HRV values should be corrected for mean heart rate is another important issue. There is some evidence that the relationship between behavioural parameters and HRV parameters changed in a few cases when mean HR was accounted for in the mixed model as opposed to plain correlations between the behaviour patterns and HRV parameters that did not correct for mean HR (König von Borstel *et al.*, 2011b). As HRV partly depends on HR, it would probably be more correct to account for HR, since it cannot be kept at a fixed rate.

Salivary Cortisol

One currently accepted indicator of stress is the elevation of concentrations of cortisol, 'the stress hormone'. For example, Schmidt *et al.* (2010c) reported increases of 2–3 ng/ml in horses following ridden training sessions of 20–40 minutes and increases of 4.1–6.5 ng/ml following road transportation of 1–8 hours (Schmidt *et al.*, 2010b). In the former study, the increase occurred 5–15 minutes after training; in the latter, the highest concentration was recorded at the end of transportation. Faecal cortisol metabolites can be used to assess long-term stress non-invasively (Schmidt *et al.*, 2009), but more transient increases in cortisol release are easily measured in plasma and saliva (Figure 15.2), since unbound, biologically available plasma cortisol rapidly diffuses through the cells of the salivary glands. Close correlations have been found between free cortisol in plasma and salivary cortisol concentrations in species including the horse (Peeters *et al.*, 2011). Research also suggests that the time taken for plasma and salivary cortisol concentrations to increase post-stressor is comparable (Hughes and Creighton, 2007). Baseline cortisol concentrations tend to increase with age (Hall *et al.*, 2014) and training (Fazio *et al.*, 2006), so it is essential to take baseline measures against which changes can be assessed (and to record all details of the horses concerned to enable valid conclusions to be drawn). Increases in cortisol concentration show a correlation with the scale and duration of the stressor.

Times of saliva sampling should, where possible, be set at regular intervals throughout the study to facilitate comparison, with samples taken prior to set trials (at 30, 15 and

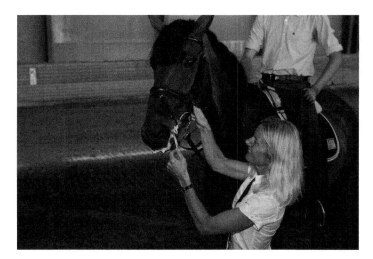

Figure 15.2 Saliva can be sampled for laboratory analysis of cortisol concentrations. (Photo courtesy of Kasia Olczak.)

0 minutes pre-trial) and at post-trial intervals (at 0, 5, 15, 30 and 60 minutes). Even where cost of laboratory analyses limits the frequency of sampling, it should continue until 60 minutes post-study to facilitate comparison between studies. That said, it remains difficult to compare reported concentrations between studies, because there can be factor differences even for samples analysed in the same lab using the exact same method. Saliva is generally collected by means of cotton rolls (e.g. salivettes, Sarstedt, UK) that are clamped within artery forceps to prevent horses swallowing them. These are inserted in the mouth and the horse is allowed to chew on them. The salivettes are then frozen at −20 °C until laboratory analysis using an enzyme-linked immunosorbent assay (ELISA). Alternatively, direct enzyme immunoassay, without extraction, has been validated for equine saliva. Generally, inter- and intra-assay coefficients of variability are reported to demonstrate the reliability of the findings.

Infra-Red Thermography (IRT)

Thermography has been used to detect early, pre-clinical signs of disease in both medical and veterinary applications and to monitor changes in body surface temperature that relate to underlying circulation and metabolism. Thermal imaging cameras detect radiation in the infrared range of the electromagnetic spectrum that is generally perceived as heat (in the range of 9000–14 000 nanometers) and produce visible images of that radiation. Further discussion of previous applications of this technology, its limitations and future potential, can be found in the review by McCafferty (2007).

Changes in skin temperature have also been associated with emotional/stress-related responses in humans and other animal species and there is currently considerable interest in the potential for IRT as a non-invasive, immediate means of objective assessment. Rapid changes in blood flow due to sympathetic activation and stimulation of the hypothalamic-pituitary-adrenocortical (HPA) axis are thought to be associated with the stress response and will affect the amount of radiated heat produced. These changes in surface temperature can be measured non-invasively using IRT (Stewart *et al.*, 2007). However, if the potential for IRT to provide an immediate, non-invasive measurement of stress in the ridden horse is to be realised, several factors must be considered. Some basic guidelines, as derived from previous clinical and other studies, should be adhered to.

A controlled environment is vital to ensure that the accuracy/successful use of thermographic scanning and the guidelines provided in previous clinical studies (e.g. Eddy *et al.*, 2001) are relevant for subsequent use in other applications. Ideally, a draught-free environment with low-level lighting and an ambient temperature of less than 30°C was advised (Eddy *et al.*, 2001). Clearly, this objective is unrealistic in most applications involving ridden horses/field testing, but where possible, readings should be taken in a constant environment (e.g. within an indoor arena or barn). Readings should not be taken in direct/bright sunlight, draughty/windy conditions or high ambient temperatures (above 30°C). Environmental temperature (and humidity, if excessive) should be recorded at each IRT reading to determine the potential effect of ambient conditions on subsequent data. For example, a temperature logger (such as the Lascar EL-USB-2) could be set to record at intervals corresponding with IRT sampling times. This will ensure that potential correlations between ambient and changed body–surface temperatures are not attributable to environmental factors. This is crucial to obtain reliable measurements.

Eye temperatures in horses are also measured by IRT (Figure 15.3). Temperature fluctuations are common, even within just a few seconds, due to environmental factors (sun, wind, evaporation, presence of tears and cleanliness of the external tear duct, which is the location of the highest 'eye' temperature) and simply the way horses are handled prior to measurement. Practices such as rugging, cooling (e.g. hosing the horse's legs or body), duration of complete rest, and intake of food and water, which all affect core temperature, can also affect eye temperature. It was noted by Eddy *et al.* (2001) that, for surface temperature measurement, the horse should have a clean, dry coat that had not been groomed within 2 hours before the scan for thermographic images to be accurate and clear. Also, no topical agents should have been applied and exercise and sedation should be avoided because of their effects on peripheral blood flow (Eddy *et al.*, 2001). In a review of the value of infrared thermography for research on mammals by McCafferty (2007), the need to take account of coat features such as colour, thickness and moisture content as sources of error in surface temperature readings is emphasised. All these

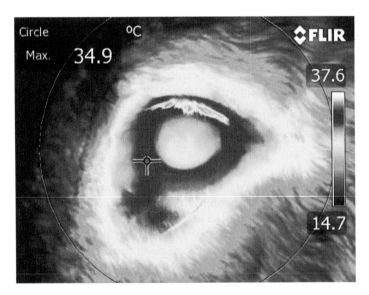

Figure 15.3 Infra-red thermography of the eye detects radiation in the infrared range of the electromagnetic spectrum and produces visible images of that radiation.

variables must be reported as should the details of whether the horses were housed or otherwise at the time of recording the eye temperatures. Ideally, eye temperature should be correlated with rectal temperature, which is the current reference standard.

Changes in temperature of the eye and surrounding area may offer the best potential for accurate monitoring of stress responses, as these have been associated with aversive procedures in some species, and this area is less affected by coat variations. For example, acute stress responses of cows during disbudding were recorded (eye temperature, behaviour, HR and HRV) (Stewart *et al.*, 2008). Eye images were collected using a FLIR Systems ThermaCam S60 infrared camera, at a distance of about 0.5 metres, 90° angle from the left eye only. The maximum temperature from a specified area (eye and immediately adjacent area described as being within the area of the medial posterior palpebral border of the lower eyelid and the lacrimal caruncle) was recorded every 38 seconds for 40 minutes. When disbudding of cattle was carried out without anaesthetic, a decrease in eye temperature from baseline was recorded (−0.27 °C) between 2–5 minutes post treatment. This was followed by an increase in eye temperature during the last 10 minutes of the sampling procedure of approximately 0.6 °C (Stewart *et al.*, 2008). The authors note that the magnitude and duration of the initial drop in eye temperature following disbudding without an anaesthetic was comparable to that found following a fright in cattle (Schaefer *et al.*, 2006).

An initial drop in eye temperature has been recorded in a horse undergoing a visual startle test (opening an umbrella adjacent to the horse) (Yarnell, 2012). The temperature of the left eye was recorded using a FLIR Thermovision A40M thermal camera and changes were recorded over a period of 5 seconds (−1 second from presentation of umbrella to +4 seconds post presentation). This camera has a thermal sensitivity of 0.08 °C at 30 °C with a range of −40 °C to 500 °C and captures thermal images in sequence at 30 frames per second. Continuous thermal images were obtained from a distance of 1 ± 0.5 metres and an angle of 90°. Clearly, this limits the utility of thermal imaging if the animal of interest has engaged in a flight response. The speed and duration of the response shown here indicate that subtle temperature changes that occur in response to stressors can easily be missed. The magnitude of the drop shown here is greater than that found in cattle by Stewart *et al.* (2008) (−1.8 °C, from 34.4 °C to 32.6 °C within one second of stimulus presentation) with a subsequent increase of 1.1 °C to 33.7 °C, but in this case related to a visual startle response rather than pain. The duration of the response appears to relate to the duration of the stressor. Although 10 horses were included in this study, eye-temperature data were obtained from only the horse that did not display immediate avoidance behaviour (Yarnell, 2012).

Currently, reliable and repeatable eye temperatures can be recorded only if taken from a set distance of between 1 and 2 metres and at an angle of 90°. It is also useful to provide the following details of the temperatures (°C): range, maximum, mean maximum and standard deviation. Temperatures should be collected from a specified area – for example, Stewart *et al.* (2008) targeted the eye and immediately adjacent area, described as being within the area of the medial posterior palpebral border of the lower eyelid and the lachrymal caruncle. This needs further investigation/confirmation in the horse.

Studies should include an example of this delineation and indicate the precise location of maximum temperature. A good example can be found in Valera *et al.* (2012), where images are provided showing the location and value of the maximum temperature recorded, in addition to values for atmospheric temperature and relative humidity taken at the same time as the image. The area of the eye that has been recorded as the location of maximum temperature, the lachrymal caruncle, has also been associated with responses to pain and stress (Valera *et al.*, 2012). This is probably the optimal location for monitoring affective state in the horse, but we can establish this only if maximum temperature location is clearly indicated in future studies. The maximum temperature of each eye should be recorded within this area and, if no significant difference is found between right and left eye, mean maximum eye temperature can be used. When specific values, including range and mean (± standard deviation), are reported they facilitate detailed comparisons between studies and enable a comprehensive picture to be compiled from results.

Current evidence suggests that eye temperature has the potential to provide an objective, non-invasive measure of 'stress', but it still requires underpinning with currently accepted measures (HR, HRV, salivary cortisol) for its validity to be fully established. Correlations between maximum eye temperature and salivary cortisol responses in horses have been found (Cook *et al.*, 2001; Yarnell *et al.*, 2013), although Valera *et al.* (2012) note that some variation is apparent. More detailed comparisons of the timing, duration and extent of the temperature change and the autonomic (sympathetic) and hypothalamic-pituitary-adrenal responses are required to fully interpret IRT data, and comparison with previously validated measures is necessary.

The correlation found between eye temperature and core body temperature also needs further investigation. A review of psychological stress-induced rises in core body temperature in humans and other animals (Oka *et al.*, 2001) discusses increases of 0.6–2 °C in response to a range of different stressors. Thermographic eye temperature was found to be associated with core body temperature in ponies, and the potential for using IRT eye temperature as a quick and non-invasive method of predicting fever onset was suggested by Johnson *et al.* (2011). Comparable increases of both eye and core body temperature were found by Hall *et al.* (2011) when horses were lunged in training equipment (Pessoa), and differences in eye temperature of approximately 1.5 °C and a mean increase in core body temperature of 0.35 °C were recorded following the tightening of the equipment. Physiological changes in response to stress appear to result in body temperature changes in varying degrees and further investigation is also required to identify whether these relate to physical or psychological stress responses or both. We suggest that core body temperature is monitored, where possible, and data included in future studies so that this may provide an additional objective measure.

More accurate interpretations of behaviour can be made when physiological data are collected. Maximum eye temperature was found to correlate with training scores in a study that primarily investigated ridden-horse behaviour, with higher eye temperatures being associated with more anxious behaviour (Hall *et al.*, 2014). Given the speed at which surface temperatures change in response to acute stressors, monitoring these changes could potentially identify specific behavioural signs indicating stress. Some IRT equipment can collect continuous images (video option) and the technology is becoming more accessible, both in terms of size/portability and cost. One such model, the MOBIR® M8 thermal camera, was used in the above study to investigate the association between ridden-horse behaviour and physiological measures of stress (Hall *et al.*, 2014). This thermal camera can record still and video images and the results from each were compared. Static images of the eye were taken from a distance of one metre with the horse at an angle of 90° and the video footage was analysed using Guide Ir Analyser software. The eye temperatures gathered using static images at a controlled distance were significantly higher than those obtained from the video footage. The distance from the horse, associated movement and variable angle will all have impacted on the temperatures recorded from this video footage. Neither still nor video readings from the camera were possible in bright sunlight. Further development is required for this technology to be applied in 'field' conditions. Also, although we have not yet found an effect of exercise *per se* on eye temperature, this factor warrants further investigation.

As noted above, it is imperative that all variables with the potential to affect the temperature readings are recorded.

Validation of Equipment

Of utmost importance to every study is the validation of all equipment to be used when designing the study. Unfortunately, in very few studies is there currently a report of how readings from the equipment used compare with alternative measures of surface temperature (to be reliable and repeatable). This is really an important consideration as the results will determine whether comparative and/or actual temperatures are meaningful. The range of equipment now available (which is increasingly affordable and easy to use) provides data that are unlikely to be consistent or comparable with earlier models (or during different conditions with the same model), since even the length of time the camera has been switched on can affect the readings. This suggests that it would be worthwhile to repeat validation trials throughout the study to confirm the reliability of readings taken.

Specifications of all equipment used must be included in all future studies, stating sensitivity, range and image-capture rate (frames/second when appropriate). The use of IRT to monitor body-surface temperature has certain advantages over other methods, such as temperature loggers: temperatures obtained via sensors attached to the surface being monitored may be compromised by the insulating properties of the equipment; and non-contact/laser thermometers record the temperature at a single point only. However, the limitations of IRT as outlined above must also be considered, but if we are to fully explore the potential for body-surface temperature changes to be used as a means of assessing stress in the horse, high-specification equipment is necessary, even if it is more expensive. Temperature changes reported in other species (associated particularly with emotional responses) have been small and rapid and could not be captured by many thermal cameras. While IRT has real potential for assessing stress, a great deal of work

remains to be done before results using this method can be relied upon and applied more widely.

Measurement of Human–Horse Interactions

Measurements are crucial to science, but assessing interactions within a dyad means that the responses of both must be assessed simultaneously. Measuring interactions between horses and riders/trainers is particularly challenging, because biofeedback from the horse may affect the rider's behaviour and *vice versa*. Numerous innate and acquired variables in both parties affect the results. Some early examples are measurements of rein tension (Clayton *et al.*, 2005; Manfredi *et al.*, 2005; 2009; Warren-Smith *et al.*, 2005b; Heleski *et al.*, 2009; Kuhnke *et al.*, 2010; Christensen *et al.*, 2011b), leg pressure (Nevison *et al.*, 2011) and pressure from the seat (de Cocq *et al.*, 2010a; Clayton *et al.*, 2013). These studies were conducted to take some of the guesswork out of equitation, to identify what works and what does not and to ensure that, wherever possible, techniques that compromise horse welfare are addressed. Ultimately, this will help us define best practice. With the emergence of smart textiles that will help us study the human–horse interface (McGreevy *et al.*, 2014b), it is likely that what cannot yet be measured will be revealed.

Rein-Tension Measurements

Rein-tension measurements offer tremendous hope for the future of equitation science, not least because the instrumentation is becoming affordable and robust (Figure 15.4). The place of rein-tension measurements in coaching and undergraduate education is well recognised.

The accuracy of what *can* be measured using rein-tension meters is still being debated. Recording rein tension for analysis and display requires that the instrumentation converts the analogue tension into digital form and there is some inherent loss of data

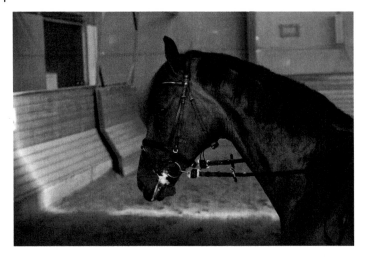

Figure 15.4 Rein-tension measurement is now reliable and affordable and will continue to play a central role in equitation science, coaching and undergraduate education. (Photo courtesy of Kasia Olczak.)

in the process. For example, display of the values is limited by the number of digital bits available to form the digital values representing the analogue-based tension (Staller, 2005). With an increased number of bits, results have greater resolution and precision. Quantisation error (the difference between the original signal and the digitised signal) is also inherent in analogue-to-digital conversions of time-variant signals (Staller, 2005). The impact of these errors on our current understanding of rein-mediated interactions is unclear, and until this is clarified, researchers should continue to record the limitations of their instrumentation.

Range and Sampling Rate

It is important that rein-tension meters can measure the full range of tensions encountered in the reins of the ridden horse if they are to be used to address questions of horse welfare. The capabilities of tension meters used varied within studies, as did the range of tensions reported in the ridden horses. The highest recorded tension was 104 N by Clayton *et al.* (2005). Young, inexperienced horses that have not habituated to bit pressure will voluntarily tolerate tensions of up to 11 N (Christensen *et al.*, 2011b), suggesting that tensions greater than this cause discomfort.

Sampling rate is another important factor in measuring rein tension. Presumably, physical rein tension is changing continuously while the digital signal is being recorded at set intervals. If the sampling rate is too infrequent, critical changes in rein tension may be missed. Clayton *et al.* (2011) confirmed Clayton *et al.*'s (2005) report that the horse's stride produced a regular pattern of peaks in rein tension, because the rider's hand does not follow the movement faithfully. In Starke *et al.*'s (2012) study, the horses' shortest mean stride duration of 683 ms was when trotting in a straight line. This provides a stride frequency of approximately 1.5 Hz (cycles per second) or 40 beats per minute. In contrast, stride frequencies reported by Clayton were 55 strides per minute for walk (Clayton, 1995), 79 strides per minute for trot (Clayton, 1994a) and 99 strides per minute for canter (Clayton, 1994b). There are two peaks for every stride cycle in walk and trot (frequency 1.8 Hz and 2.6 Hz respectively) and one per stride cycle in canter (frequency 1.7 Hz) (Clayton *et al.*, 2005).

Both horse and rider can affect rein tension by muscular contraction. Desmedt and Godaux (1977) demonstrated that, in humans, motor unit discharge rates can be up to 120 Hz during contractions associated with throwing objects, but that these may be less than 30 Hz in slow contractions. Horses are capable of fast movement, so the equine motor unit firing rates and consequent muscle movements will be more rapid. Tension meters should sample rein tension frequently, because muscle contractions by both horse and rider can change rein tension.

Validation and Calibration

The accuracy of the strain gauges within rein-tension meters may be affected by humidity and temperature changes, exactly the kind of conditions that will change as horses warm up during ridden work. All rein-tension meters must therefore be validated under practical conditions to ensure that they are measuring within the agreed error range.

Clayton *et al.* (2003) first described a method of calibration that has been used in many studies since. A known range of weights, reflecting the range of tensions expected to be recorded (currently approximately 0–11 kg), was suspended from the reins. It is unclear, however, if conducting calibration thus in the vertical plane will measure tension in a more horizontal plane without affecting accuracy, and researchers should consider alternative calibration techniques. Accurate and adaptable calibration systems must be incorporated into the design of rein-tension devices. Until we can verify calibration techniques and be confident that gauges are not adversely affected by changes in humidity and temperature, we must recognise that, at best, we are reporting approximations.

Wireless

Now that rein-tension meters can record via wireless and provide real-time feedback to researchers, coaches and riders, less equipment is needed on the horse. There should also be a capacity to link with real-time video surveillance so that data can be matched to observed events. This would make it easier to provide focused feedback to riders. It is important that this linked facility can be turned on and off remotely to control data collection and allow event markers to be placed on the recording.

Limitations and Future Requirements

Technology in this area will no doubt continue to develop and manufacturers should consider recommendations relating to range and sampling rate, as well as ease and accuracy of validation and calibration. Minimising weight, wireless communication and control are vital. Smart textiles would be one way to measure tension within the material of the reins themselves. Calibrating, validating and reading data could be made easier and this would enhance analysis and identifying patterns. It is worth noting that rein tension *per se* does not relate directly to pressure in the horse's mouth and providing real-time biofeedback to the rider and/or trainer in this area remains elusive.

Pressure-Sensing Instruments for Use Under Rider and/or Saddle

Pressure-sensing technology, adapted from medical and mechanical applications, and pressure-measuring devices to determine saddle fit have been available for some time (Harman, 1994; Jeffcott *et al.*, 1999). Several researchers have contributed information from these instruments that have informed the design and fit of horse equipment (Baltacis *et al.*, 2006; Byström *et al.*, 2010; Fruehwirth *et al.*, 2004; Hofmann *et al.*, 2006; Kotschwar *et al.*, 2010a;b; Latif *et al.*, 2010; Meschan *et al.*, 2007; Monkemoller *et al.*, 2005; Nyikos *et al.*, 2005; von Peinen *et al.*, 2010; Werner *et al.*, 2002; Winkelmayr *et al.*, 2006). More recently, attempts have been made to use technology to measure changes in pressure on the horse's back from the rider's seat and legs (Belock *et al.*, 2012; Byström *et al.*, 2009; 2010; Clayton *et al.*, 2013; de Cocq *et al.*, 2008; 2009a,b; 2010a,b; Geutjens *et al.*, 2008; Nevison *et al.*, 2011; Nevison and Timmis, 2013; Peham, 2008; Peham *et al.*, 2004; von Peinen *et al.*, 2009).

Currently Used Pressure Sensors

Various types of pressure sensor are used in these saddle-pressure pads (Figure 15.5). Several manufacturers supply saddle-pressure-measuring systems based on piezo-resistive sensors, which detect pressure changes by

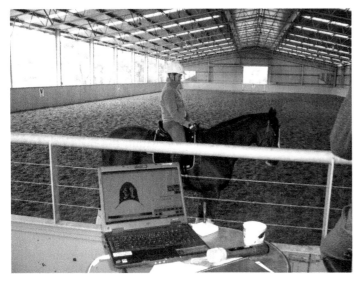

Figure 15.5 Saddle-pressure pads are revealing the complex interactions between the saddle and the horse's back. (Photo courtesy of Lesley Hawson.)

recording changes in the resistance that occurs when the sensor is deformed. Pullin *et al.* (1996) and de Cocq *et al.* (2006) have raised concerns about the accuracy of these sensors when used to measure pressures on horses' backs. Jansson *et al.* (2012) reported that such sensors suffer a reduction in load output when exposed to increasing humidity, which is just what is found under the saddle of a ridden horse.

The most popular system adopted by equine researchers in recent literature uses a capacitive sensor, which records the capacitance between two closely associated membranes. When a force changes the relative distance between the two membranes, there is a corresponding change in the capacitance (Puers, 1993), which is converted to an electrical signal that is recorded. These sensors require low power, and are more sensitive and less prone to drift or hysteresis than the piezoresistive sensors (Puers, 1993). Unfortunately, they are also prohibitively expensive, at least in saddle-pressure-pad format.

Pressure-Measurement Challenges

The area between a ridden horse's back and the rider's seat is complicated by several interacting curved and deformable surfaces. These include the horse's back muscles, the rider's buttocks and the skeletal protuberances of both, resulting in multi-directional forces moving at different velocities defined by the horse's movement, the rider's weight and the rider's capacity to synchronise with the horse's movement (Lagarde *et al.*, 2005). Usually, several layers of materials of different densities are crammed into the space under the rider's seat. These include leather or an equivalent hard-wearing synthetic layer covering the seat of the saddle, structural materials associated with the frame, shock-absorbing material, such as flocking, foam and/or air sacs, and an external cover that contacts the horse's back. Riders often use at least one more layer of external material between the saddle and the horse's back, and all this is topped by a rider (Hawson *et al.*, 2013).

These layers create more shearing, rotational and normal forces impacting on the horse's back, but both sensors discussed can detect only forces/pressures acting perpendicularly to the sensor. As the surface of the horse's back is not only curvilinear but also moving independently of the sensor mat, it is likely that we have not been capturing the tangential forces/pressures associated with shear, and therefore underestimating the total force acting on the horse's back in all data on saddle- or seat-pressure collected to date.

Even so, data presented on the moving horse are complex and challenging to analyse. Most researchers have reported ranges, peaks and means of pressures under the saddle in terms of total area as well as under sections of the saddle, and while this research has produced useful measures for saddle fit, it is obvious that more sophisticated analytical systems must be applied to identify changes in pressure on the horse's back associated with movement, and ultimately to decipher cues riders may be delivering through bodyweight redistribution.

The pressure-sensing technologies employed in saddle-pressure pads are the same as those used in many smartphones and touch screens, so consumer-driven demand for better technologies will also lead to improvements in saddle-pressure-pad products. Ideally these measuring devices will be connected by wireless and yield real-time data on screen that can be analysed dynamically. To match a variety of horse shapes, sensor pads must be thin and deformable, yet sufficiently robust to survive the rigours of riding. The sensors themselves must be accurate and reliable in this environment and there should be no cross-talk between sensors. Calibration should be automated and fast. Data analysis must become sophisticated enough to capture the complexities of the interaction between horse, saddle and rider. Ultimately, cost, accuracy and ease of use will impact on the potential for this technology to improve measurements of saddle fit and rider-seat pressure.

Calibration and Validation Protocols

There are two issues here. First, how each type of sensor is calibrated and how calibrations and other quality-control standards are reported. Second, how the different types of sensor compare with each other under standardised conditions, so the data-sets of different researchers can be appropriately contrasted in meta-analyses.

Conclusion

Research in equitation science must adopt consistent and robust methodology if it is to be useful in assessing horse welfare. There is a long tradition of performance assessment within equestrianism, based on behavioural responses and assumptions about how behaviour should be interpreted. Research has shown that some of these assumptions may be flawed and that further investigation is called for, and the framework presented here is intended to help share basic protocols with future researchers in equitation science and inform the future direction of equestrianism. The methods used are still at an early stage of development and it is imperative that we aim for robust and consistent methods, so that results obtained from future studies are valid and comparable. Equestrian practitioners can help by ensuring that the studies undertaken are of value and that findings will be taken on board. We believe that our recommendations will provide an important step in underpinning equitation science research and that the potential impact of future research will be enhanced. This framework should be updated regularly as new technology and software, including tools for individual riders and trainers, emerge.

16

The Future of Equitation Science

Introduction

Equitation science is established as a scientific area embracing a broad portfolio. The number of presentations given at the annual conferences of the International Society of Equitation Science (ISES) is steadily increasing and covers a wide range of topics in relation to training, human–animal interactions, housing and management (Table 16.1; see also www. equitationscience.com to access abstracts from ISES conferences).

The profile of equitation science has increased significantly during the past decade, due to an emphasis on measuring objective, quantifiable aspects of horse–human interactions. Science refers to a system of acquiring knowledge from testable explanations and predictions, and scientific methods are based on gathering measurable evidence subject to specific principles of reasoning. A scientist usually follows several steps:

1) formulate a question;
2) perform background research/make preliminary observations;
3) construct a hypothesis;
4) test the hypothesis by performing a carefully designed experiment with an adequate number of test subjects;
5) analyse the data with sound methodology;
6) arrive at justifiable conclusions; and, finally
7) communicate the results. (Research methods were described in detail in Chapter 15, Research Methods in Equitation Science.)

The quest for knowledge through a scientific approach should be fundamentally honest. Caution must be taken by equitation scientists to avoid bias in experimental set-up and interpretation of results, which can arise because equitation scientists are drawn to research in the first place by their love of horses. Equitation scientists must remain conscious of the effects of psychological pressure they may experience when arriving at incompatible perceptions, which can potentially occur with regard to the cognitive abilities of horses. Confirmation bias can then arise from cognitive dissonance, which means that information that confirms beliefs or hypotheses may be favoured. We need to be wary of anthropomorphism, which is an obstacle, if we are serious in our quest for the truth about horses. Communication of results also requires careful consideration: Do the results *suggest* or *prove*? Can the experiment be replicated?

We should also be mindful that just gathering quantifiable measurements does not necessarily mean that we obtain a simple answer to our research question. For example, horses that have habituated to high levels of rein tension due to incorrect application of negative reinforcement may show no clear behavioural and physiological responses when exposed to strong rein tension, compared to horses that have been ridden with less tension. Clearly, that does not mean that the habituated horse does not find the tension aversive; it may simply have learned not to

Equitation Science, Second Edition. Paul McGreevy, Janne Winther Christensen,
Uta König von Borstel and Andrew McLean.
© 2018 John Wiley & Sons Ltd. Published 2018 by John Wiley & Sons Ltd.
Companion website: www.wiley.com/go/mcgreevy/equitation

Table 16.1 The number of presentations at the annual conferences of the International Society of Equitation Science is steadily increasing (source: www.equitationscience.com).

Year	Country	Number of oral presentations	Number of poster presentations
2005	Australia	8	–
2006	Italy	16	11
2007	USA	17	6
2008	Ireland	48	51
2009	Australia	27	20
2010	Sweden	36	38
2011	The Netherlands	34	63
2012	Scotland	35	72
2013	USA	34	22
2014	Denmark	35	57
2015	Canada	30	29
2016	France	29	69

respond because there is no way out. This is an important challenge within equitation science. Similarly, we must consider the interplay between scientific scrutiny and ethical assessment that must take place when we aim to enhance the horse's welfare in its interactions with humans. Scientific evaluation and ethical assessment should complement one another; science without ethical assessment can be problematic, but so can ethical assessment without scientific study.

Areas and Anticipated Limitations for Further Research

The anticipated limitations on further research relate chiefly to the crudeness of the tools we use to measure small changes, such as cues from the rider's seat or elusive qualities such as the horse's affective state. Though we currently lack the wherewithal to make these measurements, we can look forward to the day when it will be possible. Then, we will have the knowledge to refine our understanding of individual differences between horses, and truly match horses with riders, while retaining a focus on the need for rider improvement.

New Technologies

Technology has made marked advances in equitation since the invention of the bridle, so it is logical to assume that the 21st century's technological advances will enable equitation to take a further great stride forward. That said, the quest for the next great technological advance must be matched by a quantum leap in good horsemanship.

The development of tensiometers (for the reins) and pressure pads (for the seat, legs, spurs and whips) will reveal rider interventions that may compromise horse welfare. The right equipment will allow us to measure, analyse and describe the correct and humane use of devices and practices in equitation, without which the public image of equitation in general is potentially jeopardised. The sustainability of the industry can be assured only if the appeal of horse-riding as a sport and leisure activity for animal-lovers is retained (Endenburg, 1999).

Technological advances, such as applied tension and pressure-detecting technologies (Chapter 15, Research Methods in Equitation Science) will also help educate riders of all levels in how best to apply the core principles of learning theory. By reducing confusion among riders and therefore conflict in horses, such technology forms a foundation for continuing advances in training practices and the design of equipment that will allow equitation science to make horse-riding safer (Waran *et al.*, 2002; McGreevy and McLean, 2005). Electronic devices are the most impartial means of establishing the effectiveness of less orthodox coaching and riding tools, such as imaging techniques. These new technologies may also prove to be the best means of elucidating the behavioural qualities that characterise humans who are said to have 'horse sense'. By helping to upskill humans who lack this sense, improvements in coaching and equipment will also reduce the rate of euthanasia because of unacceptable horse behaviour – so-called behavioural wastage (Hayek *et al.*, 2005).

Tension- and pressure-detecting technologies could be used to measure the qualities of effective coaching, not just effective signalling to the horse. They may also provide objective information for riders who are geographically isolated. For example, because Australia is removed geographically from Europe, its elite competition riders struggle to readily access elite levels of coaching. The validation of novel measuring and feedback technology will be the first step towards elite riders accessing real-time feedback from remote coaches.

Mathematical models may allow equitation scientists to compare horses and, over time, the efficacy of training systems (McGreevy *et al.*, 2009b) (Figure 16.1). This will assist the development of empirically sound coaching plans. Such models also have the potential to expose individual and breed differences in reactivity levels and identify sensory lateralisation in particular horses (McGreevy and Rogers, 2005) that may counter asymmetries in certain riders.

There is significant potential for so-called smart textiles in the design of devices that measure pressure, tension, moisture and heat at the human–horse interface (McGreevy *et al.*, 2014b). Research methodologies arising from theoretical and experimental physics laboratories, combined with wireless technology, can be

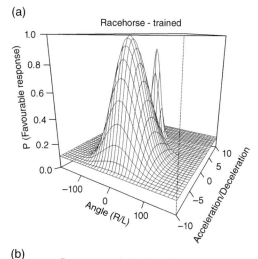
(a)

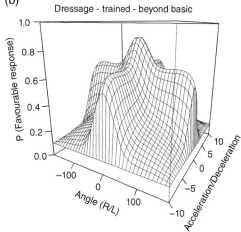
(b)

Figure 16.1 (a) An example of a response surface for a racehorse with only rudimentary foundation training and a highly probable high-speed forward response shown as a peak in sensitivity to acceleration cues. (b) An example of a response surface for a highly trained dressage horse, showing multiple peaks for given speeds and high responsiveness to *slow*, *stop* and *step-back* signals.

readily adapted to capture metrics that relate to numerous variables in equine structure and function. Activities, such as breathing, the extension and flexion of joints, limb kinematics and cardiac function, can be used to monitor physiological and behavioural conditioning (training). One day, such metrics may not only support veterinary diagnostics but also play a role in safeguarding sport-horse welfare, especially in elite contexts where horses may be pushed to their functional limits.

It is important to note that smart textiles rely on integrated sensors to sense exogenous stimuli and react to them. So, beyond the equitation science laboratory, the emergence of smart materials and polymers may enhance the effectiveness of, or challenge us to completely rethink, traditional items of equestrian gear, thus enhancing equitation. The integration of smart textiles in all sorts of extant and emergent equipment for everyday equestrians could lead to equipment that responds appropriately to the demands of a whole range of equestrian activities. Rethinking equitation through the use of smart textiles seems to have merit in that it is a novel means of both investigating and addressing problems that compromise the welfare and performance of horses.

One domain that merits particularly close scrutiny is the development of materials to be placed in the mouths of horses. Since the first models of bits as a means of restraint and control, a plethora of bits, bridles and devices has been used to deliver discomfort and pain to horses. However, devising a novel source of stimuli aversive to the horse is not an adequate response to a training deficit. Horses that do not trial conflict behaviours (and thus successfully resolve the escalated discomfort of such devices) usually habituate rapidly. The new bit is then less effective in producing a desired response and once more the rider is driven to pull harder on the reins. Thus begins an unhappy escalation.

The minimal space in which a bit can be placed inside the mouth may catalyse the search for a novel means of head control. So instead of using bits, we may explore the use of other means of applying pressure to the head. For example, the current range of bitless bridles may germinate innovations that allow riders to communicate clearly with their horses while being as humane as possible. Whatever devices emerge, the pressure from them will have to be applied fairly low down the head so that some leverage along the axis of the nose can effect a turn. We can imagine how bland and, therefore, ineffective any pressure would be if it were applied, say, near the ears. Equitation science will be able to measure and evaluate the effectiveness of such bitless bridles and identify which horses are the best candidates for various pieces of traditional and novel gear. It will eventually explore inherent breed and individual differences in head and mouth sensitivity, so that conflict can be avoided from the outset.

Animal welfare science must address the possibility of learned helplessness in horses used in sport or leisure that is a consequence of any radical restraining technique. This will provide physiological measures of the stress that accompanies this state. In addition, horse welfare will improve if we can identify horses that are simply not capable of a response. For example, an 'onboard' device that measures fatigue and exhaustion may one day allow riders to know when to quit before inducing a cycle of over-training. The same approach may allow judges and veterinarians to monitor the welfare of horses in competition. This sort of advance has the potential to ensure that fatigued horses are not pushed or beaten in the name of sport. Of course, competitive endurance riding already provides a model of such a system, which is meant to ensure that fatigued horses are not pushed beyond certain limits. This means that endurance competitors are relatively advanced in their knowledge of diet, farriery, welfare and physiology.

Ethology

The ethological aspects of equitation science will continue as rich seams for research into defining the enhanced relationship some people have with their horses, and the ways in which this connection may go beyond learning theory alone. Once we have established the variability and consistency of cues used in inter-specific communication and know exactly how classical conditioning can replace one cue with another, we can coach those less blessed with horse sense. Looking for ethological salience as we unravel the complexities and jargon of various coaching systems will allow as many stakeholders as possible to access the most critical information for the benefit of the horse.

As we saw in Chapter 2, Ethology and Cognition, there is still much to discover about the way in which horses learn from the environment, from each other and from human interactions (Murphy and Arkins, 2007; Brubaker and Udell, 2016). For example, context-specific learning needs further investigation (e.g. the effect on performance of a novel environment or the direction from which a horse approaches an obstacle). Furthermore, it is suggested that horses somehow percolate training and come back to work after a break with evidence of having made great leaps in their learning, almost as if the training needs to be interrupted to fully mature as a result of neuronal change, growth and vascularisation. It would be interesting to investigate more fully how training contingencies mature or decline with gaps in training. For example, individual horse progress could be plotted on a weekly basis to see how much learning is retained from one week to the next.

Learning theory, too, is far from complete when we consider the context of the ridden horse. The lessons from the rodent model of avoidance learning may be of limited use when explaining equestrians' application of negative reinforcement. There are also many questions remaining about positive reinforcement and how it can be administered to horses. Apart from the importance of timing, the quality of delivered rewards in horse-training has yet to be fully explored, especially for in-hand work. We should never assume that the results to date are in any way the full story. There may be practical ways of delivering jackpots to ridden horses that do not slow them down or prompt them to wait for more rewards.

It is becoming clear that ethological considerations may collide with learning theory to explain deficits in trainability. Training and performance differences between stereotypers (such as crib-biters and weavers) and other horses merit a thorough longitudinal investigation, so that the long-term effects of stereotypy on learning can be evaluated (Roberts *et al.*, 2015). This may help to create further incentives for horse owners to avoid management styles that trigger the emergence of stereotypies in predisposed horses. While ongoing research efforts are likely to identify specific risk factors for all equine stereotypies (Bachmann *et al.*, 2003; Wickens and Heleski, 2010; Hothersall and Casey, 2012), they should be used to refine stable management rather than to select horses that tolerate existing practices. When developing their stereotypies, crib-biters and weavers can be regarded as useful sentinels of sub-optimal husbandry, sentinels that should alert us to problems that are being encountered by all resident horses, not just those that produce a stereotypic response to the challenge.

As clinical equine behavioural medicine matures, we will become better at identifying individuals that are at high risk for certain disorders and managing them accordingly. We should also become more skilled at identifying horses that have true learning deficits rendering them likely to show dangerous or sustained stress responses. The impact of such advances on human safety will be significant.

Eventually, the racing industry may become more involved in equitation science as the physiology of the horse at exercise becomes less mysterious and trainers are left asking, 'What is the will to win?' The significance of emotions may then vie with cardiac output and gaseous exchange as behavioural qualities to be measured and selected for. And we may also see more scrutiny of the evidence of communication among horses competing within a group.

Nutrition

The deleterious effects of low-forage diets on the time-budgeting and health of horses have been recognised for many years (Kiley-Worthington 1987; McGreevy *et al.*, 1995a,b). More recently, the effects of increased starch loads on restlessness (Freire *et al.*, 2009), gastric ulceration (Nadeau *et al.*, 2000; Luthersson *et al.*, 2009) and behaviour (Nicol *et al.*, 2005; Bulmer *et al.*, 2015) have been highlighted. It appears that we still have some way to go in delivering appropriate nutrition to stabled horses, animals that often have the most pent-up and potentially dangerous energy. Feed with a high starch content results in higher glycaemic responses (i.e. increases in blood glucose) compared to fibre-based diets (Lacombe *et al.*, 2004). Thus, while fat- and fibre-based diets may result in calmer patterns of behaviour (Hothersall and Nicol, 2009), there is no evidence that dietary supplements such as tryptophan-containing products influences equine behaviour (Malmkvist and Christensen, 2007; Noble *et al.*, 2016). Further research is needed in this area to document the potential impact of diet on behavioural responses and consequently riding safety.

Genetics

Temperament characteristics of elite horses should be measured and characterised more fully. This will promote our understanding of breed traits that favour certain equestrian activities and selection for these where desirable and possible. An exploration of temperament and laterality tests as predictors of reactivity and suitability for certain sports and work may reduce behavioural wastage. The emergence of equine clones (Figure 16.2) will allow us to dissect the influences of nature and nurture on performance. However, a long-term perspective should be retained in any breeding programme that is based on any suite of tests for reactivity or temperament, so that the effects of selection for one set of traits can be tested in case it brings along any unwanted baggage (i.e. undesirable, unexpected traits).

Conclusion

Much of our traditional riding and stable management practices are at odds with the physical and behavioural adaptations of the horse; some horses cope, some do not. Equitation presents significant ethological challenges and, in many cases, training fails to adequately reflect the physical abilities and learning capacity of the horse. Riders often run into difficulties when they assume that the horse knows what the rider wants to achieve. All too often discord between

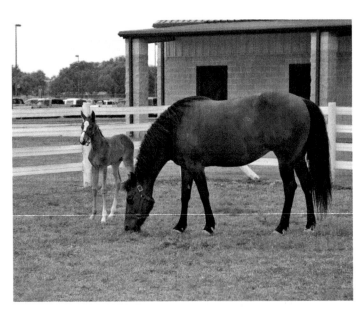

Figure 16.2 Paris Texas, one of the world's first cloned horses. (Photo courtesy of Eric Palmer, Texas A&M University, March 2005.)

horse and human emerges from the rider's inability to identify or accept his or her role in confusing the horse by issuing conflicting signals. Against this backdrop, we recognise that most horses are extremely tolerant – but just because we *can* do something to a horse does not make it an ethically sound practice. Just as dogs can be trained to salivate in response to electric shocks, we should not assume that just because a horse can be trained to offer a particular response, it enjoys giving that response.

The practical application of learning theory and ethology to equitation science has exposed the vagaries of terminology applied and translated from the research laboratory situation. Learning theory supplies a relevant and useful toolbox for trainers and riders, but current laboratory-based definitions do not always align with the practical training situation. It is crucial always to be mindful that training is essentially an exploitative event and that there is no ubiquitous training modality; all have advantages and pitfalls and learning outcomes may be influenced by arousal, attachment and affective states. It is therefore essential that riders are trained in the optimal use of reinforcement and, clearly, correct use of learning theory should be established as a 'first principle' in equestrian coaching.

Equitation science improves performance in sport horses because of more accurate operant conditioning, classical conditioning and shaping. But our greatest responsibility is never to forget that the horse's welfare is paramount: it is a privilege to ride horses and remarkable that the possibility exists. Therefore, every horse-trainer should maintain an open mind about possible limitations in horse-learning and confusion arising from training methods. This is especially important when the vast range of required responses in the trained horse is compared with the limited number of sites on the animal's body for eliciting those responses. Given that we are dealing with an animal that, so far at least, appears unable to extrapolate, we must always be mindful of the potentially confusing effects of applying pressure signals in common or overlapping sites on its body to elicit different responses. It is critical that we acknowledge how much of the global behavioural wastage tragedy is a result of our unclear interactions and the impossible expectations humans place on horses. What is needed, therefore, is a reappraisal and restructuring of contemporary horse-training within the framework of established and empirically tested principles of learning. And that is the purpose of equitation science.

Glossary of the Terms and Definitions and of Processes Associated with Equitation

Many of the glossary definitions offered below were presented at the First International Equitation Science Symposium as a collaboration by Paul McGreevy, Andrew McLean, Natalie Waran, Amanda Warren-Smith and Debbie Goodwin. Underlined words have separate entries in this glossary.

Above the bit: A posture characteristic of a hyper-reactive ridden horse exhibiting conflict behaviour, in which the horse attempts to escape an aversive situation by raising its head, quickening its pace, shortening its neck and stride and bracing its back, which becomes dorsally concave.

Accepting the bit: The way a horse responds to the bit in particular and to cues in general. During locomotion and transitions, the horse's mouth remains closed, soft in the jaw and with relaxed lips. A horse that accepts the bit does not shorten or lengthen its neck or alter its head position during travelling and transitions. Accepting the bit is generally accompanied by relaxation of the neck and body.

Against the hand: When a horse does not *stop/slow* or *step-back* from the bit correctly. Consequently, the rein contact feels heavy to the rider. This is usually accompanied by a hyper-reactive (hollow) posture in which the neck shortens or lengthens during locomotion or transitions. There may be an element of learned helplessness in this behaviour. A horse may also be described as being against one of the rider's hands, in which case it is heavy on one rein only (lugging), demonstrating a diminished response to the *turn* signal of that rein.

Against the leg: A description of a horse that is not straight in its body and is continually flexing its thorax (*see* Flexion) against one of the rider's legs. Such a horse drifts or attempts to drift sideways. The horse may also be against both legs (i.e. not going forward).

Agonistic behaviour: Any form of behaviour associated with aggression, including threats, displays and submission.

Aid: A stimulus that elicits a learned response in horses. We prefer the terms cues or signals. Traditionally, the aids were divided into two groups: natural aids and artificial aids. This distinction is misleading as it refers to what is 'naturally' available to the rider, but it neither identifies nor correlates with the two learning modalities through which the horse acquires its responses to the aids (*see* Cue).

Approach conditioning: A habituation technique that reduces flight behaviours using the natural tendency of horses to investigate and approach unknown objects, in combination with systematic desensitisation. The horse is encouraged to approach the feared object while a second trainer/controller causes the object to retreat as the horse approaches.

Equitation Science, Second Edition. Paul McGreevy, Janne Winther Christensen, Uta König von Borstel and Andrew McLean.
© 2018 John Wiley & Sons Ltd. Published 2018 by John Wiley & Sons Ltd.
Companion website: www.wiley.com/go/mcgreevy/equitation

The horse may then be signalled to stop before it reaches its fear threshold, so that the object retreats even further. The horse is then signalled to catch up. As soon as the horse slows its approach, it is deliberately stopped and this is repeated until the horse comes as close as possible to the object. The horse usually becomes increasingly motivated to investigate the object.

Associative learning: This involves the relationship between at least two events that are paired. There are two types of associative learning: classical and operant.

Avoidance learning: If an animal receives a signal before an aversive stimulus is about to occur, then – according to the principles of classical conditioning – after a few occurrences, the signal will elicit the avoidance behaviour. This type of learning occurs very quickly and is highly persistent, even when the original aversive stimulus no longer occurs. Avoidance behaviour is self-reinforcing, because relief functions as a reinforcer.

Balanced seat: The position of a mounted rider that requires the minimum of muscular effort to remain in the saddle and which interferes least with the horse's movements and equilibrium. It is generally understood that the balanced seat allows delivery of the <u>cues</u> in the most effective manner. The rider has equal weight on both seat bones and feet. (*See* <u>Independent seat</u>.)

Bars of the mouth (diastema): Area of the horse's mandible between the incisors and the molars that is free of teeth and in which the bit lies.

Baulk: Refuse to move forward, usually because of the presence of an object or obstacle (as in jumping) that the horse finds aversive. (*See* also <u>Napping</u>.)

Behind the bit: A head-and-neck-posture that is generally described as an <u>evasion</u> and which involves the horse persistently drawing its nose towards its chest, sometimes allowing the reins to become slack. This occurs in training because of mistakes made in <u>negative reinforcement</u>

or due to the use of restraining devices (such as draw reins) that force the neck to be shortened. In this situation, the horse gives two different responses to one signal (i.e. slowing or dorsoventral <u>flexion</u>) and thus frequently develops <u>conflict behaviour</u>. This posture thwarts the development of <u>impulsion.</u> The horse is generally heavy in the feel of the reins or has no contact during locomotion and <u>transitions</u> and, when this occurs, its *stop/slow* and *step-back* responses are diminished.

Behind the leg: A horse that lacks self-maintained speed and <u>rhythm</u> and requires the rider to continually deliver leg cues with each <u>stride</u> or each alternate stride.

Bend (lateral bend): The lateral curvature of the body that arises principally by the flexing at four sites on the horse's vertebral column: the cervical region in general, and the thoracic (tenth thoracic vertebra), lumbar (first lumbar vertebra) and sacral (third sacral vertebra) regions. Bend allows the horse to step into its foretracks with its hindfeet on a curved line or circle. Bend is usually accompanied by lateral, longitudinal and vertical <u>flexion</u> and is an accepted correct feature of all work on curved lines and all <u>lateral movements</u>.

Bit: An apparatus usually consisting of metal or other hard substance or a combination of both. It is positioned in the diastema of the horse's mouth and connected to the reins. Through tension in the reins, the bit places pressure on the lips, tongue and bars of the horse's mouth that results in the horse learning to *stop/slow*, *step-back* and *turn*, through the processes of <u>negative reinforcement</u> and <u>classical conditioning</u>.

Bitting: Accustoming a horse to having a <u>bit</u> in its mouth or the selection of the most appropriate bit for a horse.

Blocking: A form of interference with classical conditioning that arises when an animal has learned that a given stimulus predicts a certain event and, as a result, fails to learn new associations (i.e. a second stimulus may not become a conditional stimulus, because learning has been blocked by the presence of the first conditional stimulus).

Blow-up: When a ridden or handled horse becomes hyper-reactive during training and exhibits behaviours ranging from mild tension to bucking or breaks from the gait in which it is meant to be travelling. It is most common in early training and exposure to novel environments. It is generally a symptom of conflict behaviour.

Bolting: (a) Accelerating, usually to a gallop out of stimulus control (*see* Running (away)) and showing a lack of response to the *stop/slow* cues. This is a manifestation of conflict behaviour. Sometimes referred to as 'running blind'. (b) Eating (concentrated food) too rapidly.

Bounding: A hyper-reactive leaping movement where the horse springs from the hindlegs to the forelegs.

Break gait: The random change from one gait to another that is not under stimulus control.

Break in: Basic foundation training of a young horse to respond to cues and signals that control its rhythm and tempo, direction and posture for whatever purpose it may be required. We prefer 'foundation training' to 'breaking in'.

Bridle lameness: An irregularity of gait under-saddle that has the appearance of lameness. Mostly seen in the trot, it arises as a result of a long-term training error in which the rider maintains greater tension on a single rein, which inhibits the mobility of the ipsilateral foreleg of the horse. Bridle lameness may also arise from persistent rising on the same or incorrect diagonal at trot. There is usually an associated crookedness to the longitudinal axis of the body.

Broken neck (over-bent): The appearance of the neck of a horse in which there is (usually) a sudden change in angle (a break in the curve) in the vicinity of the third cervical vertebra. This is usually a result of persistent use of side reins that are too short, especially during early training, or draw reins that cause the neck to be too flexed and the nasal planum to be behind the vertical. Horses with broken necks generally exhibit conflict behaviours and tend to flex their necks to light rein tension rather than give the *stop/slow* or *step-back* responses.

Bronco: An unbroken or minimally trained wild horse, or one maintained in this state for rodeos.

Bucking: A sudden humping or arching of the back with the head and neck lowered, usually kicking out with the hindlegs or jumping/bounding forward/sideways with an arched back and ears laid back. Bucking is a manoeuvre that evolved to dislodge predators. Persistent bucking is a manifestation of conflict behaviour to the rein and leg cues.

Cadence: The period of suspension of the horse's limbs within a particular gait. With increased collection, the cadence is enhanced. Cadence is the result of the combined effect of correct training that a horse shows when it moves with well-marked regularity, impulsion, balanced and rhythmic strides. Cadence gives the horse the appearance of springing off the ground so the feet lift clear of the ground and float to the next step.

Champing (US): *See* Mouthing.

Cinch bound (US): Hyper-reactive behaviour (occasionally bucking) or instability, when the cinch/girth is tightened.

Classical conditioning: The process whereby an animal learns to associate external events, for example, the animal is presented with a neutral stimulus (e.g. a sound), which is followed by a biologically important stimulus (e.g. an aversive stimulus such as a shock, or a pleasant stimulus such as food). In equitation, classical conditioning is the process where learned responses are elicited from more subtle versions of the same signal or to entirely new signals (e.g. when a horse learns to react to voice commands, visual cues, or cues from the rider's seat).

Clicker training: An application of secondary reinforcement where the secondary reinforcer is an auditory signal that the correct response has been performed and that a primary reinforcer (usually food) is about to be delivered.

Cognition: The mechanisms by which animals acquire, process, store and act on information from the environment. The study of cognition covers many topics, such as perception, learning, memory and communication.

Cold-back: <u>Hyper-reactive behaviour</u> (occasionally <u>bucking</u>) or instability, when the saddle is placed on the back or when the horse is mounted.

Cold-jawed (US tough-mouthed): *See* <u>Hard-mouthed.</u>

Collected walk/trot/canter: Where each step of the <u>stride</u> of the gait is shorter and higher rather than longer. The horse should remain <u>on the bit</u>, the hindquarters should be <u>engaged</u> (lowered), with the horse showing activity, <u>impulsion</u> and <u>lightness</u>. Collected paces should develop from the correct training of the horse over time, so that it is physically able to maintain true <u>collection</u>.

Collection: The progressive development of increased carrying power of the horse where the steps become shorter and higher. Collection is derived from the progressive physical and mental development of the horse through <u>Impulsion</u>, <u>Engagement</u> and <u>Throughness</u>. The poll and withers are carried higher, the hindquarters lowered and the hindfeet step further forward with higher and shorter steps. Collection gives the appearance that the hindquarters carry more weight than in the working paces; however, research shows minimal alteration of the horse's centre of mass. Collection develops from repeated gait, tempo and <u>stride-length transitions</u> when the horse is in <u>self-carriage</u>. The combined effect of the transitions and the inertia of the animal is that over time the horse's physique changes. The propulsion of the body is then in a more upward and forward direction, giving greater <u>cadence</u> to the strides and increased <u>lightness</u> of the forehand. Collection can occur in the walk, trot or canter. So, for example, in a collected canter, the strides are shorter and the horse's frame is shorter and compressed. *See also* <u>False collection.</u>

Conflict behaviour: Stress-induced behavioural changes that arise from conflicting motivations, especially when avoidance reactions are prevented. Conflict behaviour may be agonistic behaviours, redirected aggression or displacement activities. If the stressor is recurrent, conflict behaviour may become repetitive and ritualised. Stereotypes and self-mutilation may develop from severe, chronic or frequent stressors. In equitation, conflict behaviours may be caused by application of simultaneous opposing signals (such as *go* and *stop/slow*), such that the horse is unable to offer any learned responses sufficiently and is forced to endure discomfort from relentless rein tension and leg pressures. Similarly, conflict behaviour may result from incorrect negative reinforcement, such as the reinforcement of inconsistent responses or lack of pressure removal.

Conformation: Features of the external morphology (i.e. the relative musculoskeletal dimensions) of a horse that interests trainers, riders, breeders and exhibitors, not least because they can affect the horse's performance.

Connection: The <u>contact</u> of the rein, seat and leg. This contact may be absent (no connection), correct (an easily habituated light connection) or too strong (unendurable pressure).

Contact: The <u>connection</u> of the rider's hands to the horse's mouth, of the legs to the horse's sides and of the seat to the horse's back via the saddle. The topic of contact with both hand and leg generates considerable confusion related to the pressure that the horse should endure if the contact is deemed to be correct. In ethical equitation, contact to the rein and rider's leg involves a light pressure (approximately 200 g) to the horse's lips/tongue and body, respectively. Although a light contact is the aim, there are brief moments (seconds or parts of a second) when contact may need to be stronger, particularly at the start of training, or in retraining, to overcome <u>resistances</u> from the horse. A heavy contact may cause progressive habituation leading to diminished reactions to rein and leg signals as a result of incorrect negative reinforcement and/or simultaneous application of pressure cues.

Contiguous: Adjoining or touching. Stimuli that are closely associated by time and space with specific behaviours. For example, when a reinforcement (release of rein tension) should immediately follow a response (*step-back*).

Contingent: Dependent upon: contingent outcomes are those directly linked to a causal behaviour. For example, pressing a switch turns a light on. The light is contingent upon the switch.

Contralateral: That is on the opposite side, as opposed to <u>ipsilateral</u>.

Counter-bending, counter-flexing, counter-canter: The practice of bending or flexing the horse to the <u>outside</u> of the circle or away from the direction of the direct turn. Counter-canter arises when the horse is cued to canter with the <u>contralateral</u> canter lead (e.g. to canter to the left with the right foreleg leading).

Counter-conditioning: A habituation technique based on the principles of classical conditioning that attempts to replace fear responses to a stimulus with more desirable responses. The term means training an animal to show a behaviour that is opposite to or fundamentally different from the one the trainer wishes to eliminate. The technique is widely used in combination with systematic desensitisation. By ensuring that the preferred behaviour is more rewarding, the animal learns to perform the new behaviour when exposed to the problematic stimulus.

Crabbing: A behaviour in ridden and in-hand horses where the horse fails to go straight and the resistance manifests as a sideways and forward (frequently alternating the direction) crab-like motor behaviour. Crabbing may also be associated with a <u>hyper-reactive</u> horse under restraint.

Cue: An event that elicits a learned response. In equitation, cues are sometimes termed <u>aids</u> or <u>signals</u>. Rein, leg, whip and spur cues are initially learned through <u>negative reinforcement</u> and then transformed to lighter cues (light rein, light leg, voice, seat) via <u>classical conditioning</u>.

Detraining: Where a stimulus is applied without the learned response being performed. The result is reduction or extinction of the likelihood of the learned response arising from the stimulus.

Diagonal: (a) Refers to a foreleg moving in unison with the contralateral hindleg, as seen in the gaits of trot (two diagonal couplets) and canter (one diagonal couplet). (b) Being on the correct diagonal refers to the rising and sitting of the rider being synchronised with the trotting horse's footfalls so that the rider sits when the <u>outside</u> foreleg and <u>inside</u> hindleg are in stance phase and rises as they begin swing phase.

Diagonal advanced placement (DAP): Where a break in the normal synchrony of the horse's gaits occurs. In DAP, the break is typically seen in the gait of trot, where the diagonal couplets lose their synchrony so that a hindfoot begins stance phase slightly before or after its contralateral foreleg counterpart. DAP is believed to be typical of the dressage movement known as piaffe; however, in other cases it is attributed to errors in training where maximal dorsoventral flexion of the cervical vertebrae (Rollkur) occurs so that the diagonal pairing of legs may be temporally split, with subsequent losses in the <u>purity of the gaits</u> and the possible emergence of <u>conflict behaviours</u> (*see* <u>Rollkur</u>).

Differential reinforcement: The use of positive and negative reinforcement in a structured manner so that only the desired behaviour is reinforced, whereas extinction (i.e. discontinuing of reinforcement of previously reinforced behaviour) is applied to other responses.

Direct rein: When the rein is 'opened' (i.e. moved laterally away from the horse's midline).

Direct turn: Where the rider increases tension on the rein to change direction by moving the hand laterally (about 4 cm) away from the horse's midline and towards the direction of turn. Turning the horse via lateral rein tension rather than by caudal rein tension enables the horse to discriminate between signals for changing direction and those for deceleration.

Discrimination: The ability of the horse to distinguish between different stimuli (e.g. situations, objects and cues/signals).

Disunited canter: An undesirable broken gait, most often seen in horses with a tendency to pace or horses that are not straight (*see* Straightness). It occurs when there is a shift from ipsilateral to contralateral coupling of forelegs and hindlegs.

Dominance/submission: Suites of behaviours in social interactions that signal rank or determine priority of access to resources (a dynamic process affected by motivation). There is a belief in horse-training that human–horse interactions are governed by dominance/submission, which implies that trainers need to be dominant over horses to train them effectively. The notion that a horse must respect a human to be effectively controlled may be at odds with equine cognition and learning theory.

Dorsal: Pertaining to, or situated on, the back of an animal, as opposed to ventral.

Double-gaited: A horse that can both trot and pace.

Downhill: An observed fault in the physique of a sport horse, where the horse appears noticeably higher at the point of the croup than at the withers.

Driving: (a) Where either a horse or a team of horses pulls a vehicle. (b) *See* Long-reining. (c) Locomotion (*see* Engagement) in which the horse is pushing forward with its hocks underneath it at the moment of pushing. The moment of push should not continue beyond the point at which the fetlock is behind the vertical line of the hock.

Engagement: Where the horse's forelegs and hindlegs are under stimulus control of the rider. Engagement arises from the effects of inter-gait and intra-gait transitions that occur in a brief timeframe and optimally in a linear increase or reduction in tempo. The brevity of the timeframe is less than or equal to three steps of the forelegs in walk and trot and three strides in canter. Classically, this process is trained over time with concomitant physique changes. Sometimes known as engaging the hocks (tarsal joints).

Escape learning: This type of learning occurs when an animal performs an operant response to terminate an aversive stimulus. The behavioural response that produces escape from the aversive stimulus is negatively reinforced by the elimination of the unpleasant stimulus.

Ethogram: A list of the type of behaviours performed by a species in a particular environment. The list includes precise, mutually exclusive descriptions of each behaviour. It is fundamental to any study of animal behaviour to define which behaviour types are being observed and recorded.

Ethology: The scientific and objective study of animal behaviour, usually with a focus on behaviour under natural conditions, and viewing behaviour in terms of evolved adaptations.

Evading the bit: Oral behaviours (such as moving the tongue backwards or out of the mouth) and neck postures (such as dorsoventral <u>flexion</u>) that enable horses to reduce the discomfort caused by bits or the extent to which riders can apply and maintain pressure. In training, these result from errors in <u>negative reinforcement</u>.

Evasions and resistances: Descriptive terms for <u>conflict behaviours</u> where evasions are similar to resistances, except that evasions refer to the more severe and violent behaviours. These terms arose because of the horse's natural tendency to avoid pressure/pain by learning through <u>negative reinforcement</u> to perform any attempted behaviour that results in lessening of pressure/pain. The problem with these terms is that they imply malevolent and calculated behaviour on the part of the horse, whereas these behaviours are more likely to be the result of errors in <u>negative reinforcement</u>.

Extension/extended strides: Strides that are longer than typical or working paces in each gait. In equitation, extended paces arise only from <u>collected</u> paces. For the average horse, in the extended walk and trot, the hindtrack should begin its stance phase approximately 2–3 hoofprints in front of the foretracks, and in extended canter the inside hindfoot should begin its stance phase approximately 1 m in front of the inside foretrack.

Extinction: The disappearance of a previously learned behaviour when the behaviour is no longer reinforced. Extinction can occur in all types of behavioural conditioning, but it is most often associated with operant conditioning. When implemented consistently over time, extinction results in the eventual decrease of the undesired behaviour but, in the short-term, the animal may exhibit a pre-extinction burst.

Extinction burst: (Synonymous with <u>Spontaneous recovery</u>). A sudden and temporary increase in the frequency or magnitude of a behaviour, followed by the eventual decline and extinction of the behaviour targeted for elimination.

Extinction bursts are more likely to occur when the extinction procedure is in the early stages.

Falling in/falling out: Losses of <u>straightness</u> associated with the horse drifting in or out of the circle. It is similar to <u>lugging</u>, but denotes the slower gaits.

False collection: Forcing a horse into an apparently collected <u>outline</u> through the simultaneous actions of the rein and leg or with the use of gadgets and pulleys rather than the progressive development of <u>collection</u> over time through training. False collection frequently results in <u>conflict behaviour</u>, because concurrent *stop* and *go* signals cause confusion and pain.

Flexion: (a) Longitudinal: the dorsoventral lowering, lengthening and relaxing of the horse's neck and back where the horse's poll is carried at the height of its withers. In reality, this is not a flexion but an extension and should be redefined as longitudinal extension. This is a fundamental quality of being <u>on the bit</u>. (b) Lateral: the lateral bending of the atlanto-occipital junction and including the first three cervical vertebrae of the horse's neck. This is primarily a shaped quality of correct turning and in the well-trained horse is thus involved whenever the <u>turn</u>, circles or the turn-position is required, such as in <u>lateral movements</u>. The extent of lateral flexion negatively correlates with the size of the circle. Lateral flexion is a secondary precursor to being <u>on the bit</u>, where the <u>nasal planum</u> is maintained at around 6 degrees in front of the vertical axis, and the poll is at the highest point. This is also known as vertical flexion. Lateral flexion is also a precursor to a 'lateral bend' (*see* <u>Bend</u>).

Flooding (response prevention): A behaviour modification technique where the animal is exposed to an overwhelming amount of a fear-eliciting stimulus for a prolonged period while avoidance responses are prevented, until the animal's apparent resistance ceases. The method is generally not recommended because there are severe risks associated with it (e.g. injuries due to exaggerated fear reactions).

Forehand (forequarters): Those parts of the horse that lie in front of the rider (i.e. the head, neck, shoulders, withers and forelegs).

Foundation training: The basic training of a young horse to respond to cues that control its gait, tempo, direction and posture for whatever purpose may be required. Foundation training may also include habituation to saddle and rider.

Freeze: The sudden alert motionless stance of a horse associated with a highly attentive reaction to an external stimulus.

Gait: The continuous cycle of a specific sequence of strides that denote walk (four beats), trot (two beats), canter (three beats) and gallop (four beats).

Gallop: A four-beat gait that provides maximum speed. Generally, the gallop is transverse where the leading hindleg and leading foreleg are on the same side of the body. A rotary gallop may also be seen when the horse is anxious under-saddle. In a rotary gallop, the leading foreleg and hindlegs are on opposite sides of the body.

Generalisation: Transferring a learned response to a different stimulus (i.e. a horse may respond similarly to two different objects or cues because it perceives them as similar).

Girth shy: *See* Cinch bound.

Go: The acceleration response in horse-training that provides forward motion. The *go* response is trained via negative reinforcement using the rider's legs under-saddle and using anterior lead-rein tension when working a horse in-hand. Through classical conditioning, these responses are converted first to lighter versions of the leg or lead-rein and then to the cues of seat, position and, perhaps, voice.

Good mouth: *See* Soft mouth.

Green: (a) An inexperienced horse with no training or one that has undergone foundation training but is not fully trained.

(b) A racehorse that has yet to undergo a time trial.

Habit: When a learned response is consolidated as a result of long-term potentiation (LTP).

Habituation: The waning of a response to a repeated stimulus that is not caused by fatigue or sensory adaptation. Habituation techniques include systematic desensitisation, counter-conditioning, over-shadowing, stimulus blending and approach conditioning.

Half-halt: A subtle, sequential application of the seat, leg and rein cue that is separated in time by one beat of the rhythm of the gait. The half-halt is intended to increase the attention and balance of the ridden horse.

Halt: When the horse is stationary and, in dressage, this means that the horse should be standing with his weight evenly distributed bilaterally, in other words, standing square.

Hanging: *See* Lugging.

Hard/tough-mouthed: A term that describes horses that have habituated to rein tension. This outcome is generally a result of incorrect negative reinforcement and can result in learned helplessness and conflict behaviours.

Heavy, heavy-mouthed: A term that describes a horse that has been trained with incorrect rein signals such that it will be accustomed to always being ridden with heavy tension in the reins at all times and will have deficits in its deceleration responses with no persistence of the speed of the gait (i.e. no self-carriage).

Hitch: (a) To tether a horse. (b) A defect in the gait noted in the hindlegs, which seem to skip at the trot.

Hollow: Undesirable contraction of the vertebral column, so that the head comes up and the neck and back become slightly concave. The strides of the horse generally become faster and shorter ('choppy'). Habitual hollowness is usually a result of incorrect negative reinforcement and is frequently associated with conflict behaviours.

Horse-breaking: *See* Break in.

HPA axis (Hypothalamic–Pituitary–Adrenal axis): An organ system comprising the hypothalamus, the pituitary gland and the adrenal gland. The activation of the HPA axis is heightened when an animal is challenged with a stressor, and HPA axis products, such as cortisol, can serve as a physiological indicator of stress in animals.

Hyperflexion (of the neck) (Low Deep and Round/Rollkur): A training technique in which the horse is trained to carry its head low with its cervical vertebrae maximally flexed (chin closer to the chest) in the belief that the hindquarters are engaged and that the activity and power of the hindlegs is improved. To critics, the technique is seen as a form of false collection and it may have welfare implications.

Hyper-reactive behaviour: Behaviours characteristic of an activated HPA axis and associated with various levels of arousal. Such behaviours typically involve the horse having a hollow posture and leg movements with increased activity and tempo, yet shorter strides. Hyper-reactive behaviours are quickly learned and relatively resistant to extinction because of their adaptiveness in the equid ethogram. Behavioural evidence of hyper-reactivity ranges from postural tonus to responses such as shying, bolting, bucking and rearing.

Hypersensitive: (a) The genetic tendency in an animal to be more sensitive than average. (b) A learned response where an animal has become sensitised to a stimulus.

Impulsion: The locomotory effect of an immediate acceleration response of a horse from a signal/cue. In a correctly trained horse, impulsion manifests as moving forward energetically with a self-maintained rhythm, straightness and outline when signalled to do so. Impulsion is the earliest step in the progressive development of collection where, in contemporary dressage, the horse is believed to progressively carry more weight on its hindquarters. Three types of impulsion have been described: (1) *Instinctive:* the inherited tendency to have more or less impulsion; (2) *Mechanical:* develops from instinctive impulsion and improves with work and gymnastic training; (3) *Transmitted:* that given to the horse by the rider in collecting the horse. True impulsion, in which the horse conveys itself calmly under a light rein and without constant pressure from the rider, is distinct from states of general excitement in which the horse pulls at the bit and requires forceful restraint to be controlled.

In front of the leg: A desirable quality in equitation describing a horse with a correctly trained *go* response, such that it is neither slowing nor accelerating of its own volition (i.e. it self-maintains its rhythm).

Independent seat: The ability of a rider to maintain a secure, firm and balanced position on a horse's back, without relying on the reins or stirrups. (*See* Balanced seat.)

Indirect rein: When the rein is 'closed' (i.e. moved laterally toward the horse's midline).

Indirect turn: Where the rider increases tension on a rein to change direction or line by moving the hand laterally (about 4 cm) towards the horse's midline.

In-hand: The trainer works from the ground rather than from the saddle, positioned beside and/or behind the horse and controlling it with rein, voice and training whip. In-hand work allows the horse to acquire signal response entities of *go* and *stop* as a prelude to foundation training, or during retraining or when training advanced movements.

Inside/outside: Identifies either side of the horse as it is being schooled. These require some clarification as to whether we are referring to the relative position in the arena, to the curvature of the path or to the bend of the horse (e.g. inside leg usually refers to the leg of the rider or horse nearest to the centre of the circle the horse is following, or on the bent side, which can be the outside of the arena as in renvers).

Inter-gait transition: Transitions from one gait to another, such as from walk to trot or canter to walk.

Intra-gait transition: Transitions within the gait, such as from one stride length to another or from one movement to another.

Ipsilateral: That is on the same side, as opposed to contralateral.

ISES: International Society for Equitation Science.

ISES training principles: A series of 10 horse-training principles that arise from equine cognition, ethology and learning theory. These principles provide benchmarks for ethical horse training.

Jog: (a) A slow, short-striding trot, usually associated with heightened arousal and involving short choppy steps and constant tendencies to accelerate as the horse is attempting to flee an aversive situation. Habitual jogging can be associated with conflict behaviours and result in diminished responses to the *slow/stop/ step-back* signals. (b) In harness-racing, the term given to the exercise conducted on non-hopple days (Hobble = restraint, hopple = harness). (c) A slow trot used mainly in Western pursuits.

Join-up: An element of round-pen training (popularised by US trainer Monty Roberts), in which the horse learns under some circumstances to remain close to the human.

Lateral: Towards the left or right side of the body, as opposed to medial.

Lateral movements: Any of the training exercises (such as leg-yield, shoulder-in, travers, renvers and half-pass) that involve the horse having longitudinal bend and travelling with the forelegs and hindlegs on three or four different tracks with the aim of improving its engagement and suppleness.

Leadership: According to one tenet of natural horsemanship, the horse must accept the human as a leader to respond correctly in training. This assumption may be contradicted by learning theory and, because of its inherent anthropomorphism, the significance of the idea of leadership in equitation calls for further study.

Leaning on the bit: A sign of habituation to bit pressure that manifests with the horse persistently tensioning the rein(s) as though relying on the rider to support the weight of its head. This arises through incorrect negative reinforcement and can be associated with conflict behaviours and learned helplessness.

Learned helplessness: A state in which an animal has learned not to respond to pressure or pain. Arises from prolonged exposure to environments or aversive situations that deny the possibility of avoidance or control. It may occur from inappropriate application of negative reinforcement or positive punishment, which results in the horse being unable to obtain relief from or avoid the aversive stimuli. If this continues over a period, the horse will no longer make responses that were once appropriate, even if they would be appropriate under the current conditions.

Learning theory: Learning theories are conceptual frameworks describing how information is absorbed, processed and retained during learning.

Leg-yield: The simplest and most recently described of lateral movements in which the horse moves both forwards and sideways from the rider's single leg signal. Leg-yield is usually trained before more complex lateral manoeuvres. In leg-yield, the horse is almost straight, except for slight lateral flexion away from the direction of travel.

Lightness: A desirable quality that reflects self-carriage and the horse's self-maintenance of rhythm, straightness and outline. Lightness involves the bringing into action by the rider and the use by the horse of only those muscles necessary for the intended movement. Activity in any other muscle groups can create resistance and thus detract from the lightness.

Long and low: Where the horse travels with its poll extended and carried lower than its withers and its neck slightly dorsoventrally flexed while attempting to achieve more <u>looseness</u>.

Longitudinal flexion: *See* <u>Flexion</u>.

Long-reining: A method of training the horse using two reins, each attached to the horse's bit and returning to the trainer, who moves behind and/or beside the horse, as if <u>driving</u> it without being attached to any vehicle or load. Long-reining is sometimes used as a prelude to foundation training, retraining or in the training of advanced movements.

Long-term potentiation (LTP): The strengthening (or *potentiation*) of specific neural networks that lasts for an extended period; it is commonly regarded as the cellular basis of habit formation and memory.

Loose training: The horse is typically loose-schooled in the outer lane of an arena and frequently encounters grid exercises or series of fences for jumping on predetermined distances and stride patterns.

Looseness: A term used in dressage when a horse is relaxed and has well-trained basic responses so that the locomotion of the horse is swinging and elastic.

Lope: The Western version of a very slow canter, this is a smooth, slow gait in which the head is carried low.

Lugging, pulling: A term, mostly used in horse-racing, which refers to a <u>straightness</u> problem where the horse drifts sideways, particularly at the gallop. In doing so, the horse becomes heavy on the rein on the side away from which it is drifting. A horse that habitually lugs does so as a result of incorrect <u>negative reinforcement</u>, because the rider holds the heavy rein tighter as he or she attempts to maintain a straight line; in other words, the horse is failing to respond to the *<u>turn</u>* cue.

Lunge (also longe): Exercising a horse in circles with the trainer in the middle of the circle using a long lead-rein or rope. Lungeing is used to <u>habituate</u> a horse to the saddle during <u>foundation training</u>, to train <u>obedience</u>, to warm up a horse and to tire a <u>hyper-reactive</u> horse.

Medial: Relating to the median plane or midline of the body; situated towards or nearer to the median plane, as opposed to <u>lateral</u>.

Medium walk/trot/canter: Stride length between that for the <u>working</u> and <u>extended</u> versions of those gaits. For example, in the medium canter, the stride length is between the working canter and extended canter.

Mouthing (US champing): (a) Mouthing/Champing is where the horse gently moves the bit with the tongue, which is sometimes encouraged by use of a bit with 'keys' attached to the mouthpiece to facilitate saliva flow and keep the mouth moist. (b) The process of habituating a horse to a <u>bit</u> in its mouth and learning to respond to the *<u>stop/slow</u>*, *<u>step-back</u>* and *<u>turn</u>* signals of the reins.

Movement: Combinations of basic responses of *go*, *stop/slow*, stride-length changes, tempo changes, direct and indirect turns of forelegs, turns of hindlegs, flexion and bend that result in movements such as leg-yield, shoulder-in, travers, renvers, pirouette, passage and piaffe.

Napping, propping: When a horse fails to respond appropriately to the rider's signals, as in refusing to go forwards, running sideways, <u>spinning</u> or running backwards. This <u>conflict behaviour</u> could also result in attempts at rearing.

Nasal: Pertaining to the nose. Sometimes used as an orientation term to locate a part of the head that lies more towards the nostrils than the dorsum.

Nasal planum: This denotes the line along the bridge of the nose.

Natural horsemanship: A system of horse-training developed by Pat Parelli that has its basis in North American horsemanship. It is based on an interpretation of the natural ethogram of the horse. Natural horsemanship focuses on concepts of dominance/submission, respect and leadership, which are currently controversial in definition and application and may be at odds with equine cognition and learning theory.

Natural outline: Where the horse under-saddle or in-hand carries its head and neck freely without any force from the rider or trainer.

Neck rein: To turn or steer a horse by tension of the rein against the neck.

Negative punishment (Subtraction punishment): The removal of something pleasant (such as food) to decrease the probability of an undesired response and thus delete that response.

Negative reinforcement (Subtraction reinforcement): The removal of an aversive stimulus (such as pressure) to reward a desired response and thus increase the probability of that response.

Non-associative learning: A change in the strength of response to a stimulus due to repeated exposure to that stimulus. Non-associative learning can be divided into habituation (i.e. a reduction in response), dishabituation (i.e. recovery of the original response) and sensitisation (i.e. an increase in response).

Obedience: In traditional horsemanship, compliance with the cues. In equitation science, a more objective definition is the horse's immediate initiation of the required response to a light cue.

Object permanence: The capacity to perceive that an object still exists, even after it has been removed/obscured from the perceptual field.

Observational learning: Learning that emerges in an individual after watching another, rather than on the basis of direct experience.

Off the bit: The horse does not have contact or connection to the rider's hands through the reins. This is usually referred to as being above the bit or behind the bit (i.e. there is a lack of at least one of the three prerequisites for on the bit).

On the bit: The self-maintained neck-and-head position of the horse in correct training, where vertical flexion of the cervical vertebrae and atlanto-occipital joint (also known as poll flexion or roundness) results in the nasal planum being approximately 12 degrees in front of the vertical at walk or 6 degrees in other gaits. In dressage, this posture is assumed to improve the balance of the ridden horse (relocating extra weight to the hindquarters) and its willingness to respond to the signals transmitted by the rider through the reins, seat and rider's legs. There are three precursors to the horse being on the bit. The first is longitudinal flexion, followed by lateral flexion and finally vertical flexion. To most people, 'on the bit' means that the horse travels with its neck arched and with its nasal planum near vertical (roundness). However, a vertical nose does not necessarily mean that the horse is on the bit. On the bit is believed to be necessary in horse-training because, as a result of vertical flexion, the centre of gravity shifts posteriorly towards the rider's centre of gravity. There are various forms of false roundness where the horse is forced by the rider's hands or with the use of mechanical devices to flex his cervical vertebrae.

On the forehand: An undesirable form of locomotion that involves the horse carrying an inappropriate proportion of its weight on its forequarter, a posture that runs counter to impulsion, collection and self-carriage. Usually seen in young or poorly schooled horses where the withers appear lower than the croup of the horse during locomotion.

Opening/closing rein: *See* Direct/Indirect rein/turn.

Operant conditioning (Instrumental conditioning): The process whereby an animal learns from the consequences of its responses, that is, either through positive or negative reinforcement (which will increase the likelihood of a behaviour), or through positive or negative punishment (which will decrease the likelihood of a behaviour).

Operant contingency: The three-part series of events in response learning. It involves a cue, a response and a reinforcement.

Out behind: *See* Trailing hindquarters.

Outline (US Shape, frame): An aspect of the horse's posture that refers to the alterations in the curvature of the vertebral column and so encompasses the degree of flexion of the neck and poll and the associated flexion of the lumbo-sacral region. (*See* on the bit, roundness).

Outside: *See* Inside/outside.

Over-bent (broken-neck): Where the horse assumes a posture in which its nasal planum is described as being behind the vertical. Usually caused by faults in negative reinforcement, such as unrelenting pressure from the rider's hands on the bit.

Overface: Undertaking a task during riding or training that is beyond the horse's capacity or experience (i.e. where the trainer demands unachievable increments during shaping).

Overshadowing: The effect of two signals of different intensity being applied simultaneously, such that only the most intense or relevant stimulus will result in a learned response. It can explain why animals sometimes fail to associate the intended cue with the desired behaviour in favour of a different stimulus that was perceived at the same time and was more relevant to the animal. The term overshadowing also denotes a habituation technique where habituation to a stimulus is facilitated by the simultaneous presentation of two stimuli (such as applying lead rein cues/tension at the same time as exposure to clippers).

Over-tracking: Associated with engagement of the hindlimbs to the point where the footfall of the hindlimb reaches forward and overlays or surpasses the track of the ipsilateral forelimb.

Pace/pacing: Sometimes referred to as a gait. Also denotes a two-time lateral gait in which the ipsilateral hindleg and the foreleg are synchronous in swing and stance phase.

Pig-rooting: A conflict behaviour involving lowering the head and arching the back and with a kick out or bounding of the back legs (a minor form of bucking). It is often a prelude to bucking.

Positive punishment (Addition punishment): The addition of something unpleasant to punish an undesired response and thus decrease the probability of that response. Incorrect use of positive punishment can lower an animal's motivation to trial new responses, desensitise the animal to the punishing stimulus and create fearful associations.

Positive reinforcement (Addition reinforcement): The addition of something pleasant (such as food or a pleasant tactile interaction) to reward a desired response and thus increase the probability of that response.

Primary (unconditioned) reinforcer: A resource or stimulus that the animal is attracted to and that can serve to strengthen instrumental responding.

Pulling: Reflects the resistance of a horse to bit pressure; this is seen when a horse pulls the reins and shows no deceleration.

Punishment: The process in which a punisher follows a particular behaviour so that the frequency (or probability) of that behaviour decreases. (*See* also Positive punishment and Negative punishment.)

Purity of the gaits: The regular temporal sequence of the natural footfalls of the gaits of the horse. These are considered fundamental to the sport and practice of dressage (FEI, 2008). When these are not present due to incorrect negative reinforcement or the simultaneous application of *go* and *stop/slow* pressures, hyper-reactive behaviours may emerge and conflict behaviours may develop.

Rapping, touch up: Inappropriate strategy used to sensitise the legs in an attempt to improve jumping performance in the horse; various irritant substances are applied to the anterior aspects of the third metacarpal or cannon of the forelimbs such that the horse will try harder to avoid hitting a fence when jumping.

Rearing: A sudden postural change in a horse so that it stands only on its hindlegs. Rearing is both an innate counter-predator manoeuvre and an intra-specific social behaviour, usually between stallions or colts. Habitual rearing in horses usually accompanies other conflict behaviours.

Refusal: A conflict behaviour that is typically associated with the approach to jumping an obstacle during which the horse suddenly stops. A precursor to or a form of napping.

Rein back: A series of steps backwards with the legs in diagonal pairs. It is initially trained by the decelerating effects of the reins and later cued via classical conditioning by leg position of the rider.

Reinforcer: An environmental change that increases the likelihood that an animal will make a particular response (i.e. the *addition* of a reward, a positive reinforcer, or *removal* of an aversive stimulus, a negative reinforcer). (*See* also Primary (unconditioned) reinforcer, and Secondary reinforcement.)

Reinforcement: The process in which a reinforcer follows a particular behaviour so that the frequency (or probability) of that behaviour increases. (*See* also Positive reinforcement and Negative reinforcement.)

Reinforcement schedule: The frequency of the reinforcers used in training. The schedule may be continuous, intermittent or declining.

Resistance: *See* Conflict behaviour, Evasions and resistances.

Respect: A term used in general horsemanship and natural horsemanship that emphasises the significance and relevance of the hierarchy in horse–human interactions. The notion of respect may imply subjective mental states that

the horse may not possess. Furthermore, in training and retraining, the concept of respect may encourage remedies for behaviour problems that are unrelated to the original behaviour problem. Thus, from the viewpoint of learning theory, such a concept may be inappropriate and have negative welfare implications.

Response: A reaction to a stimulus. A term that defines fundamental elements of movements such as *go, stop/slow*, stride-length changes, tempo changes, direct and indirect turns of forelegs, turns of hindlegs, flexion and bend.

Rhythm: The beat of the legs within a particular gait. The quality of rhythm in dressage denotes a consistent tempo, stride length and stride height. When a horse is said to maintain a rhythm, its rhythm should be self-maintained.

Rollkur: *See* Hyperflexion.

Round/Roundness: Synonymous with on the bit.

Round-pen (round-yard) training: The practice of causing a horse to move forward in a round-pen with various changes in direction under human stimulus control until it offers a desirable response (such as alterations of focus or slowing), at which point the sending forward is instantly terminated (negative reinforcement). Critics of this technique question the accepted interpretation of the responses of the horse undergoing this process, particularly allowing fearful behaviour because of its obvious association with humans and the high risk of spontaneous recovery.

Running (away): A hyper-reactive state in the horse characterised by acceleration and, usually, heaviness in the reins. The horse is exhibiting conflict behaviour and attempting to flee the aversive situation. Such states are usually the result of incorrect negative reinforcement and can be associated with conflict behaviour. (*See* Rushing.)

Rushing: Seen in a horse that is not under the stimulus control of the cues to *slow*, usually in relation to approaching a jumping obstacle. Often anthropomorphically interpreted as 'keenness'.

Sagittal: A vertical plane passing through the standing body from front to back. The midsagittal or median plane splits the body into left and right halves.

School: (a) An enclosed area, either covered or open, in which a horse can be trained or exercised. (b) To train a horse for whatever purpose it may be required.

Scope: The range of both the stride patterns associated with the gaits and the ability to spring or jump.

Secondary reinforcement: Making a response more likely in the future by using a stimulus that has acquired reinforcing properties on the basis of its relationship to a primary (unconditioned) reinforcer.

Self-carriage: Refers to the self-maintenance of rhythm, straightness and outline. Because of the obtrusive and aversive potential of rein tension and leg pressures, it is important that the horse travels in-hand and under-saddle free of any constant rein tension or leg pressure because of the risk of habituation to strong tactile pressures and consequent conflict behaviour or learned helplessness.

Sensitisation: A type of non-associative learning where a progressive amplification of a response follows repeated administration of a stimulus.

Shape, frame (US): See Outline.

Shaping: The successive approximation of a behaviour towards a targeted desirable behaviour through the consecutive training of one single quality of a response followed by the next. In horse-training, a shaping programme is known as a training scale.

Shying: The sudden hyper-reactive sideways leaping of the horse, either from an aversive object it encounters or as an expression of conflict behaviour that has arisen due to unresolved problems in negative reinforcement (e.g. when the contact is too strong). A shy begins with the horse turning away its forequarters followed by an acceleration response. Shying is frequently associated with other conflict behaviours and may be followed by bucking.

Signal: See Cue.

Slow gait: One of the gaits of the five-gaited breeds characterised by a prancing action in which each foot in turn is raised and then held momentarily in mid-air before descending.

Soft condition: Easily fatigued or unfit.

Soft mouth: Sensitive mouth, responsive to bit pressure.

Spinning: A sudden change in direction, akin to shying in origin and expression; it has associations with conflict behaviour.

Spontaneous recovery: The reappearance of a conditioned response that had been extinguished.

Spooky: Shies or baulks readily/frequently.

Stance phase: When the limbs are in contact with the ground.

Star-gazer: A horse that moves in-hand or under-saddle in an awkward position with its head elevated, as if looking upwards.

Step: The single complete movement of raising one foot and putting it down in another spot, as in walking, used in equitation parlance to describe the nature of the movement in an individual horse and often erroneously based on the observation of the forelimbs only.

Step-back: A single step or stride of stepping backwards. *Step-back* is trained to facilitate *stop/slow* responses because of the effect of *step-back* on the major muscles (mostly pectorals) for deceleration. A precursor to rein-back.

Stereotypy: A repeated, relatively invariant sequence of movements that has no function obvious to the observer. Stereotypies are abnormal behaviours and are generally considered a sign of impaired welfare. Stereotypic behaviour arises from frequent or chronic stress and may help the animal to cope with adverse conditions. The behaviours may persist, even if the triggering factors are eliminated. A number of stereotypic behaviours, such as box-wandering, pacing and crib-biting, are seen in horses and are erroneously referred to as stable vices.

Stimulus: Something that causes a reaction. *See also* Cue.

Stimulus blending: A technique to systematically desensitise the horse to a fear-inducing stimulus by exposing it to a similar stimulus, to which the horse has already habituated. The fear-inducing stimulus is applied simultaneously with the known, non-fear-inducing stimulus, and then systematically increased in intensity. The auditory and tactile characteristics of the two stimuli are gradually mixed, making differentiation between the two difficult. The old, benign stimulus can then be diminished and finally terminated, after which the horse will become habituated to the new stimulus.

Stimulus control: The process by which a response becomes consistently elicited by a signal or cue.

Stop/slow: The decelerating response in the trained horse that results in it ceasing or decreasing its forward movement in-hand and under-saddle. The *stop* response is most commonly trained by negative reinforcement, using the bit in the horse's mouth, stimulated by the reins in the rider's hands. Classical conditioning converts the *stop* response to lighter cues and then to the bracing of the seat. Decelerating involves activation and emphasis of different musculature from that involved in forward motion. These muscles are isolated by the *step-back* response. Therefore, it is not surprising that training the *step-back* trains the *stop* response. Slowing the horse can occur through shortening the stride or slowing the activity or tempo of the legs.

Straightness: A fundamentally desirable trait in equitation such that the hindlegs move into the line of the foretracks on lines and circles and the longitudinal axis of the vertebral column is straight. Straightness is necessary in order to achieve maximal biomechanical and motor efficiency in the horse and consequently considered a tenet of basic training. When horses are not straight, they tend to drift towards the convex side. Thus, crookedness can be seen as a symptom; the deeper problem is that the horse is not following the rider's (or trainer's) intended line.

Stress: Stress is a state characterised by the behavioural and physiological responses elicited when an individual encounters a threat to its homeostasis ('internal balance'). The threat is termed a stressor.

Stress colic: Abdominal pain that is thought to be associated with inability to cope with aversive conditions.

Stressor: Any event that disrupts homeostasis (e.g. physical and psychological threats, including lack of fulfilment of natural behavioural needs). The severity of stressors is affected by loss of control, loss of predictability, and the absence of outlets for frustration.

Stress response: The body's adaptations evolved to re-establish homeostasis. Stress responses are elicited when an animal anticipates or faces a stressor, and involves a range of endocrine and neural systems. The responses are somewhat nonspecific to the type of stressors that trigger them. Stress responses are adaptive by nature but when provoked for a long duration or repeatedly, they can cause negative effects such as increased susceptibility to diseases, gastric ulceration, abnormal behaviour, reproduction problems, and reduced performance.

Stride: (a) The set of changes occurring during a single complete locomotory cycle that includes the stance phase and the swing phase of a limb, from one landing of a particular foot to the next. A series of strides comprise a gait. (b) Used in jumping to describe a rider's appreciation of the number of whole steps a horse takes between obstacles. (c) Medium walk/trot/canter: a descriptive term for strides that are longer than at working paces, but not as long as extended paces. Medium strides are therefore part of the development of longer strides in equitation. For the average horse in medium walk and trot, the hindtracks should land approximately 10–20 cm in front of the foretracks, whereas in medium canter the hindtracks land approximately 1.5 m in front of the foretracks.

Stride length: The length of the horse's step.

Stubborn: A horse that appears unwilling to respond to <u>cues</u>, probably due to lack of motivation or habituation to signals as a result of incorrect <u>negative reinforcement</u>.

Submission: *See* <u>Dominance/submission.</u>

Swing, swinging the hindquarters: The lumbar musculature is described as swinging during collected movements. The hindquarters may move laterally and be said to swing out during lateral movements. Swinging out is also a term used to describe hindquarters that move laterally but not under stimulus control. This may indicate that the forelegs are not under the stimulus control of the reins. Thus, the forequarters also show deviations of line.

Swing phase: When the limbs are in the air phase and not in contact with the ground.

Switch off, tune out: A lack of response to any signal (altered attention and motivation levels) provided by a rider or trainer. This may be an expression of <u>learned helplessness</u>.

Systematic desensitisation: A commonly used habituation technique for the alleviation of behaviour problems caused by inappropriate arousal. In a controlled situation, the animal is first exposed to low levels of the arousing stimulus followed by an increasing gradient, until habituation occurs. An increase in the level of the stimulus is not made until the animal reliably fails to react to the previous level. In this way, the technique aims to raise the threshold for a response. The decrease in arousal can be reinforced by either negative or positive reinforcement.

Tail swishing: Lateral and dorsoventral movements of the tail symptomatic of <u>conflict</u> <u>behaviour</u> in <u>hyper-reactive</u> horses. In the absence of other irritants, tail swishing can be a clue to incorrect <u>negative reinforcement</u> of the <u>go</u> response or indicate a dislike of too-tight reins and unrelenting leg/spur pressure.

Teeth grinding: In the absence of dental or other health disorders, grinding the teeth is a response to unresolved stressors encountered during training, or a product of general management. It may be associated with incorrect <u>negative reinforcement</u> of the *stop/slow* and *step-back* responses.

Tempo: The speed of the horse's steps and <u>strides</u>.

Temporal: (a) Anatomical term pertaining to the temple region of the head. The temporal lobe of the brain is located beneath the temple. (b) Also relating to time; lasting or existing only for a time; passing, temporary. From the Latin *tempus*, which means both the temple of the head (and time).

Tension: In equitation, <u>hyper-reactivity</u> and, presumably, heightened <u>HPA axis</u> activity. Tense horses are frequently <u>hollow</u> and show various behavioural indicators of <u>stress</u>.

Throughness: In equitation, throughness initially develops when the rein/seat signals have an immediate decelerating effect on the horse's hindlegs, most notably in transitions from trot to halt and less visibly on other downward transitions. This effect causes the hindfeet to begin stance phase further forwards (cranially) and the hindquarters to lower as a consequence. As this quality develops, the horse's back is said to soften and participate in both upward and downward transitions and enables a more 'connected' way of going that is a major goal of dressage training. In the 'through' stance at halt, the hindfeet rest one hoofprint closer to the forefeet than usual. Following development of the *stop/slow* response, the go response and continuous locomotion, throughness is the final precursor to collection.

Tilting: In equitation, tilting refers to the horse that is seen to be tilting its withers or dropping its shoulder. This is typically a result of losses of straightness or bridle lameness.

Tilting nose: A posture adopted by some horses during locomotion under-saddle, such that the nose tilts to one side. It typically results from incorrect negative reinforcement of flexion principally during the training of the *turn* response (no release for the correct response or pressuring for the turn when the inside leg is on the ground and unable to respond), but also in the training of the *stop* response (no release and contact too tight).

Tonic immobility, aka freezing: An aroused state in which the horse remains immobile, sometimes in spite of stimulation from the rider.

Tracking up: During locomotion, the horse's hindhooves land in or over the tracks left by the ipsilateral forefeet.

Trailing hindquarters: In equitation, the action of the hindlegs such that, at the moment of thrust, the hindhooves are not underneath the hocks but behind them. The horse is said to be out behind and is usually also hollow. This prevents the horse from attaining impulsion and collection and typically results from too-strong rein contact.

Training scale: A progressive order of training particular qualities of responses through the process of shaping.

Transition: The change from one gait type to another, or from one stride length to another. A transition can be between gaits (inter-gait transitions), within a gait (intra-gait transitions) or from one tempo to another, as well as into and out of the halt.

Transverse: A horizontal plane passing through the standing body parallel to the ground.

Tune out: *See* Switch off.

Turn: A change in the line of locomotion by the horse through the biomechanics of abduction and adduction. The turn is initiated by the forequarters with the hindfeet following the foretracks. Turning occurs through the abduction/adduction sequences where the legs open and close more or less laterally in stance and swing phases. The turn is trained by negative reinforcement using the stimulus of the single rein, which classically conditions to lighter rein cues and then to cues of associated changes of the rider's position at the initiation of the turn. The turn cue should be applied when the turning leg is beginning the swing phase. (*See* Direct turn, and Indirect turn.)

Under-saddle: The situations in which a horse is being ridden, rather than led or driven.

Under-tracking, stepping short: During locomotion, the horse's hindhooves land on the ground in front of the tracks left by the ipsilateral forefeet.

Unlevel/uneven: In equitation, this refers to a horse that is seen to be tilting its withers or dropping its shoulder. This is typically a result of losses of straightness or bridle lameness. The term is also a euphemism for abnormal action caused by either clinical lameness or a physical abnormality that changes the action of the horse.

Ventral: Pertaining to the underside of the horse, as opposed to dorsal.

Working trot/canter: A term that refers to the normal stride length within the gaits. In the working trot, the stride length is where the hindfeet land one hoofprint over the foretracks. In working canter, the inside hindfoot typically lands 70–80 cm over the inside foretracks.

References

Adams, O.R. 1979. *Lameness in Horses*, 3rd edn. Lea & Febiger Publishing, Philadelphia.

Ahrendt, L.P., Christensen, J.W., Ladewig, J. 2012. The ability of horses to learn an instrumental task through social observation. *Applied Animal Behaviour Science*, 139, 105–113.

Ahrendt, L.P., Labouriau, R., Malmkvist, J., Nicol, C., Christensen, J.W. 2015. Development of a standard test to assess negative reinforcement learning in horses. *Applied Animal Behaviour Science*, 169, 38–42.

AIHW National Injury Surveillance Unit. 2005. Mortality Data. Bulletin 24, Flinders University, http://www.nisu.flinders.edu.au/pubs/bulletin24/bulletin24-Mortalit.html. [Accessed 9 December 2005.]

Albert A., Bulcroft, K. 1988. Pets, families, and the life course. *Journal of Marriage and the Family*, 2, 543–552.

Albright, J.L., Arave, C.W. 1997. *The Behaviour of Cattle*. CABI Publishing, Wallingford, UK.

Ali, A., Gutwein, K., Hitzler, P., Heleski, C. 2015. Assessing the influence of nose twitching during a potentially aversive husbandry procedure (ear clipping) using behavioural and physiological measures. Proceedings of the 11th Conference of the International Society for Equitation Science, Vancouver, Canada.

Andrieu, J., Henry, S., Hausberger, M., Thierry, B. 2015. Informed horses are influential in group movements, but they may avoid leading. *Animal Cognition*, 19, 451–458.

Andersson, L.S., Larhammar, M., Memic, F., Wootz, H., Schwochow, D. *et al.* 2012. Mutations in DMRT3 affect locomotion in horses and spinal circuit function in mice. *Nature*, 488(7413), 642–646.

Appleby, M.C. 1997. Life in a variable world: behaviour, welfare and environmental design. *Applied Animal Behaviour Science*, 54(1), 1–19.

Archer, J. 1997. Why do people love their pets? *Evolution and Human Behaviour*, 18, 237–259.

Archer, M. 1971. Preliminary studies on the palatability of grasses, legumes and herbs to horses. *Veterinary Record*, 89, 236.

Argue, C.K. 1994. The kinematics of piaffe, passage and collected trot of dressage horses. MS Thesis, University of Saskatchewan, Saskatoon, Canada.

Argue, C.K., Clayton, H.M. 1993a. A preliminary study of transitions between the walk and trot in dressage horses. *Acta Anatomica*, 146, 179–182.

Argue, C.K., Clayton, H.M. 1993b. A study of transitions between the trot and canter in dressage horses. *Journal of Equine Veterinary Science*, 13, 171–174.

Bachmann, I., Audigé, L., Stauffacher, M. 2003. Risk factors associated with behavioural disorders of crib-biting, weaving and box-walking in Swiss horses. *Equine Veterinary Journal*, 35, 158–163.

Equitation Science, Second Edition. Paul McGreevy, Janne Winther Christensen, Uta König von Borstel and Andrew McLean.
© 2018 John Wiley & Sons Ltd. Published 2018 by John Wiley & Sons Ltd.
Companion website: www.wiley.com/go/mcgreevy/equitation

Back, W. 2001. Intra-limb co-ordination: the forelimb and the hindlimb. In: *Equine Locomotion*, 95–153. Eds: W. Back, H.M. Clayton. W.B. Saunders, Edinburgh, UK.

Back, W., Clayton, H.M. 2001. *Equine Locomotion*. W.B. Saunders, Edinburgh, UK.

Baer, K.L., Potter, G.D., Friend, T.H., Beaver, B.V. 1983. Observation effects on learning in horses. *Applied Animal Ethology*, 11, 123–129.

Bagshaw, C.S., Ralston, S.L., Fisher, H. 1994. Behavioral and physiological effect of orally administered tryptophan on horses subjected to acute isolation stress. *Applied Animal Behaviour Science*, 40(1), 1–12.

Bailey, C.H., Chen, M. 1983. Morphological basis of long-term habituation and sensitization in Aplysia. *Science*, 220, 91–93.

Baker, A.E.M., Crawford, B.H. 1986. Observational learning in horses. *Applied Animal Behaviour Science*, 15, 7–13.

Ball, C., Ball, J., Kirkpatrick, A., Mulloy, R. 2007. Equestrian injuries: incidence, injury patterns, and risk factors for 10 years of major traumatic injuries. *The American Journal of Surgery*, 193(5), 636–640.

Baltacis, A., Hofmann, A., Schobesberger, H., Peham, C. 2006. Evaluation of pressure distribution under a fitting saddle with different saddle pads. *Journal of Biomechanics*, 39, S559–S559.

Baragli, P., Vitale, V., Banti, L., Sighieri, C. 2014. Effect of aging on behavioural and physiological responses to a stressful stimulus in horses (*Equus caballus*). *Behaviour*, 151, 1513–1533.

Baron, A., Galizio, M., 2006. The distinction between positive and negative reinforcement: Use with care. *The Behavior Analyst*, 29, 141–151.

Barrey, E. 2001. Inter-limb coordination. In: *Equine Locomotion* 78. Eds: W. Back, H.M. Clayton. W.B. Saunders, Edinburgh, UK.

Bartos, L., Bartosova, J., Starostova, L. 2008. Position of head is not associated with changes in horse vision. *Equine Veterinary Journal*, 40, 599–601.

Bassett, L., Buchanan-Smith, H.M. 2007. Effects of predictability on the welfare of captive animals. *Applied Animal Behaviour Science*, 102, 223–245.

Baum, M. 1970. Extinction of avoidance responding through response prevention (flooding). *Psychological Bulletin*, 74, 276–284.

Beausoleil, N.J., Mellor, D.J. 2014. Introducing breathlessness as a significant animal-welfare issue. *New Zealand Veterinary Journal*, 63, 44–51.

Beck, L., Madresh, E.A. 2008. Romantic partners and four-legged friends: An extension of attachment theory to relationships with pets. *Anthrozoös*, 21, 1, 43–56.

Bekoff, M. 1995. Cognitive ethology, vigilance, information gathering, and representation: Who might know what and why? *Behavioural Processes*, 35, 225–237.

Bell, R.A., Nielsen, B.D., Waite, K., Rosenstein, D., Orth, M. 2001. Daily access to pasture turnout prevents loss of minerals in the third metacarpus of Arabian weanlings. *Journal of Animal Science*, 79(5), 1142–1150.

Belock, B., Kaiser, L.J., Lavagnino, M., Clayton, H.M. 2012. Comparison of pressure distribution under a conventional saddle and a treeless saddle at sitting trot. *The Veterinary Journal*, 193, 87–91.

Bermond, B. 1997. The myth of animal suffering. In: *Animal Consciousness and Animal Ethics – Perspectives from the Netherlands*, 125–143. Eds: M. Dol, S. Kasanmoentalib, S. Lijmbach, E. Rivas, R. Van Den Bos. *Animals in Philosophy and Science Series*. Van Gorcum and Co., Assen, The Netherlands.

BHA 2008. *Use of the Whip in Horseracing*. British Horseracing Authority, London.

BHA 2009. Disciplinary: Whip use. British Horseracing Authority, London. http://www.britishhorseracing.com/insidehorseracing/about/whatwedo/disciplinary/whipuse.asp. [Accessed 18 July 2009.]

Birke, L., Hockenhull, J. 2015. Journeys together: Horses and humans in partnership. *Society and Animals*, 23, 81–100.

Björnsdottir, S., Arnason, T., Lord, P. 2003. Culling rate of Icelandic horses due to bone spavin. *Acta Veterinaria Scandinavica*, 44, 161–9.

Blackshaw, J.K., Kirk, D., Creiger, S.E. 1983. A different approach to horse handling, based on the Jeffrey method. *International Journal for the Study of Animal Problems*, 4(2), 117–123.

Blecha, F. 2000. Immune system in response to stress. In: *The Biology of Animal Stress. Basic Principles and Implications for Animal Welfare*, 111–122. Eds: G.P. Moberg, J.A. Mench. CABI Publishing, Wallingford, UK.

Boissy, A. 1995. Fear and fearfulness in animals. *Quarterly Review of Biology*, 70(2), 165–191.

Boissy, A. 1998. Fear and fearfulness in determining behavior. In: *Genetics and the Behaviour of Domestic Animals*, 67–111. Ed: T. Grandin. Academic Press, San Diego, USA.

Boot, M., McGreevy, P.D. 2013. The X files: Xenophon re-examined through the lens of equitation science. *Journal of Veterinary Behavior: Clinical Applications and Research*, 8, 367–375.

Bourjade, M., Thierry, B., Hausberger, M., Petit, O. 2015. Is leadership a reliable concept in animals? An empirical study in the horse. *PLoS One*, 10, 14.

Bourjade, M., Thierry, B., Maumy, M., Petit, O. 2009. Decision-making in Przewalski horses (*Equus ferus przewalskii*) is driven by the ecological contexts of collective movements. *Ethology*, 115, 321–330.

Boyd, L., Bandi, N. 2002. Reintroduction of Takhi, *Equus ferus przewalskii*, to Hustai National Park, Mongolia: Time budget and synchrony of activity pre- and post-release. *Applied Animal Behaviour Science*, 78(2–4), 87–102.

Bradshaw, G. 2009. Inside looking out: Neuroethological compromise effects of elephants in captivity. In: Eds: Forthman, D.L., Kane, L.F., Hancocks, D., Waldau, P.F., *An Elephant in the Room*, Tufts Centre for Animal Policy, Massachusetts, 58.

Bradshaw, J.W.S., Blackwell, E., Casey, R.A. 2009. Dominance in domestic dogs – useful construct or bad habit? *Journal of Veterinary Behavior: Clinical Applications and Research*, 4, 135–144.

Breland, K., Breland, M. 1962. The misbehavior of organisms. *American Psychologist*, 16, 681–684.

Briard, L., Dorn, C., Petit, O. 2015. Personality and affinities play a key role in the organisation of collective movements in a group of domestic horses. *Ethology*, 121, 888–902.

Brubaker, L., Udell, M.A.R. 2016. Cognition and learning in horses (*Equus caballus*): What we know and why we should ask more. *Behavioural Processes*, 126, 121–131.

Brunberg, E., Gille, S., Mikko, S., Lindgren, G., Keeling, L.J. 2013. Icelandic horses with the Silver coat colour show altered behaviour in a fear-reaction test. *Applied Animal Behaviour Science*, 146, 72–78.

Buckley, P. 2007. Health and performance of Pony Club horses in Australia. PhD thesis. CSU, Wagga Wagga, NSW.

Bulmer, L., McBride, S., Williams, K., Murray, J.-A. 2015. The effects of a high-starch or high-fibre diet on equine reactivity and handling behaviour. *Applied Animal Behaviour Science*, 165, 95–102.

Burn, C.C., Pritchard, J.C., Whay, H.R. 2009. Observer reliability for working equine welfare assessment: Problems with high prevalences of certain results. *Animal Welfare*, 18, 177–187.

Byström, A., Rhodin, M., von Peinen, K., Weishaupt, M.A., Roepstorff, L. 2009. Basic kinematics of the saddle and rider in high-level dressage horses trotting on a treadmill. *Equine Veterinary Journal*, 41, 280–284.

Byström, A., Stalfelt, A., Egenvall, A., von Peinen, K., Morgan, K., Roepstorff, L. 2010. Influence of girth strap placement and panel flocking material on the saddle-pressure pattern during riding of horses. *Equine Veterinary Journal*, 42, 502–509.

Caanitz, H. 1996. Ausdrucksverhalten von Pferden und Interaktion zwischen Pferd und Reiter zu Beginn der Ausbildung. DVM-thesis, Klinik für Pferde der Tierärztlichen Hochschule Hannover und dem Tierhygienischen Institut Freiburg.

Cabib, S. 2006. The neurobiology of stereotypy. II: The role of stress. In: *Stereotypic Animal Behaviour: Fundamentals and Applications to Welfare*, 2nd edn, 227–255. Eds: G. Mason, J. Rushen. CABI Publishing, Wallingford, UK.

Casey, V., McGreevy, P.D., O'Muiris, E., Doherty, O. 2013. A preliminary report on estimating the pressures exerted by a crank noseband in the horse. *Journal of Veterinary Behavior: Clinical Applications and Research*, 8, 479–484.

Castellucci, V.F., Blumenfeld, H., Goelet, P., Kandel, E.R. 1989. Inhibitor of protein synthesis blocks long-term behavioral sensitization in the isolated gill-withdrawal reflex of Aplysia. *Journal of Neurobiology*, 20, 1–9.

Ceroni, D. 2007. Support and safety features in preventing foot and ankle injuries in equestrian sports. *International Sportmed Journal*, 8, 166–178.

Chalmers, H.J., Farberman, A., Bermingham, A., Sears, W., Viel, L. 2013. The use of a tongue tie alters laryngohyoid position in the standing horse. *Equine Veterinary Journal*, 45(6), 711–714.

Chamove, A.S., Crawley-Hartrick, O.J.E., Stafford, K.J. 2002. Horse reactions to human attitudes and behavior. *Anthrozoös*, 15, 323–331.

Chance, P. 1993. *Learning and Behaviour*. Brooks & Cole, Belmont, USA.

Chateau, H., Degueurce, C., Denoix, J-M. 2004. Evaluation of three-dimensional kinematics of the distal portion of the forelimb in horses walking in a straight line. *American Journal of Veterinary Research*, 65, 447–455.

Chaya, L., Cowan, E., McGuire, B. 2006. A note on the relationship between time spent in turnout and behaviour during turnout in horses (*Equus caballus*). *Applied Animal Behaviour Science*, 98, 155–160.

Christensen, J.W. 2007. Fear in horses: Social influence, generalisation and reactions to predator odour. PhD thesis, Faculties of Agriculture and Life Sciences, University of Aarhus and University of Copenhagen, Denmark.

Christensen, J.W. 2013. Object habituation in horses: The effect of voluntary versus negatively reinforced approach to frightening stimuli. *Equine Veterinary Journal*, 45, 298–301.

Christensen, J.W. 2016. Early-life exposure with a habituated mother reduces fear reactions in foals. *Animal Cognition*, 19, 171–179.

Christensen, J.W., Rundgren, M. 2008. Predator odour *per se* does not frighten domestic horses. *Applied Animal Behaviour Science*, 112, 136–145.

Christensen, J.W., Ladewig, J., Søndergaard, E., Malmkvist, J. 2002. Effects of individual versus group stabling on behaviour in domestic stallions. *Applied Animal Behaviour Science*, 75, 233–248.

Christensen, J.W., Keeling, L.J., Nielsen, B.L. 2005. Responses of horses to novel visual, olfactory and auditory stimuli. *Applied Animal Behaviour Science*, 93, 53–65.

Christensen, J.W., Rundgren, M., Olsson, K. 2006. Training methods for horses: Habituation to a frightening stimulus. *Equine Veterinary Journal*, 38, 439–443.

Christensen, J.W., Malmkvist, J., Nielsen, B.L., Keeling, L.J. 2008a. Effects of a calm companion on fear reactions in naïve test horses. *Equine Veterinary Journal*, 40, 46–50.

Christensen, J.W., Zharkikh, T., Ladewig, J. 2008b. Do horses generalise between objects during habituation? *Applied Animal Behaviour Science*, 114, 509–520.

Christensen, J.W., Søndergaard, E., Thodberg, K., Halekoh, U. 2011a. Effects of repeated regrouping on horse behaviour and injuries. *Applied Animal Behaviour Science*, 133, 199–206.

Christensen, J.W., Zharkikh, T.L., Antoine, A., Malmkvist, J. 2011b. Rein tension acceptance in young horses in a voluntary test situation. *Equine Veterinary Journal*, 43(2), 223–238.

Christensen, J.W., Zharkikh, T.L., Chovaux, E. 2011c. Object recognition and generalisation during habituation in horses. *Applied Animal Behaviour Science*, 129, 83–91.

Christensen, J.W., Ahrendt, L.P., Lintrup, R., Gaillard, C., Palme, R., Malmkvist, J. 2012. Does learning performance in horses relate to fearfulness, baseline stress hormone, and social rank? *Applied Animal Behaviour Science*, 140, 44–52.

Christensen, J.W., Beekmans, M., van Dalum, M., Van Dierendonck, M.C. 2014. Effects of hyperflexion on acute stress responses in ridden dressage horses. *Physiology & Behavior*, 128, 39–45.

Christensen, J.W., Munk, R., Hawson, L., König von Borstel, U., Roepstorff, L., Egenvall, A. 2015. Subjective scoring of rideability by professional riders – is it linked to rein tension and occurrence of conflict behaviour? Proceedings of the 11th International Conference of the International Society of Equitation Science, 28.

Clarke, J., Nicol, C.J., Jones, R., McGreevy, P.D. 1996. Effects of observational learning on food selection in horses. *Applied Animal Behaviour Science*, 50, 177–184.

Clayton, H.M. 1989. Terminology for the description of equine jumping kinematics. *Journal of Equine Veterinary Science*, 9, 341–348.

Clayton, H.M. 1994a. Comparison of the stride kinematics of the collected, working, medium and extended trot in horses. *Equine Veterinary Journal*, 26, 230–234.

Clayton, H.M. 1994b. Comparison of the collected, working, medium and extended canters. *Equine Veterinary Journal Supplement*, 17, 16–19.

Clayton, H.M. 1995. Comparison of the stride kinematics of the collected, medium and extended walk in horses. *American Journal of Veterinary Research*, 56, 849–852.

Clayton, H.M. 1997. Classification of collected trot, passage and piaffe using stance phase temporal variables. *Equine Veterinary Journal Supplement*, 23, 54–57.

Clayton, H.M. 2004. The mysteries of self-carriage. *USDF Connection*, September, 14–17.

Clayton, H.M. 2005. Bitting: The inside story. *USDF Connection*, December, 28–32.

Clayton, H.M., Belock, B., Lavagnino, M., Kaiser, L.J. 2013. Forces and pressures on the horse's back during bareback riding. *The Veterinary Journal*, 195(1), 48–52.

Clayton, H.M., Kaiser, L.J., Lavagnino, M., Stubbs, N.C. 2010. Dynamic mobilisations in cervical flexion: Effects on intervertebral angulations. *Equine Veterinary Journal*, 42, 688–694.

Clayton, H.M., Lanovaz, J.L., Schamhardt, H.C., van Wessum R. 1999. The effects of a rider's mass on ground reaction forces and fetlock kinematics at the trot. *Equine Veterinary Journal Supplement*, 30, 218–221.

Clayton, H.M., Larson, B., Kaiser, L.J., Lavagnino, M. 2011. Length and elasticity of side reins affect rein tension at trot. *The Veterinary Journal*, 188, 291–294.

Clayton, H.M., Sha, D.H., Stick, J.A., Robinson, P. 2007a. 3D kinematics of the interphalangeal joints in the forelimb of walking and trotting horses. *Veterinary and Comparative Orthopaedics and Traumatology*, 20, 1–7.

Clayton, H.M., Sha, D., Stick, J., Elvin, N. 2007b. 3D kinematics of the equine metacarpophalangeal joint at walk and trot. *Veterinary and Comparative Orthopaedics and Traumatology*, 20, 86–91.

Clayton, H.M., Singleton, W.H., Lanovaz, J.L., Cloud, G.L. 2003. Measurement of rein tension during horseback riding using strain-gauge transducers. *Experimental Techniques*, 27, 34–36.

Clayton, H.M., Singleton, W.H., Lanovaz, J.L., Cloud, G.L. 2005. Strain gauge measurement of rein tension during riding: A pilot study. *Equine and Comparative Exercise Physiology*, 2(3), 203–205.

Colborne, G.R., Heaps, L.A., Franklin, S.H. 2009. Horizontal movement around the hoof's centre of pressure during walking in a straight line. *Equine Veterinary Journal*, 41(3), 242–246

Cook, N.J., Schaefer, A.L., Warren, L. 2001. Adrenocortical and metabolic responses to ACTH injection in horses: An assessment by salivary cortisol and infrared thermography of the eye. *Canadian Journal of Animal Science* (abstract of technical paper), 81, 621.

Cooper, J.J., McDonald, L., Mills, D.S. 2000. The effect of increasing visual horizons on stereotypic weaving: implications for the social housing of stabled horses. *Applied Animal Behaviour Science*, 69(1), 67–83.

Cooper, J., McGreevy, P. 2002. Stereotypic behaviour in the stabled horse: causes, effects and prevention without compromising horse welfare. In: *The Welfare of Horses*, 99–124. Ed: N. Waran. Kluwer Academic Publishers, Dordrecht, The Netherlands.

Cornelisse, C.J., Holcombe, S.J., Derksen, F.J., Berney, C., Jackson, C.A. 2001a. Effect of a tongue-tie on upper airway mechanics in horses during exercise. *American Journal of Veterinary Research*, 62(5), 775–778.

Cornelisse, C.J., Rosenstein, D.S., Derksen, F.J., Holcombe, S.J. 2001b. Computed tomographic study of the effect of a tongue-tie on hyoid apparatus position and nasopharyngeal dimensions in anesthetized horses. *American Journal of Veterinary Research*, 62(12), 1865–1869.

Cothran, E.G., MacCluer, J.W., Weitkamp, L.R., Bailey, E. 1987. Genetic differentiation associated with gait within American Standardbred horses. *Animal Genetics*, 18, 285–296.

Creighton, E. 2007. Equine learning behaviour: Limits of ability and ability limits of trainers. *Behavioural Processes*, 76, 43–44.

Darwin, C. 1872. *The Expression of Emotions in Man and Animals*. Republished 2002. Oxford University Press, New York.

Davies, H.M.S. 1996. The effects of different exercise conditions on metacarpal bone strains in Thoroughbred racehorses. *Pferdeheilkunde*, 12(4), 666–670.

de Cartier d'Yves, A., Ödberg, F.O. 2005. A preliminary study on the relation between subjectively assessing dressage performances and objective welfare parameters. In: Proceedings of the 1st International Equitation Science Symposium, Broadford, Victoria. Eds: P. McGreevy, A. McLean, N. Waran, D.

Goodwin, A. Warren-Smith. Post-Graduate Foundation in Veterinary Science, Sydney, 89–110.

de Cocq, P., Clayton, H.M., Terada, K., Muller, M., van Leeuwen, J.L. 2009a. Usability of normal force distribution measurements to evaluate asymmetrical loading of the back of the horse and different rider positions on a standing horse. *The Veterinary Journal*, 181, 266–273.

de Cocq, P., Prinsen, H., Springer, N.C.N., van Weeren, P.R., Schreuder, M. *et al.* 2009b. The effect of rising and sitting trot on back movements and head-neck position of the horse. *Equine Veterinary Journal*, 41, 423–427.

de Cocq, P., Duncker, A.M., Clayton, H.M., Bobbert, M.F., Muller, M., van Leeuwen, J.L. 2010a. Vertical forces on the horse's back in sitting and rising trot. *Journal of Biomechanics*, 43, 327–631.

de Cocq, P., Mooren, M., Dortmans, A., Van Weeren, P.R., Timmerman, M. *et al.* 2010b. Saddle and leg forces during lateral movements in dressage. *Equine Veterinary Journal*, 42, 644–649.

de Cocq, P., Muller, M., van Leeuwen, J. 2008. Horse-rider interaction: A simple model for different riding techniques at trot. *Comparative Biochemistry and Physiology a-Molecular & Integrative Physiology*, 150, S81–S82.

de Cocq, P., van Weeren, P.R., Back, W. 2006. Saddle pressure measuring: Validity, reliability and power to discriminate between different saddle-fits. *The Veterinary Journal*, 172, 265–273.

de la Guérinière, F.R. 1992. Ecole de Cavalerie. Xenophon Press, Ohio, USA. First imprinted 1733. J. Collombat, Paris.

Deacon, T.W. 1990. Fallacies of progression in theories of brain-size evolution. *International Journal of Primatology*, 11, 193–236.

DeAraugo, J., McLean, A., McLaren, S., Caspar, G., McLean, M., McGreevy, P. 2014. Training methodologies differ with the attachment of humans to horses. *Journal of Veterinary Behavior: Clinical Applications and Research*, 9(5), 235–241.

Decarpentry, General, 1949. *Academic Equitation* (Translated by N. Bartle, 1971). J.A. Allen & Co Ltd, London.

Dennett, D.C. 1996. *Kinds of Minds*, 13. Orion Books Ltd., London.

Desmedt, J.E., Godaux, E. 1977. Ballistic contractions in man: characteristic recruitment pattern of single motor units of the tibialis anterior muscle. *Journal of Physiology*, 264, 673–693.

Deuel, N.R., Lawrence, L.M. 1987. Effects of urging by the rider on equine gallop stride limb contacts. *Proceedings of the Equine Nutrition and Physiology Symposium*, 10, 487–494.

Deuel, N.R., Park, J-J. 1990. The gait patterns of Olympic dressage horses. *International Journal of Sport Biomechanics*, 6, 198–226.

Devenport, J.A., Patterson, M.R., Devenport, L.D. 2005. Dynamic averaging and foraging decisions in horses (*Equus caballus*). *Journal of Comparative Psychology*, 119(3), 352–358.

Diehl, K.D., Egan, B., Tozer, P. 2002. Intensive, early handling of neonatal foals: mare–foal interactions. In: Proceedings of the Havermeyer Foundation Horse Behavior and Welfare Workshop, Holar, Iceland, 23–26.

Doherty, O., Casey, V., McGreevy, P. Arkins, S. 2017. Noseband use in equestrian sports – an international study. *PLoS ONE*, 12, e0169060.

Döhne, D., Klein, M., König von Borstel, U. 2014. Influence of reinforcement technique and husbandry-related factors on horses' reaction to training of a frightening task. Proceedings of the 10th International Equitation Science Conference August 6–9, Velje, Denmark, 71.

Dorey, N.R., Conover, A.M., Udell, M.A.R. 2014. Interspecific communication from people to horses (*Equus ferus caballus*) is influenced by different horsemanship training styles. *The Journal of Comparative Psychology*, 128, 337–342.

Dougherty, D.M., Lewis, P. 1991. Stimulus generalization, discrimination-learning, and peak shift in horses. *Journal of the Experimental Analysis of Behavior*, 56, 97–104.

Drevemo, S., Fredricson, I., Hjerten, G., McMiken, D. 1987. Early development of gait asymmetries in trotting Standardbred colts. *Equine Veterinary Journal*, 19, 189–191.

Dudink, S., Simonse, H., Marks, I., de Jonge, F.H., Spruijt, B.M. 2006. Announcing the arrival of enrichment increases play behavior and reduces weaning stress-induced behaviors of piglets directly after weaning. *Applied Animal Behaviour Science*, 101, 86–101.

Duvall-Antonacopoulos, N.M., Pychyl, T.A. 2008. An examination of the relations between social support, anthropomorphism and stress among dog owners. *Anthrozoös*, 21(2), 139–142.

Eddy, A.L., Van Hoogmoed, L.M., Snyder, J.R. 2001.The role of thermography in the management of equine lameness. *The Veterinary Journal*, 162, 172–181.

EFA. 2003. Endurance horse fatalities at the 2002 World Equestrian Games. www.efanational.com/default.asp?id=359. [Accessed 11 January 2008.]

Egenvall, A., Christensen, J.W., Munk, R., Hawson, L., Roepstorff, L. 2015. Can we detect rider-related differences in roll and pitch motion of the equine back in professional riders riding the same horses? Proceedings of the 11th International Conference of the International Society of Equitation Science, 67.

Egenvall, A., Eisersiö, M., Roepstorff, L. 2012. Pilot study of behavior responses in young riding horses using 2 methods of making transitions from trot to walk. *Journal of Veterinary Behavior: Clinical Applications and Research*, 7, 157–168.

Ehrenhofer, M.C.A., Deeg, C.A., Reese, S., Liebich, H-G., Stangassinger, M., Kaspers, B. 2002. Normal structure and age-related changes of the equine retina. *Veterinary Ophthalmology*, 5, 39–47.

Eisersiö, M., Rhodin, M., Roepstorff, L., Egenvall, A. 2015. Rein tension in 8 professional riders during regular training sessions. *Journal of Veterinary Behavior: Clinical Applications and Research*, 10, 419–426.

Eisersiö, M., Roepstorff, L., Weishaupt, M.A., Egenvall, A. 2013. Movements of the horse's mouth in relation to horse-rider kinematic variables. *The Veterinary Journal*, 198, e33–838.

Elgersma, A., Wijnberg, I., Sleutjens, J., van der Kolk, J., van Weeren, R., Back, W. 2010. A pilot study on objective quantification and anatomical modelling of *in vivo* head and neck positions commonly applied in training and competition of sport horses. *Equine Veterinary Journal*, 42, 436–443.

Endenburg N. 1999. Perceptions and attitudes towards horses in European societies. The role of the horse in Europe. *Equine Veterinary Journal Supplement*, 28, 38–41.

Eng, J. 2003. Sample size estimation: How many individuals should be studied? *Radiology*, 227, 309–313.

Engell, M.T., Clayton, H.M., Egenvall, A., Weishaupt, M.A., Roepstorff, L. 2016. Postural changes and their effects in elite riders when actively influencing the horse versus sitting passively at trot. *Comparative Exercise Physiology*, 12, 27–33.

Epley, N., Waytz, A., Cacioppo, J.T. 2007. On seeing human: A three-factor theory of anthropomorphism. *Psychological Review*, 114(4), 864–886.

Evans, D., Jeffcott, L., Knight, P. 2006. Performance-related problems and exercise physiology. In: *The Equine Manual*, 2, 1059–1104. Eds: A.J. Higgins, J.R. Snyder. W.B. Saunders, London.

Evans, K.E., McGreevy, P.D. 2006. The distribution of ganglion cells in the equine retina and its relationship to skull morphology. *Anatomia, Histologia, Embryologia*, 35, 1–6.

Evans, D.L., McGreevy, P.D. 2011. An investigation of racing performance and whip use by jockeys in Thoroughbred races. *PLoS ONE*, 6(1), e15622.

Ewers, J.C. 1955. The horse in Blackfoot Indian culture – with comparative material from other western tribes. Bureau of American Ethnology, Smithsonian Institution, Bulletin 159, 62. Government Printing Office, Washington, DC.

Faber, M., Johnston, C., Schamhardt, H., van Weeren, R., Roepstorff, L., Barneveld, A. 2001a. Basic three-dimensional kinematics of the vertebral column of horses trotting on a treadmill. *American Journal of Veterinary Research*, 62(5), 757–764.

Faber, M., Johnston, C., Schamhardt, H.C., van Weeren, P.R., Roepstorff, L., Barneveld, A. 2001b. Three-dimensional kinematics of equine spine during canter. *Equine Veterinary Journal Supplement*, 33, 145–149.

Faber, M., Schamhardt, H.C., van Weeren, P.R. 1999. Determination of 3D spinal kinematics without defining a local vertebral coordinate system. *Journal of Biomechanics*, 32, 1355–1358.

Faber, M., Schamhardt, H.C., van Weeren, P.R., Johnston, C., Roepstorff, L., Barneveld, A. 2000. Basic three-dimensional kinematics of the vertebral column of horses walking on a treadmill. *American Journal Veterinary Research*, 61, 399–406.

FAO. 2003. FAO Statistical Database Website. Food and Agriculture Organisation, Rome, Italy (FAOSTATS: http://apps.fao.org).

Farley, C.T., Taylor, C.R. 1991. A mechanical trigger for the trot–gallop transition in horses. *Science*, 253, 306–308.

Faverot de Kerbrech, F. 1891. *The Methodical Training of the Saddle Horse after the Last Method of Baucher, Recounted by one of his Pupils*. Jean-Michel Place, Paris.

Fazio, E., Calabrō, G., Medica, P., Messineo, C., Ferlazzo, A. 2006. Serum cortisol levels of Quarter horses: Circadian variations and effects of training and western riding events. In: Ed: A. Lindner, *Management of lameness causes in sport horses*. Conference on Equine Sports Medicine and Science, Cambridge, UK. Wageningen Academic Publishers, 175–179.

Fédération Equestre International (FEI). 2006. Report of the FEI Veterinary and Dressage Committee's Workshop. The use of over-bending ('Rollkur') in FEI Competition, 31 January, during the FEI Veterinary Committee meeting at the Olympic Museum, Lausanne, Switzerland.

Fédération Equestre Internationale (FEI). 2007. Abuse of horses. In: *General Regulations*, 22nd edn. Lausanne, Switzerland.

Fédération Equestre Internationale (FEI). 2008. *Rules for Dressage Events*, 22nd edn. Lausanne, Switzerland.

Fédération Equestre International (FEI) (Ed). 2012. Rules for dressage events. 24th edn. [Online] http://www.fei.org/disciplines/dressage/rules [Accessed 21 March 2013].

Feh, C., de Mazières, J. 1993. Grooming at a preferred site reduces heart rate in horses. *Animal Behaviour*, 46, 1191–1194.

Fenner, K., Yoon, S., White, P., Starling, M.J., McGreevy, P.D. 2016. The effect of noseband tightening on horses' behaviour, eye temperature, and cardiac responses. *PLoS ONE*, 11(5), e0154179.

Fielding, D. 1991. The number and distribution of equines in the world. In: *Donkeys, Mules and Horses in Tropical Agricultural Development*, 62–66. Eds: D. Fielding, R.A. Pearson. Centre for Tropical Veterinary Medicine, University of Edinburgh, UK.

Fisher, J.A. 1990. The myth of anthropomorphism. In: *Interpretation and Explanation in the Study of Animal Behavior*. Eds: M. Bekoff, D. Jamieson, vol. I: *Interpretation, Intentionality, and Communication*. Westview Press, Boulder, Colorado, USA.

Fiske, J.C., Potter, G.D. 1979. Discrimination reversal learning in yearling horses. *Journal of Animal Science*, 49, 583–588.

Fjordbakk, C.T., Chalmers, H.J., Holcombe, S.J., Strand, E. 2013. Results of upper airway radiography and ultrasonography predict dynamic laryngeal collapse in affected horses. *Equine Veterinary Journal*, 45, 705–710.

Flakoll, B. 2016. Twitching in veterinary procedures: How does this technique subdue horses? Proceedings of the 12th Conference of the International Society for Equitation Science, Saumur, France, 83.

Flannery, B. 1997. Relational discrimination learning in horses. *Applied Animal Behaviour Science*, 54, 267–280.

Flegal, K.M., Carroll, M.D., Kuczmarski, R.J., Johnson, C.L. 1998. Overweight and obesity in the United States: Prevalence and trends, 1960–1994. *International Journal of Obesity*, 22, 39–47.

Forkman, B. 1996. The foraging behaviour of Mongolian gerbils: A behavioural need or a need to know? *Behaviour*, 133, 129–143.

Forkman, B., Boissy, A., Meunier-Salaün, M.-C., Canali, E., Jones, R.B. 2007. A critical review of fear tests used on cattle, pigs, sheep, poultry and horses. *Physiology & Behaviour*, 92, 340–374.

Fraley, R.C., Heffernan, M.E., Vicary, A.M., Brumbaugh, C.C. 2011. The Experiences in Close Relationships–Relationship Structures questionnaire: A method for assessing attachment orientations across relationships. *Psychological Assessment*, 23, 615–625.

Francis-Smith, K., Wood-Gush, D.G.M. 1997. Coprophagia as seen in Thoroughbred foals. *Equine Veterinary Journal*, 9, 155–157.

Franklin, S.H., Naylor, J.R., Lane, J.G. 2002. The effect of a tongue-tie in horses with dorsal displacement of the soft palate. *Equine Veterinary Journal Supplement*, 34, 430–433.

Fraser, A.F. 1992. *The Behaviour of the Horse*. CABI Publishing, Wallingford, UK.

Fredricson, I., Dalin, G., Drevemo, S., Hjerten, G., Nilsson, G., Alm, L.O. 1975. Ergonomic aspects of poor racetrack design. *Equine Veterinary Journal*, 7, 63–65.

Freire, R., Clegg, H.A., Buckley, P., Friend, M.A., McGreevy, P.D. 2009. The effects of two different amounts of dietary grain on the digestibility of the diet and behaviour of intensively managed horses. *Applied Animal Behaviour Science*, 117(1–2), 69–73.

Freud, S. 1930. *Civilization and its Discontents*. Republished 1989. Norton, New York.

Freymond S.B., Briefer, E.F., Zollinger, A., Gindrat-von Allmen, Y., Wyss, C., Bachmann, I. 2014. Behaviour of horses in a judgement bias test associated with positive or negative reinforcement. *Applied Animal Behaviour Science*, 158, 34–45.

Fruehwirth, B., Peham, C., Scheidl, M., Schobesberger, H. 2004. Evaluation of pressure distribution under an English saddle at walk, trot and canter. *Equine Veterinary Journal*, 36, 754–757.

Fureix, C., Beaulieu, C., Argaud, S., Rochais, C., Quinton, M. *et al.* 2015. Investigating anhedonia in a non-conventional species: Do some riding horses *Equus caballus* display symptoms of depression? *Applied Animal Behaviour Science*, 162, 26–36.

Fureix, C., Jego, P., Sankey, C., Hausberger, M. 2009. How horses (*Equus caballus*) see the world: Humans as significant 'objects'. *Animal Cognition*, 12, 643–654.

Fureix, C., Menguy, H., Hausberger, M. 2010. Partners with bad temper: Reject or cure? A study of chronic pain and aggression in horses. *PLoS ONE*, 5(8), e12434.

Galef, B.G., Giraldeau, L.-A. 2001. Social influences on foraging in vertebrates: Causal mechanisms and adaptive functions. *Animal Behaviour*, 61, 3–15.

Gamelin, F.X., Berthoin, S., Bosquet, L. 2006. Validity of the Polar S810 Heart Rate Monitor to measure R-R intervals at rest. *Medical Science Sports Exercise*, 38, 887–893.

Garcia, J., Koelling, R.A. 1966. Relation of cue to consequence in avoidance learning. *Psychonomic Science*, 4(1), 123–124

Gardyn, R. 2002. Animal magnetism. *American Demographics*, 24, 30–37.

Garner, J.P., Mason, G.J. 2002. Evidence for a relationship between cage stereotypes and behavioural disinhibition in laboratory rodents. *Behavioural Brain Research*, 136(1), 83–92.

German National Equestrian Federation. 1992. *The German Driving and Riding System: Book 2*. Kenilworth, UK.

German National Equestrian Federation. 1997. *The Principles of Riding – The Official Instruction Handbook of the German National Equestrian Federation*. Kenilworth, UK.

German National Equestrian Federation (FN). 2012. Grundausbildung für Reiter und Pferd. Band 1. [Foundation training for rider and horse, vol, 1]. FN-Verlag, Warendorf, Germany 280 pp.

Geutjens, C.A., Clayton, H.M., Kaiser, L.J. 2008. Forces and pressures beneath the saddle during mounting from the ground and from a raised mounting platform. *The Veterinary Journal*, 175, 332–337.

Giese, C., Gerber, V., Howald, M., Bachmann, I., Burger, D. 2014. Stress parameters and behaviour of horses in walkers with and without the use of electricity. *Schweizer Archiv fur Tierheilkunde*, 156(4), 163–169. Epub 2014/04/02. Stressbelastung und Verhalten von Pferden in stromfuhrenden gegenuber nicht stromfuhrenden Fuhranlagen.

Go, L.M.,Barton, A., Ohnesorge, B., 2014a. Objective classification of different head and neck positions and their influence on the radiographic pharyngeal diameter in sport horses. *BMC Veterinary Research*, 10, 118.

Go, L.M., Barton, A., Ohnesorge, B., 2014b. Pharyngeal diameter in various head and neck positions during exercise in sport horses. *BMC Veterinary Research*, 10, 117.

Go, L., Barton, A.K., Ohnesorge, B., 2014c. Evaluation of laryngeal function under the influence of various head and neck positions during exercise in 58 performance horses. *Equine Veterinary Education*, 26, 4147.

Gomez Alvarez, C.B., Rhodin, M., Bobber, M.F., Meyer, H., Weishaupt, M.A. *et al.* 2006. The effect of head and neck position on the thoracolumbar kinematics in the unridden horse. *Equine Veterinary Journal Supplement*, 36, 445–451.

Goodwin, D. 1999. The importance of ethology in understanding the behaviour of the horse. *Equine Veterinary Journal Supplement*, 28, 15–19.

Goodwin, D. 2007. Equine learning behaviour: What we know, what we don't and future research priorities. *Behavioural Processes*, 76(1), 17–19.

Goodwin, D., Davidson, H.P.B., Harris, P. 2002. Foraging enrichment for stabled horses: Effects on behaviour and selection. *Equine Veterinary Journal*, 34(7), 686–691.

Goodwin, D., Davidson H.P.B., Harris, P. 2005. Sensory varieties in concentrate diets for stabled horses: effects on behaviour and selection. *Applied Animal Behaviour Science*, 90, 337–349.

Goodwin, D., Hughes, C.F. 2005. Equine play behaviour. In: *The Domestic Horse: The evolution, development and management of its behaviour*, 150–157. Eds: D. Mills, S. McDonnell. Cambridge University Press, Cambridge.

Górecka-Bruzda, A., Jastrzębska, E., Muszyńska, A., Jędrzejewska, E., Jaworski, Z. *et al.* 2013. To jump or not to jump? Strategies employed by leisure and sport horses. *Journal of Veterinary Behavior: Clinical Applications and Research*, 8(4), 253–260.

Górecka-Bruzda, A., Suwala, M., Jezierski, T. 2012. Typical artefacts in equine heart rate. Annual Meeting of the International Society for Equitation Science, Edinburgh, UK, 66.

Graf, P., König von Borstel, U., Gauly, M. 2014. Practical considerations regarding the implementation of a temperament test into horse performance tests: results of a large-scale test run. *Journal of Veterinary Behaviour*, 9, 329–340.

Gramsbergen, A. 2001. The neurobiology of locomotor development. In: *Equine Locomotion*, 37. Eds: W. Back, H.M. Clayton. W.B. Saunders, Edinburgh, UK.

Grandin, T. 2007. The Use of the Wheat Pressure Box on Horses (Equine Restraint System). http://www.grandin.com/behaviour/tips/equine.restraint.html. [Accessed 18 September 2007.]

Gray, J.A. 1987. *The Psychology of Fear and Stress*, 2nd edn. Cambridge University Press, Cambridge.

Greenebaum, J. 2004. It's a dog's life: Elevating status from pet to 'fur baby' at yappy hour. *Society and Animals*, 12, 117–137.

Griffin, T.M., Kram, R., Wickler, S., Hoyt, D.F. 2004. Biomechanical and energetic determinants of the walk-trot transition in horses. *Journal of Experimental Biology*, 207, 4215–4223.

Grimmett, A., Sillence, M.N. 2005. Calmatives for the excitable horse: A review of L-tryptophan. *The Veterinary Journal*, 170(1), 24–32.

Grisone, F. 1550. *Gliordini di cavalcare*. Translated and edited by Elizabeth Mackenzie Tobey and Federica Brunori.

Published by ACMRS (Arizona Center for Medieval and Renaissance Studies) Tempe, Arizona, 2014.

Grzimek, B. 1952. Versuche über das Farbsehen von Pflanzenessern. *Z. Tierpsychol.* 9, 23–39.

Gust, D., Gordon, T., Brodie, A., McClure, H. 1996. Effects of companions in modulating stress associated with new group formation in juvenile rhesus macaques. *Physiology & Behavior*, 59, 941–945.

Haag, E.L., Rudman, R., Houpt, K.A. 1980. Avoidance, maze learning and social dominance in ponies. *Journal of Animal Science*, 50(2), 329–335.

Hahn, C. 2004. Behavior and the brain. In: *Equine Behaviour – A Guide for Veterinarians and Equine Scientists*, 55–84. Ed: P.D. McGreevy. W.B. Saunders, Edinburgh, UK.

Hall, C.A. 2007. The impact of visual perception on equine learning. *Behavioural Processes*, 76, 29–33.

Hall, C., Burton, K., Maycock, E., Wragg, E. 2011. A preliminary study into the use of infrared thermography as a means of assessing the horse's response to different training methods. *Journal of Veterinary Behavior*, 6, 291–292.

Hall, C.A., Cassaday, H.J., Derrington, A.M. 2003. The effect of stimulus height on visual discrimination in horses. *Journal of Animal Science*, 81, 1715–1720.

Hall, C.A., Cassaday, H.J., Vincent, C.J., Derrington, A.M. 2005. The selection of coloured stimuli by the horse. 1. In: BSAS Conference (September 20–21): Applying Equine Science, Research into Business, Royal Agricultural College, Cirencester, UK.

Hall, C.A., Goodwin, D., Heleski, C., Randle, H., Waran, N. 2007. Is there evidence of 'Learned Helplessness' in horses? In: Proceedings of the 3rd International Equitation Science Symposium, Michigan. Eds: D. Goodwin, C. Heleski, P. McGreevy, A. McLean, H. Randle, C. *et al.*, MSU, Michigan, USA, p. 8.

Hall, C., Heleski, C. 2017. The role of the ethogram in equitation science. *Applied Animal Behaviour Science*, 190, 102–110.

Hall, C., Kay, R., Yarnell, K. 2014. Assessing ridden horse behaviour: Professional judgment and physiological measures. *Journal of Veterinary Behavior: Clinical Applications and Research*, 9, 22–29.

Hall, C., Nuws, N., White, C., Taylor, L., Owen, H., McGreevy, P. 2013. Assessment of ridden horse behaviour. *Journal of Veterinary Behavior*, 8, 74–81.

Halliday, E., Randle, H. 2013. The horse and rider bodyweight relationship within the UK horse-riding population. *Journal of Veterinary Behavior: Clinical Applications and Research*, 8(2), e8–e9.

Hampson, B.A., Morton, J.M., Mills, P.C., Trotter, M.G., Lamb, D.W., Pollitt, C.C. 2010. Monitoring distances travelled by horses using GPS tracking collars. *Australian Veterinary Journal*, 88, 176–181.

Hamra, J.G., Kamerling, S.G., Wolfsheimer, K.J., Bagwell, C.A. 1993. Diurnal variation in plasma ir-beta-endorphin levels and experimental pain thresholds in the horse. *Life Sciences*, 53, 121–129.

Hanggi, E.B. 1999. Categorization learning in horses (*Equus caballus*). *Journal of Comparative Psychology*, 113, 243–252.

Hanggi, E.B. 2003. Discrimination learning based on relative size concepts in horses (*Equus caballus*). *Applied Animal Behaviour Science*, 83, 201–213.

Hanggi, E.B., Ingesoll, J.F. 2009, Long-term memory for categories and concepts in horses (*Equus caballus*). *Animal Cognition*, 12, 451–462.

Hannum, R.D., Rosellini, R.A., Seligman, M.E.P. 1976. Learned helplessness in the rat: Retention and immunization. *Developmental Psychobiology*, 12, 449–454.

Harman, A.M., Moore, S., Hoskins, R., Keller, P. 1999. Horse vision and the explanation of visual behaviour originally explained by the 'ramp retina'. *Equine Veterinary Journal*, 31(5), 384–390.

Harman, J.C. 1994. Practical use of a computerized saddle pressure-measuring device to determine the effects of saddle pads on the horse's back. *Journal of Equine Veterinary Science*, 14, 606–611.

Hartmann, E., Christensen, J.W., Keeling, L.J. 2011. Training young horses to social separation: Effect of a companion horse on training efficiency. *Equine Veterinary Journal*, 43, 580–584.

Hartmann, E., Søndergaard, E., Keeling, L.J. 2012. Keeping horses in groups: A review. *Applied Animal Behaviour Science*, 136, 77–87.

Hartmann, E., Hopkins, R.J., Blomgren, E., Ventorp, M., von Brömssen, C., Dahlborn, K. 2015. Daytime shelter use of individually kept horses during Swedish summer. *Journal of Animal Science*, 93, 802–810.

Hartmann, E., Christensen, J.W., McGreevy, P.D., 2017. Dominance and leadership: Useful concepts in human–horse interactions? *Journal of Equine Veterinary Science* (open access) https://doi.org/10.1016/j.jevs.2017.01.015.

Haselgrove, M., Aydin, M., Pearce, J.M. 2004. A partial reinforcement extinction effect despite equal rates of reinforcement during Pavlovian conditioning. *Journal of Experimental Psychology – Animal Behaviour Processes*, 30, 240–250.

Hausberger, M., Bruderer, U., Le Scolan, N., Pierre, J.S. 2004. Interplay between environmental and genetic factors in temperament/personality traits in horses (*Equus caballus*). *Journal of Comparative Psychology*, 118(4), 434–446.

Hausberger, M., Muller, C., Gautier, E., Jego, P. 2007a. Lower learning abilities in stereotypic horses. *Applied Animal Behaviour Science*, 107(3–4), 299–306.

Hausberger, M., Muller, C., Gautier, E., Jego, P., 2007b. Lower learning abilities in stereotypic horses. *Applied Animal Behaviour Science*, 107(3–4), 299–306.

Hausberger, M., Roche, H., Henry, S., Visser, E.K. 2008. A review of the human–horse relationship. *Applied Animal Behaviour Science*, 109, 1–24.

Haussler, K.K., Stover, S.M., Willits, N.H. 1999. Pathologic changes in the lumbosacral vertebrae and pelvis in Thoroughbred racehorses. *American Journal of Veterinary Research*, 60(2), 143–153.

Hawson, L.A., McLean, A.N., McGreevy, P.D. 2010a. The roles of equine ethology and applied learning theory in horse-related human injuries. *Journal of Veterinary Behavior: Clinical Applications and Research*, 5, 324–338.

Hawson, L.A., McLean, A.N., McGreevy, P.D. 2010b. Variability of scores in the 2008 Olympics dressage competition and implications for horse training and welfare. *Journal of Veterinary Behavior: Clinical Applications and Research*, 5, 170–176.

Hawson, L.A., McLean, A.N., McGreevy, P.D. 2013. A retrospective survey of riders' opinions of the use of saddle pads in horses. *Journal of Veterinary Behavior*, 8, 74–81.

Hayek, A.R., Jones, B., Evans, D.L., Thomson, P.C., McGreevy, P.D. 2005. Epidemiology of horses leaving the Thoroughbred and Standardbred racing industries. In: Proceedings of the 1st International Equitation Science Symposium, Broadford, Victoria, 84–89. Eds: P. McGreevy, A. McLean, N. Waran, D. Goodwin, A. Warren-Smith. Post-Graduate Foundation in Veterinary Science, Sydney.

Hearst, E., Jenkins, H. 1974. *Sign-tracking: The stimulus-reinforcer relation and directed action*. Psychonomic Society, Austin, Texas.

Heffner, H.E., Heffner, R.S. 1983. The hearing ability of horses. *Equine Practice*, 5, 27–32.

Heffner, H.E., Heffner, R.S. 1984. Sound localisation in large mammals: Localisation of complex sounds by horses. *Behavioral Neuroscience*, 98, 541–555.

Heffner, H.E., Heffner, R.S. 1992. Auditory perception. In: *Farm Animal and the Environment*, 159–184. Eds: C. Phillips, D. Piggens. CABI Publishing, Wallingford, UK.

Heffner, R.S., Heffner, H.E. 1986. Localisation of tones by horses: Use of binaural cues and the superior olivary complex. *Behavioral Neuroscience*, 100, 93–103.

Heinecke, S. 2014. Fit fürs Fernsehen? Die Medialisierung des Fernsehens als Kampf um Gold und Sendezeit. [Fit for television? The mediatization of television as competition for gold and broadcasting time.] PhD-thesis, LMU Munich; Publisher: Herbert-von-Halem, 504.

Heird, J.C., Whitaker, D.D., Bell, R.W., Ramsey, C.B., Lokey, C.E. 1986a. The effects of handling at different ages on the subsequent learning ability of 2-year-old horses. *Applied Animal Behaviour Science*, 15, 15–25.

Heird, J., Lokey, C., Cogan, D. 1986b. Repeatability and comparison of two maze tests to measure learning ability in horses. *Applied Animal Behaviour Science*, 16, 103–119.

Heleski, C., Bauson, L., Bello, N. 2008. Evaluating the addition of positive reinforcement for learning a frightening task: A pilot study with horses. *Applied Animal Welfare Science*, 11(3), 213–222.

Heleski, C.R., McGreevy, P.D., Kaiser, L.J., Lavagnino, M., Tans, E. *et al.* 2009. Effects on behavior and rein tension on horses ridden with or without martingales and rein inserts. *The Veterinary Journal*, 181(1), 56–62.

Heleski, C., Wickens, C., Minero, M., DallaCosta, E., Wu, C. *et al.* 2015. Do soothing vocal cues enhance horses' ability to learn a frightening task? *Journal of Veterinary Behavior: Clinical Applications and Research*, 10, 41–47.

Helton, W.S., Feltovich, P.J., Velkey, A.J. 2009. Skill and expertise in working dogs: a cognitive science perspective. In: *Canine Ergonomics: The Science of Working Dogs*, 171–178. Ed.: W.S. Helton. CRC Press, Boca Raton, Florida, USA.

Hemmings, A., McBride, S.D., Hale, C.E. 2007. Perseverative responding and the aetiology of equine oral stereotypy. *Applied Animal Behaviour Science*, 104, 143–150.

Hendriksen, P., Elmgreen, K., Ladewig, J. 2011. Trailer-loading of horses: Is there a difference between positive and negative reinforcement concerning effectiveness and stress-related signs? *Journal of Veterinary Behavior: Clinical Applications and Research*, 6, 261–266.

Hennessy, K., Quinn, K., Murphy, J. 2007. Different expectations between producers (vendors) and purchasers may lead to wastage and welfare concerns for the horse. In: Proceedings of the 3rd International Equitation Science Symposium, Michigan, 20.

Eds: D. Goodwin, C. Heleski, P. McGreevy, A. McLean, H. Randle, *et al.* MSU, Michigan.

Henriquet, M. 2004. *Henriquet on Dressage.* (translated by Hilda Nelson). J.A. Allen & Co Ltd, London.

Henry, S., Briefer, S., Richard-Yris, M-A., Hausberger, M. 2007. Are 6-month-old foals sensitive to dam's influence. *Developmental Biology*, 49, 514–521.

Henry, S., Hemery, D., Richard, M-A., Hausberger, M. 2005. Human–mare relationships and behaviour of foals toward humans. *Applied Animal Behaviour Science*, 93, 341–362.

Henry, S., Richard-Yris, M-A., Hausberger, M. 2006. Influence of various early human–foal interferences on subsequent human–foal relationship. *Developmental Psychobiology*, 48, 712–718.

Henry, S., Richard-Yris, M-A., Tordjman, S., Hausberger, M. 2009. Neonatal handling affects durable bonding and social development. *PLoS ONE*, 4, e5216.

Henry, S., Zanella, A., Sankey, C., Richard-Yris, M-A., Marko, A., Hausberger, M. 2012. Adults may be used to alleviate weaning stress in domestic foals (*Equus caballus*). *Physiology & Behavior*, 106, 428–438.

Henshall, C., McGreevy, P.D. 2014. The role of ethology in round-pen horse training – A review. *Applied Animal Behaviour Science*, 155, 1–11.

Herbermann, E. 1980. *Dressage Formula.* J.A. Allen & Co Ltd, London.

Heuschmann, G. 2007. *Tug of War: Classical versus 'Modern' dressage.* Trafalgar Square, Vermont, USA.

Heyes, C.M. 1994. Social learning in animals: Categories and mechanisms. *Biological Reviews*, 69, 207–231.

Higgins, A.J., Wright, I.M. 1995. *The Equine Manual.* Baillière Tindall, London.

Hinchcliff, K.W., Couetil, L.L., Knight, P.K., Morley, P.S., Robinson, N.E. *et al.* 2015. Exercise induced pulmonary hemorrhage in horses: American College of Veterinary Internal Medicine Consensus Statement. *Journal of Veterinary Internal Medicine*, 29, 743–758.

Hinde, R.A. 1987. *Individuals, Relationships and Culture.* Cambridge University Press, Cambridge, UK.

Hiney, K.M., Nielsen, B.D., Rosenstein, D. 2004. Short-duration exercise and confinement alters bone mineral content and shape in weanling horses. *Journal of Animal Science*, 82, 2313–2320.

Hinnemann, J., van Baalen, C. 2003. *The Simplicity of Dressage.* J.A. Allen & Co Ltd, London.

Hintz, R.L. 1980. Genetics of performance in the horse. *Journal of Animal Science*, 51, 582–594.

Hofmann, A., Baltacis, A., Schobesberger, H., Peham, C. 2006. Evaluation of pressure distribution under a too-wide saddle with different saddle pads. *Journal of Biomechanics*, 39, S559–S560.

Holcomb, K.E., Tucker, C.B., Stull, C.L. 2013. Physiological, behavioral, and serological responses of horses to shaded or unshaded pens in a hot, sunny environment. *Journal of Animal Science*, 91, 5926–5936.

Holcombe, S.J., Berney, C., Cornelisse, C.J., Derksen, F.J., Robinson, N.E. 2002. Effect of commercially available nasal strips on airway resistance in exercising horses. *American Journal of Veterinary Research*, 63(8), 1101–1105.

Holmström, M., Fredricson, I., Drevemo, S. 1994. Biokinematic differences between riding horses judged as good and poor at the trot. *Equine Veterinary Journal Supplement*, 17, 51–56.

Holmström, M., Fredricson, I., Drevemo, S. 1995. Biokinematic effects of collection on the trotting gaits in the elite dressage horse. *Equine Veterinary Journal*, 27, 281–287.

Hölzel, W., Hölzel, P., Plewa, M. 1995. *Dressage Tips and Training Solutions.* Kenilworth Press, Addington, UK.

Hood, J., McDonald, C., Wilson, B., McManus, P., McGreevy, P. 2017. Whip Rule Breaches in a Major Australian Racing Jurisdiction: Welfare and Regulatory Implications. *Animals*, 7(3), doi:10.3390/ani7010004.

Hothersall, B., Casey, R. 2012. Undesired behaviour in horses: A review of their development, prevention, management and association with welfare. *Equine Veterinary Education*, 24(9), 479–485.

Hothersall, B., Nicol, C. 2007. Equine learning behaviour: Accounting for ecological constraints and relationships with humans in experimental design. *Behavioural Processes*, 76, 45–48.

Hothersall, B., Nicol, C. 2009. Role of diet and feeding in normal and stereotypic behaviors in horses. *Veterinary Clinics of North America – Equine Practice*, 25, 167–181.

Houpt, K.A. 2000. Equine welfare. In: *Recent Advances in Companion Animal Behavior Problems*. Ithaca, NY: International Veterinary Information Services.

Houpt, K.A. 2007. Imprinting training and conditioned taste aversion. *Behavioural Processes*, 76, 14–16.

Houpt, K.A., Houpt, T.R. 1988. Social and illumination preferences of mares. *Journal of Animal Science*, 66, 2159–2164.

Houpt, K.A., Houpt, T.R. 1992. Social and illumination preferences of mares. *Equine Practice*, 14, 11–16.

Houpt, K.A., Houpt, T.R., Johnson, J.L., Erb, H.N., Yeon, S.C. 2001. The effect of exercise deprivation on the behaviour and physiology of straight-stall confined pregnant mares. *Animal Welfare*, 10(3), 257–267.

Houpt, K.A., Keiper, R. 1982. The position of the stallion in the equine hierarchy of feral and domestic ponies. *Journal of Animal Science*, 54, 945–950.

Houpt, K.A., Marrow, M., Seeliger, M. 2000. A preliminary study of the effect of music on equine behaviour. *Journal of Equine Veterinary Science*, 20(11), 691–737.

Houpt, K.A., Parsons, M.S., Hintz, H.F. 1982. Learning ability of orphan foals, of normal foals and of their mothers. *Journal of Animal Science*, 55, 1027–1032.

Houpt, K.A., Wolski, T.R. 1982. *Domestic Animal Behavior for Veterinarians and Animal Scientists*. Ames University Press, Iowa, USA.

Howery, L.D., Bailey, D.W., Laca, E.A. 1999. Impact of spatial memory on habitat use. In: *Grazing Behavior of Livestock and Wildlife*, 91–100. Eds: K.L. Lunchbaugh, K.D.

Sanders, J.C. Mosley. University of Idaho, Moscow, ID, USA.

Hoyt, D.F., Taylor, C.R. 1981. Gait and the energetics of locomotion in horses. *Nature*, 292, 239–240.

Hughes, T.J., Creighton, E. 2007. Measuring cortisol as an indicator of stress response in domestic horses. *Journal of Equine Studies*, 4, 26–28.

Hume, D. 1757. *The Natural History of Religion*. Republished 1956. Stanford University Press, Stanford, CA.

Hussain, M.Z. 1971. Desensitization and flooding (implosion) in the treatment of phobias. *The American Journal of Psychiatry*, 127, 1509–1514.

Hutson, G.D. 2002. *Watching Racehorses: A Guide to Betting on Behavior*. Clifton Press, Melbourne, Australia.

Innes, L., McBride, S. 2008. Negative versus positive reinforcement: An evaluation of training strategies for rehabilitated horses. *Applied Animal Behaviour Science*, 112, 357–368.

ISES (The International Society for Equitation Science), 2017. Principles of learning theory in equitation. http://equitationscience.com/equitation/principles-of-learning-thoery-in-equitation [Accessed 19.01.2018].

Iwata, B.A. 2006. On the distinction between positive and negative reinforcement. *The Behavior Analyst*, 29, 121–123.

Jansen, F., Van der Krogt, J., Van Loon, K., Avezzú, V., Guarino, M. et al. 2009. Online detection of an emotional response of a horse during physical activity. *The Veterinary Journal*, 181, 38–42.

Jansen, T., Forster, P., Levine, M.A., Oelke, H., Hurles, M. et al. 2002. Mitochondrial DNA and the origins of the domestic horse. *Proceedings of the National Academy of Science*, 99(16), 10905–10910. Epub 2002 July 18.

Jansson, K.S., Michalski, M.P., Smith, S.D., LaPrade, R.F., Wijdicks, C.A. 2012. Tekscan pressure sensor output changes in the presence of liquid exposure. *Journal of Biomechanics*, 46, 612–614.

Jeffcott, L.B., Dalin, G. 1980. Natural rigidity of the horse's backbone. *Equine Veterinary Journal*, 12, 101–108.

Jeffcott, L.B., Holmes, M.A., Townsend, H.G.G. 1999. Validity of saddle pressure measurements using force-sensing array technology – Preliminary studies. *The Veterinary Journal*, 158, 113–119.

Jezierski, T., Jaworski, Z., Gorecka, A. 1999. Effects of handling on behaviour and heart rate in Konik horses: Comparison of stable and forest reared young stock. *Applied Animal Behaviour Science*, 62, 1–11.

Johnson, S.R., Rao, S., Hussey, S.B., Morley, P.S., Traub-Dargatz, J.L. 2011. Thermographic eye temperature as an index to body temperature in ponies. *Journal of Equine Veterinary Science*, 31, 63–66.

Jones, B., Goodfellow, J., Yeates, J., McGreevy, P.D. 2015. A critical analysis of the British Horseracing Authority's review of the use of the whip in horseracing. *Animals*, 5(1), 138–150.

Jones, B., McGreevy, P.D. 2010. Ethical equitation: Applying a cost-benefit approach. *Journal of Veterinary Behavior: Clinical Applications and Research*, 5(4), 196–202.

Jørgensen, G.H.M., Bøe K.E. 2007. A note on the effect of daily exercise and paddock size on the behaviour of domestic horses (*Equus caballus*). *Applied Animal Behaviour Science*, 107, 166–173.

Jørgensen, G.H.M., Fremstad, K.E., Mejdell, C.M., Boe, K.E. 2011. Separating a horse from the social group for riding or training purposes: a descriptive study of human–horse interactions. *Animal Welfare*, 20, 271–279.

Jung, C.G. 1968. *Man and His Symbols*. Dell Publishing Co., Laurel Edition, New York.

Kandel, E.R. 2006. *In Search of Memory: The Emergence of a New Science of Mind*. W.W. Norton & Co. New York.

Kandel, E.R., Schwartz, J.H., Jessell, T.M. 2000. *Principles of Neural Science*, 4th edn. McGraw-Hill, New York.

Kattelans, A. 2012. Eine Untersuchung zum Einfluss der Kopf-Hals-Haltungen auf Gelenkwinkel der Hintergliedmaße mit dem Bewegungsanalysesystem Simi und dem Tekscan®-HoofTM-System. DVM-thesis, University of Veterinary Medicine, Hanover.

Keay, K., Bandler, R. 2008. Emotional and behavioural significance of the pain signal and the role of the midbrain periaqueductal gray (PAG). In: *The Senses: A Comprehensive Reference*. Eds: Allan I. Basbaum, Akimichi Kaneko, Gordon M. Shepherd, Gerald Westheimer. *Pain*, 5, 627–634. M. Catherine Busnell, Allan I. Basbaum. Academic Press, San Diego, USA.

Keeling, L.J., Blomberg, A., Ladewig J. 1999. Horseriding accidents: when the human–animal relationship goes wrong! In: 33rd International Congress of the International Society for Applied Ethology, Lillehammer, Norway, 86.

Keeling, L.J., Jonare, L., Lanneborn. L. 2009. Investigating horse–human interactions: The effect of a nervous human. *The Veterinary Journal*, 181, 70–71.

Keiper, R.R., Sambraus, H.H. 1986. The stability of equine dominance hierarchies and the effects of kinship, proximity and foaling status on hierarchy status. *Applied Animal Behaviour Science*, 16, 121–130.

Kendal, R.L., Coolen, I., Van Bergen, Y., Laland, K.N. 2005. Trade-offs in the adaptive use of social and asocial learning. *Advances in the Study of Behaviour*, 35, 333–379.

Kieffer, N.M. 1968. *Heritability of Cutting in Horses. Horse Short Course*. Texas A&M University, College Station, USA, 46.

Kienapfel, K. 2011. And what are the opinions of the horses? – on the expressive behaviour of horses in different neck positions. *Pferdeheilkunde*, 27, 372–380.

Kienapfel, K. 2015. The effect of three different head-neck positions on the average EMG activity of three important neck muscles in the horse. *Journal of Animal Physiology and Animal Nutrition*, 99, 132–138.

Kienapfel, K., Link, Y., König von Borstel, U. 2014. Prevalence of different head-neck positions in horses shown at dressage competitions and their relation to conflict behaviour and performance marks. *PLoS ONE* 9, e103140.

Kienapfel, K., Preuschoft, H. 2011. What affects hyperflexion of the neck? The influence of the head-neck position on stretching of the soft tissue. *Pferdeheilkunde*, 27, 358 *et seq.*

Kienapfel, K., Preuschoft, H. 2014. Activity patterns of trunk muscles in walk, trot and canter and their relation to different head-and-neck positions. Proceedings of the 10th International Equitation Science Conference, Vejle, Denmark, 45.

Kiley-Worthington, M. 1987. *The Behaviour of Horses in Relation to Management and Training*. J.A. Allen & Co Ltd, London.

King, S.R.B. 2002. Home range and habitat use of free-ranging Przewalski horses at Hustai National Park, Mongolia. *Applied Animal Behaviour Science*, 78(2–4), 103–113.

Kingsley, M., Lewis, M.J., Marson, R.E. 2005. Comparison of Polar 810s and an ambulatory ECG system for RR interval measurement during progressive exercise. *International Journal of Sports Medicine*, 26, 39–44.

König von Borstel, U. 2013. Assessing and influencing personality for improvement of animal welfare: A review. *CAB Reviews*, 8, e 1–27.

König von Borstel, U., Krauskopf, K. (2016) Relationship between rideability and tactile sensitivity assessed via algometer and von-Frey filaments. Proceedings of the 12th International Equitation Science Conference, Nantes, France, June 23–25, 2016.

König von Borstel, U., Krienert, N. 2012b. Influence of familiarity with the rider and type of work on horses' fear reactions. Proceedings of the 8th International Equitation Science Conference in Edinburgh, UK, July 18–20th, 153.

König von Borstel, U. and Keil, J. (2012) Horses' behaviour and heart rate in a preference test for shorter and longer riding bouts. *Journal of Veterinary Behavior-Clinical Applications and Research*, 7, 362–374

König von Borstel, U., Glißman, C. 2014. Alternatives to conventional evaluation of rideability in horse performance tests: Suitability of rein tension and behavioural parameters. *PLoS ONE*, 9, e87285.

König von Borstel, U., McGreevy, P.D. 2014. Behind the vertical and behind the times. *The Veterinary Journal*, 202(3), 403–404.

König von Borstel, U., Claesson-Lundin, M., Duncan, I.J.H., Keeling, L.J. 2010a. Fear reactions in trained and untrained horses of dressage and showjumping breeding lines. *Applied Animal Behaviour Science*, 125, 124–131.

König von Borstel, U., Kassebaum, L., Ladewig, K., Gauly, M. 2010b. Person-hour expenditures in equine housing systems: A comparison of single-stalls, group housing, and group housing with automated feeding systems. *Züchtungskunde*, 82(6), 417–427.

König von Borstel, U., Pasing, S., Gauly, M. 2011a. Towards a more objective assessment of equine personality using behavioural and physiological observations from performance test training. *Applied Animal Behaviour Science*, 135, 277–285.

König von Borstel, U., Euent, S., Graf, P., König, S., Gauly, M. 2011b. Equine behavior and heart rate in temperament tests with or without rider or handler. *Physiology & Behavior*, 104, 454–463.

König von Borstel, U., Pasing, S., Gauly, M., Christmann, L. 2013. Status quo of the personality trait evaluation in horse breeding: Judges' assessment of the situation and strategies for improvement. *Journal of Veterinary Behavior: Clinical Applications and Research*, 8, 326–334.

König von Borstel, U., Peinemann, V., Glissmann, C., Euent, S. 2012. Willing to work? Suitability of different riding situations in evaluation of equine personality. 8th International Equitation Science Conference, Edinburgh, UK, 129

König von Borstel, U., Kienapfel, K., Wilkins, C., Evans, D., McLean, A., McGreevy, P. 2015. Hyperflexing horses' necks: A meta-analysis and cost-benefit evaluation. Proceedings of the 11th International Equitation Science Conference, Vancouver, Canada, August 5–8, 2015.

König von Borstel, U., Erdmann, C., Maier, M., Garlipp, F. 2016a. Relationships between health problems and husbandry, use and management of horses: an analysis based on health-insured horses. Proceedings of the 12th International Equitation Science Conference, Nantes, France, June 23–25, 43.

König von Borstel, U., Erdmann, C., Maier, M., Garlipp, F. 2016b. Relationships between behaviour problems (stereotypies and dangerous behaviour) and husbandry, use and management of horses. Proceedings of the 12th International Equitation Science Conference, Nantes, France, June 23–25, 110.

Küllmar, A., König von Borstel, U. 2015. A pilot study on horses' behaviour and distance travelled in a 'Paddock Trail' husbandry system. Proceedings of the 3rd International Equine Science Meeting, Nürtingen, Germany. 37.

Korte, S.M. 2001. Corticosteroids in relation to fear, anxiety and psychopathology. *Neuroscience Biobehaviour Review*, 25, 117–142.

Kotschwar, A.B., Baltacis, A., Peham, C. 2010a. The influence of different saddle pads on force and pressure changes beneath saddles with excessively wide trees. *The Veterinary Journal*, 184(3), 322–325.

Kotschwar, A.B., Baltacis, A., Peham, C. 2010b. The effects of different saddle pads on forces and pressure distribution beneath a fitting saddle. *Equine Veterinary Journal*, 42(2), 114–118.

Kratzer, D.D., Netherland, W.M., Pulse, R.E., Baker, J.P. 1977. Maze learning in quarter horses. *Journal of Animal Science*, 46, 896–902.

Krause, J., Ruxton, G.D. 2002. *Living in Groups*. Oxford: Oxford University Press.

Krueger, K. 2007. Behaviour of horses in the 'roundpen technique'. *Applied Animal Behaviour Science*, 104, 162–170.

Krueger, K., Flauger, B., Farmer, K., Maros, K. 2011. Horses (*Equus caballus*) use human local enhancement cues and adjust to human attention. *Animal Cognition*, 14, 187–201.

Krueger, K., Farmer, K., Heinze, J. 2014a. The effects of age, rank and neophobia on social learning in horses. *Animal Cognition*, 17(3), 645–655.

Krueger, K., Flauger, B., Farmer, K., Hemelrijk, C. 2014b. Movement initiation in groups of feral horses. *Behavioural Processes*, 103, 91–101.

Kubiak, M., Vogt, A., Sauter, H., Christensen, J.W., König von Borstel, U. 2016. Gebisslose Zäumungen versus Trensenzäumungen – wie hoch ist die maximale Zügelkraft, der sich Pferde freiwillig in Erwartung einer Futterbelohnung aussetzen? Symposium on Bitless Bridles of the Leisure Riders'. Drivers' and Endurance Riders' Association, Fulda, Germany, 31 October.

Kuhnke, S., Dumbell, L., Gauly, M., Johnson, J.L., McDonald, König von Borstel, U. 2010. A comparison of rein tension of the rider's dominant and non-dominant hand and the influence of the horse's laterality. *Comparative Exercise Physiology*, 7(2), 57–63.

Kuhnke, S., König von Borstel, U. 2016a. A comparison of methods to determine equine laterality in thoroughbreds. Proceedings of the 12th International Equitation Science Conference, Nantes, France, June 23–25, 67.

Kuhnke, S., König von Borstel, U. 2016b. A comparison of rein tension with methods to determine equine laterality. Proceedings of the 12th International Equitation Science Conference, Nantes, France, June 23–25, 49.

Kyrklund, K. 1998. *Dressage with Kyra: The Kyra Kyrklund Training Method*. Trafalgar Square Publishing, Vermont, USA.

Lacombe, V.A., Hinchcliff, K.W., Kohn, C.W., Devor, S.T., Taylor, L.E. 2004. Effects of feeding meals with various soluble-carbohydrate content on muscle glycogen synthesis after exercise in horses. *American Journal of Veterinary Research*, 65, 916–923.

Ladewig, J. 2000. Chronic intermittent stress: a model for the study of long-term stressors. In: *The Biology of Animal Stress. Basic Principles and Implications for Animal Welfare*, 159–169. Eds: G.P. Moberg, J.A. Mench. CABI Publishing, Wallingford, UK.

Ladewig, J. 2003. Of mice and men: Improving welfare through clinical ethology. Wood-Gush memorial lecture, ISAE congress, Abano-terme, Italy.

Ladewig, J., Søndergaard, E., Christensen, J.W. 2005. Ontogeny: Preparing the young horse for its adult life. In: *The Domestic Horse.*

The Origins, Development, and Management of Its Behaviour, 139–149. Eds: D.S. Mills, S.M. McDonnell. Cambridge University Press, Cambridge.

Lagarde, J., Kelso, J.A.S., Peham, C., Licka, T. 2005. Coordination dynamics of the horse-rider system. *Journal of Motor Behavior*, 37, 418–424.

Lagerweij, E., Nelis, P.C., Wiegant, V.M., van Ree, J.M. 1984. The twitch in horses: A variant of acupuncture. *Science*, 225(4667), 1172–1174.

LaHoste, G.J., Mormede, P., Rivet, J-M., LeMoal, M. 1998. Differential sensitisation to amphetamine and stress responsivity as a function of inherent laterality. *Brain Research*, 453, 381–384.

Lampe, J.F., Andre, J. 2012. Cross-modal recognition of human individuals in domestic horses (*Equus caballus*). *Animal Cognition*, 15, 623–630.

Lansade, L., Bertrand, M., Boivin, X., Bouissou, M-F. 2004. Effects of handling at weaning on manageability and reactivity of foals. *Applied Animal Behaviour Science*, 87, 131–149.

Lansade, L., Bertrand, M., Bouissou, M-F. 2005. Effects of neonatal handling on subsequent manageability, reactivity and learning ability of foals. *Applied Animal Behaviour Science*, 92, 143–158.

Lansade, L., Bouissou, M-F., Boivin, X. 2007. Temperament in pre-weanling horses: Development of reactions to humans and novelty, and startle responses. *Developmental Psychology*, 49(5), 501–513.

Lansade, L., Bouissou, M-F., Erhard, H.W. 2008. Fearfulness in horses: A temperament trait stable across time and situations. *Applied Animal Behaviour Science*, 115, 182–200.

Lashley, M.J., Nauwelaerts, S., Vernooij, J.C.M., Back, W., Clayton, H.M. 2014. Comparison of the head and neck position of elite dressage horses during top-level competitions in 1992 versus 2008. *The Veterinary Journal*, 202, 462–465.

Latif, S.N., von Peinen, K., Wiestner, T., Bitschnau, C., Renk, B., Weishaupt, M.A. 2010. Saddle pressure patterns of three different training saddles (normal tree, flexible tree, treeless) in Thoroughbred racehorses at trot and gallop. *Equine Veterinary Journal*, 42, 630–636.

Le Doux, J.E. 1994. Emotion, memory and the brain. *Scientific American*, 270(6), 32–39.

Le Scolan, N., Hausberger, M., Wolff, A. 1997. Stability over situations in temperamental traits of horses as revealed by experimental and scoring approaches. *Behavioural Processes*, 41, 257–266.

Lea, S.E.G. 1984. In what sense do pigeons learn concepts? In: *Animal Cognition*, 263–276. Eds: H.L. Roitblat, T.G. Bever, H.S. Terrace. Lawrence Erlbaum Associates, NJ, USA.

Lea, S.E.G., Kiley-Worthington, M. 1996. Can animals think? In: *Unsolved Mysteries of the Mind*, 211–244. Ed: V. Bruce. Psychology Press Ltd., Hove, East Sussex.

Leach, D.H., Cymbaluk, N.F. 1986. Relationships between stride length, stride frequency, velocity and morphometrics of foals. *American Journal of Veterinary Research*, 47, 2090–2097.

Leblanc, M-A., Duncan, P. 2007. Can studies of cognitive abilities and of life in the wild really help us to understand equine learning? *Behavioural Processes*, 76, 49–52.

Lee, J., Floyd, T., Erb, H., Houpt, K. 2011. Preference and demand for exercise in stabled horses. *Applied Animal Behaviour Science*, 130(3–4), 91–100.

Lee, R., Coccaro, E. 2001. The neuropsychopharmacology of criminality and aggression. *Canadian Journal of Psychiatry*, 46(1), 35–44.

Lefebvre, D., Lips, D., Ödberg, F.O., Giffroy, J.M. 2007. Tail docking in horses: A review of the issues. *Animal*, 1, 1167–1178.

Lefebvre, L., Helder, R. 1997. Scrounger numbers and the inhibition of social learning in pigeons. *Behavioural Processes*, 40, 201–207.

Lehner, P.N. 1996. *Handbook of Ethological Methods*, 2nd edn. Cambridge University Press, Cambridge, UK.

Leiner, L., Fendt, M. 2011. Behavioural fear and heart-rate responses of horses after exposure to novel objects: Effects of habituation. *Applied Animal Behaviour Science*, 131, 104–109.

Lepore, S., Allen, K., Evans, G. 1993. Social support lowers cardiovascular reactivity to an acute stressor. *Psychosomatic Medicine*, 55, 518–524.

Leslie, J.C. 1996. *Principles of Behavioral Analysis*. Overseas Publishers Association, Amsterdam, The Netherlands.

Levine, M.A. 2005. Domestication and early history of the horse. In: *The Domestic Horse. The Origins, Development, and Management of its Behaviour*, 5–22. Eds: D.S. Mills, S.M. McDonnell. Cambridge University Press, Cambridge, UK.

Lieberman, D.A. 1993. *Learning: Behaviour and Cognition*. Brooks/Cole Publishing, Pacific Grove, California, USA.

Lindberg, A.C., Kelland, A., Nicol, C.J. 1999. Effects of observational learning on acquisition of an operant response in horses. *Applied Animal Behaviour Science*, 61(3), 187–199.

Lindsay, S.R. 2000. Adaptation and learning. In: *Handbook of Applied Dog Behaviour and Training*, vol. I, 233–288. Blackwell, Iowa, USA.

Linklater, W.L. 2007. Equine learning in a wider context – opportunities for integrative pluralism. *Behavioural Processes*, 76, 53–56.

Linklater, W.L., Cameron, E.Z., Stafford, K.J., Veltman, C.J. 2000. Social and spatial structure and range use by Kaimanawa wild horses (*Equus caballus: Equidae*). *New Zealand Journal of Ecology*, 24(2), 139–152.

Liss, S., Wolframm, I. 2011, Lack of effect of a tryptophan product on behavioural and physiological parameters of competition horses during a stressful event. Proceedings of the 7th Conference of the International Society for Equitation Science, Hooge Mierde, The Netherlands, 15.

Loch, S. 1977. *The Classical Rider: Being at One with Your Horse*. Trafalgar Square, North Pomfret, VT, USA.

Looney, T.A., Cohen, P.S. 1982. Aggression induced by intermittent positive reinforcement. *Neuroscience and Biobehavioral Reviews*, 6, 15–37.

Lorenz, K.Z. 1937. The companion in the bird's world. *Auk*, 54, 245–473.

Lovett, T., Hodson-Tole, E., Nankervis, K. 2004. A preliminary investigation of rider position during walk, trot and canter. *Equine and Comparative Exercise Physiology*, 2, 71–76.

Lovrovich, P., Sighieri, C., Baragli, P. 2015. Following human-given cues or not? Horses (*Equus caballus*) get smarter and change strategy in a delayed three-choice task. *Applied Animal Behaviour Science*, 166, 80–88.

Ludewig, A.K., Gauly, M., König von Borstel, U., 2013. Effect of shortened reins on rein tension, stress and discomfort behavior in dressage horses. *Journal of Veterinary Behavior: Clinical Applications and Research* 8, 15–16

Luthersson, N., Nielsen, K.H., Harris, P., Parkin, T.D.H. 2009. Risk factors associated with equine gastric ulceration syndrome (EGUS) in 201 horses in Denmark. *Equine Veterinary Journal*, 41, 625–630.

Macfarlane, D.J., Fogarty, B.A., Hopkins, W.G. 1989. The accuracy and variability of commercially available heart-rate monitors. *New Zealand Journal of Sports Medicine*, 17, 51–53.

Mader, D.R., Price, E.O. 1982. Discrimination learning in horses: effects of breed, age and social dominance. *Journal of Animal Science*, 50, 962–965.

Maes, L., Abourachid, A. 2013. Gait transitions and modular organization of mammal locomotion. *Journal of Experimental Biology*, 216, 2257–2265.

Maier, S.F., Seligman, M.E.P., Solomon, R.L. 1969. Pavlovian fear conditioning and learned helplessness: effects on escape and avoidance behaviour (a) the CS–US contingency and (b) the independence of the US and voluntary responding. In: *Punishment and Aversive Behaviour*. Eds: B. Campbell, R.M. Church. Holt, Rinehart and Winston, New York, 299–343.

Mair, R.G., Onos, K.D., Hembrook, J.R. 2011. Cognitive activation by central thalamic stimulation: The Yerkes-Dodson law revisited. *Dose-Response*, 9, 313–331.

Mal, M.E., Friend, T.H., Lay, D.C., Vogelsang, S.G., Jenkins, O.C. 1991. Behavioural responses of mares to short-term confinement and social isolation. *Applied Animal Behaviour Science*, 31, 13–24.

Mal, M.E., McCall, C.A. 1996. The influence of handling during different ages on a halter training test in foals. *Applied Animal Behaviour Science*, 50, 115–120.

Mal, M.E., McCall, C.A., Cummins, K.A., Newland, M.C. 1994. Influence of preweaning handling methods on post-weaning ability and manageability of foals. *Applied Animal Behaviour Science*, 40, 187–195.

Malmkvist, J., Christensen, J.W. 2007. A note on the effects of a commercial tryptophan product on horse reactivity. *Applied Animal Behaviour Science*, 107, 361–366.

Malmkvist, J., Poulsen J.M., Luthersson, N., Palme, R., Christensen, J.W., Søndergaard, E. 2012. Behaviour and stress responses in horses with gastric ulceration. *Applied Animal Behaviour Science*, 142, 160–167.

Manfredi, J., Clayton, H.M., Derksen, F.J. 2005. Effects of different bits and bridles on frequency of induced swallowing in cantering horses. *Equine and Comparative Exercise Physiology*, 2(4), 241–244.

Manfredi, J., Rosenstein, D., Lanovaz, J.L., Nauwelaerts, V., Clayton, H.M. 2009. Fluoroscopic study of oral behaviors in response to the presence of a bit and the effects of rein tension. *Comp. Exerc. Physiol.*, 6, 143–148.

Manfredi, J., Rosenstein, D., Lanovaz, J.L., Nauwelaerts, V., Clayton, H.M. 2010. Fluoroscopic study of oral behaviors in response to the presence of a bit and the effects of rein tension. *Equine and Comparative Exercise Physiology*, 6(4), 143–148.

Manning, A. 1972. *Contemporary Biology*. Edward Arnold, London.

Manteca, X., Deag, J.M. 1993. Use of physiological measures to assess individual differences in reactivity. *Applied Animal Behaviour Science*, 37, 265–270.

Maricich, S.M., Wellnitz, S.A., Nelson, A.M., Lesniak, D.R., Gerling, G.J. *et al.* 2009. Merkel cells are essential for light-touch responses. *Science*, 324(5934), 1580–1582.

Marinier, S., Alexander, A. 1994. The use of a maze in testing learning and memory in horses. *Applied Animal Behaviour Science*, 39, 177–182.

Marks, I. 1977. Phobias and obsessions: Clinical phenomena in search of a laboratory model. In: *Psychopathology: Experimental Models*, 174–213. Eds: J.D. Maser, M.E.P. Seligman. W.H. Freeman, San Francisco.

Maros, K., Gácsi, M., Miklósi, Á. 2008. Comprehension of human pointing gestures in horses (*Equus caballus*). *Animal Cognition*, 11, 457–466.

Marsbøll, A.F., Christensen, J.W. 2015. Effects of handling on fear reactions in young Icelandic horses. *Equine Veterinary Journal*, 47, 615–619.

Martin, P., Bateson, P. 1993. *Measuring Behaviour: An Introductory Guide*, 2nd edn. Cambridge University Press, Cambridge UK.

Masserman, J.H. 1950. Experimental neurosis. *Scientific American*, 182, 38–43.

McBride, S.D., Hemmings, A. 2005. Altered mesoaccumbens and nigro-striatal dopamine physiology is associated with stereotypy development in a nonrodent species. *Behavioural Brain Research*, 159, 113–118.

McBride, S.D., Hemming, A., Robinson, K. 2004. A preliminary study on the effect of massage to reduce stress in the horse. *Journal of Equine Veterinary Science*, 24, 76–81.

McCafferty, D.J. 2007. The value of infrared thermography for research on mammals: previous applications and future directions. *Mammal Review*, 37, 207–223.

McCall, C.A. 1990. A review of learning behaviour in horses and its application in horse training. *Journal of Animal Science*, 68, 75–81.

McCall, C.A. 2007. Making equine learning research applicable to training procedures. *Behavioural Processes*, 76, 27–28.

McCall, C.A., Burgin, S.E. 2002. Equine utilization of secondary reinforcement during response extinction and acquisition. *Applied Animal Behaviour Science*, 78(2–4), 253–262.

McCall, C.A., Hall, S., McElhenney, W.H., Cummins, K.A. 2006. Evaluation and comparison of four methods of ranking horses based on reactivity. *Applied Animal Behaviour Science*, 96, 115–127.

McCall, C.A., Potter, G., Friend, T., Ingram, R. 1981. Learning abilities in yearling horses using the Hebb–Williams closed field maze. *Journal of Animal Science*, 53, 928–933.

McCann, J.S., Heird, J.C., Bell, R.W., Lutherer, L.O. 1988. Normal and more highly reactive horses. I: Heart rate, respiration rate and behavioural observations. *Applied Animal Behaviour Science*, 19, 201–214.

McDonnell, S.M. 2003. *The Equid Ethogram. A Practical Field Guide to Horse Behavior*. The Blood Horse Inc, Lexington, Kentucky.

McDonnell, S.M., Haviland, J.C.S. 1995. Agonistic ethogram of the equid bachelor band. *Applied Animal Behaviour Science*, 43, 147–188.

McEwen, B.S., Sapolsky, R.M. 1995. Stress and cognitive function. *Current Opinion in Neurobiology*, 5, 205–216.

McGreevy, P.D. 1996. *Why Does My Horse…?* Souvenir Press, London.

McGreevy, P.D. 2004. *Equine Behaviour: A Guide for Veterinarians and Equine Scientists*. W.B. Saunders, Edinburgh, UK.

McGreevy, P.D. 2007. The advent of equitation science. *The Veterinary Journal*, 174, 492–500.

McGreevy, P.D. 2009. *A Modern Dog's Life*. UNSW Press, Sydney, Australia.

McGreevy, P.D., Boakes, R.A. 2007. *Carrots and Sticks – Principles of Animal Training*. Cambridge University Press, Cambridge, UK.

McGreevy, P.D., Burton, F.L., McLean, A.N. 2009a. The horse–human dyad: Can we align horse training and handling activities with the equid social ethogram? *The Veterinary Journal*, 181(1), 12–18.

McGreevy, P.D., McLean, A.N., Thomson, P.C. 2009b. SMART: Sensitivity models for animals in response to training. *The Veterinary Journal*, 181(1), 72–73.

McGreevy, P.D., Corken, R.A., Salvin, H., Black, C. 2013. Whip use by jockeys in a sample of Australian Thoroughbred races – an observational study. *PLoS ONE*, 7(3), e33398.

McGreevy, P.D., Cripps, P.J., French, N.P., Green, L.E., Nicol, C.J. 1995a. Management factors associated with stereotypic and redirected behaviour in the Thoroughbred horse. *Equine Veterinary Journal*, 27, 86–91.

McGreevy, P.D., French, N.P., Nicol, C.J. 1995b. The prevalence of abnormal behaviours in dressage, eventing and endurance horses in relation to stabling. *Veterinary Record*, 137, 36–37.

McGreevy, P.D., Harman, A., McLean, A., Hawson, L. 2010. Over-flexing the horse's neck: A modern equestrian obsession? *Journal of Veterinary Behavior: Clinical Applications and Research*, 5, 180–186.

McGreevy, P.D., Henshall, C., Starling, M.J., McLean, A.N., Boakes, R.A. 2014a. The importance of safety signals in animal handling and training. *Journal of Veterinary Behavior: Clinical Applications and Research*. 6, 382–387.

McGreevy, P., Sundin, M., Karlsteen, M., Berglin, L., Ternstrom, J. *et al.* 2014b. Problems at the human–horse interface and prospects for smart textile solutions. *Journal of Veterinary Behavior: Clinical Applications and Research*, 9, 34–42.

McGreevy, P.D., Landrieu, J-P., Malou, P.F.J. 2007. A note on motor laterality in plains zebras (*Equus burchellii*) and impalas (*Aepyceros melampus*). *Laterality*, 12(5, 449–457.

McGreevy, P.D., McLean, A.N. 2005. Behavioural problems with the ridden horse. In: *The Domestic Horse. The Origins, Development, and Management of Its Behaviour*, 196–211. Eds: D.S. Mills, S.M. McDonnell. Cambridge University Press, Cambridge, UK.

McGreevy, P.D., McLean, A.N. 2006. Ethological challenges for the working horse and the limitations of ethological solutions in training. In: Second International Equitation Science Symposium, Milan, Italy. Eds: M. Minero, E. Canali, A. Warren-

Smith, A. McLean, D. Goodwin, *et al.* Veterinary Faculty of Milano, Italy, 11.

McGreevy, P.D., McLean, A.N. 2007. The roles of learning theory and ethology in equitation. *Journal of Veterinary Behavior: Clinical Applications and Research*, 2, 108–118.

McGreevy, P.D., McLean, A.N. 2009a. Punishment in horse-training and the concept of ethical equitation. *Journal of Veterinary Behavior: Clinical Applications and Research*, 4(5), 193–197.

McGreevy, P.D., McLean, A.N., Warren-Smith, A.K., Waran, N., Goodwin, D. 2005. Defining the terms and processes associated with equitation. In: Proceedings of the 1st International Equitation Science Symposium, Broadford, Victoria. Eds: P. McGreevy, A. McLean, N. Waran, D. Goodwin, A. Warren-Smith. Post-Graduate Foundation in Veterinary Science, Sydney, 10–43.

McGreevy, P.D., Nicholas, F.W. 1999. Some practical solutions to welfare problems in dog breeding. *Animal Welfare*, 8, 329–341.

McGreevy, P.D., Nicol, C.J. 1998. The effect of short-term prevention on the subsequent rate of crib-biting in horses. *Equine Veterinary Journal Supplement. Clinical Behaviour*, 27, 30–34.

McGreevy, P.D., Oddie, C.F. 2011. Holding the whip hand – a note on the distribution of jockeys' whip-hand preferences in Australian Thoroughbred racing. *Journal of Veterinary Behavior: Clinical Applications and Research*, 6(5), 287–289.

McGreevy, P.D., Ralston, L. 2012. The distribution of whipping of Australian Thoroughbred racehorses in the penultimate 200 metres of races is influenced by jockeys' experience. *Journal of Veterinary Behavior: Clinical Applications and Research*, 7, 186–190.

McGreevy, P.D., Rogers, L.J. 2005. Motor and sensory laterality in Thoroughbred horses. *Applied Animal Behaviour Science*, 92(4), 337–352.

McGreevy, P., Warren-Smith, A., Guisard, Y. 2012. The effect of double bridles and jaw-clamping crank nosebands on facial cutaneous and ocular temperature in horses. *Journal of Veterinary Behavior: Clinical Applications and Research*, 7, 142–148.

McKinley, J. 2004. Training in a laboratory environment: Methods, effectiveness and welfare implications of two species of primate. PhD thesis, University of Stirling, Scotland, UK.

McLean, A.N. 2001. Cognitive abilities – the result of selective pressures on food acquisition? *Applied Animal Behaviour Science*, 71(3), 241–258.

McLean, A.N. 2003. *The Truth about Horses*, 48–49. Penguin, Melbourne, Australia.

McLean, A.N. 2004. Short-term spatial memory in the domestic horse. *Applied Animal Behaviour Science*, 85, 93–105.

McLean, A.N. 2005a. The mental processes of the horse and their consequences for training. PhD thesis, University of Melbourne.

McLean, A.N. 2005b. The positive aspects of correct negative reinforcement. *Anthrozoos*, 18(3), 245–254.

McLean, A.N. 2008. Overshadowing: A silver lining to a dark cloud in horse training? *Journal of Applied Animal Welfare Science*, 11(3), 236–248.

McLean, A.N. 2010. Conflict theory – the missing link in equestrian culture. Proceedings of the 6th International Equitation Science Conference, Uppsala, Sweden, 8.

McLean, A.N., 2013. Training the ridden animal: An ancient hall of mirrors. *The Veterinary Journal*, 196(2), 133–136.

McLean, A.N., Christensen, J.W. 2017. The application of learning theory in horse training. *Applied Animal Behaviour Science*, 190, 18–27.

McLean, A.N., Henshall, C., Starling, M., McGreevy, P.D. 2013. Arousal, attachment and affective states. Proc. 9th International Equitation Science Conference, Delaware, USA, 50.

McLean, A.N., McGreevy, P.D. 2004. Training. In: *Equine Behaviour – A Guide for Veterinarians and Equine Scientists*, 291–312. W.B. Saunders, Edinburgh, UK.

McLean, A.N., McGreevy, P.D. 2010a. Horse-training techniques that may defy the principles of learning theory and compromise welfare. *Journal of Veterinary Behavior: Clinical Applications and Research*, 5, 187–195.

McLean, A.N, McGreevy, P.D. 2010b. Ethical equitation: Capping the price horses pay for human glory. *Journal of Veterinary Behavior: Clinical Applications and Research*, 5, 203–209.

McLean, A.N., McLean, M.M. 2008. *Academic Horse Training: Equitation Science in Practice.* Australian Equine Behaviour Centre, Victoria, Australia.

McMillan, F.D. 2005. *Mental Health and Well-Being in Animals.* Blackwell, Iowa, USA.

Mejdell, C.M., Buvik, T., Jørgensen, G.H.M., Bøe, K.E. 2016. Horses can learn to use symbols to communicate their preferences. *Applied Animal Behaviour Science*, 184, 66–73.

Mendl, M. 1999. Performing under pressure: Stress and cognitive function. *Applied Animal Behaviour Science*, 65, 221–244.

Mendl, M., Paul, E.S. 2008. Do animals live in the present? Current evidence and implications for welfare. *Applied Animal Behaviour Science*, 113, 357–382.

Merkies, K., Sievers, A., Zakrajsek, E., MacGregor, H., Bergeron, R., von Borstel, U.K. 2014. Preliminary results suggest an influence of psychological and physiological stress in humans on horse heart rate and behaviour. *Journal of Veterinary Behavior: Clinical Applications and Research*, 9, 242–247.

Meschan, E.M., Peham, C., Schobesberger, H., Licka, T.F. 2007. The influence of the width of the saddle tree on the forces and the pressure distribution under the saddle. *The Veterinary Journal*, 173, 578–584.

Midgley, M. 1983. *Animals and Why They Matter.* University of Georgia Press, Athens, USA.

Midkiff, M.D. 1996. *Fitness, Performance and the Female Equestrian.* Macmillan, New York.

Midkiff, M.D. 2001. *She Flies without Wings: How Horses Touch a Woman's Soul.* Random House, New York.

Miklósi, Á., Kubinyi, E., Topál, J., Gácsi, M., Virányi, Z., Csányi, V. 2003. A simple reason for a big difference: Wolves do not look back at humans but dogs do. *Current Biology*, 13, 763–766.

Miller, R.M. 1991. *Imprint Training of the Newborn Foal.* Western Horseman, Colorado Springs, CO, USA.

Miller, R.M. 1995. Behavior of the horse. 1. The 10 behavioral characteristics unique to the horse. *Journal of Equine Veterinary Science*, 15(1), 13–14.

Miller, R.M. 2001. Fallacious studies of foal imprint training. *Journal of Equine Veterinary Science*, 21(3), 102–103.

Mills, D.S. 1998. Applying learning theory to the management of the horse: the difference between getting it right and getting it wrong. *Equine Veterinary Journal Supplement*, 27, 44–48.

Mills, D.S. 2005. Repetitive movement problems in the horse. In: *The Domestic Horse. The Origins, Development, and Management of its Behaviour*, 212–227. Eds: D.S. Mills, S.M. McDonnell. Cambridge University Press, Cambridge, UK.

Mills, D.S., Marchant-Forde, J.N., McGreevy, P.D., Morton, D.B., Nicol, C. *et al.* (Eds.) 2010. *The Encyclopedia of Applied Animal Behaviour and Welfare.* CAB International, UK.

Minero, M., Canali, E., Ferrante, V., Verga, M., Ödberg, F.O. 1999. Heart rate and behavioural responses of crib-biting horses to two acute stressors. *The Veterinary Record*, 145(15), 430–433.

Minetti, A.E., Ardig, O.L., Reinach, E., Saibene, F. 1999. The relationship between mechanical work and energy expenditure in horses. *Journal of Experimental Biology*, 202, 2329–2338.

Miyashita, Y., Nakajima, S., Imada, H. 2000. Differential outcome effect in the horse. *Journal of Experimental Animal Behaviour*, 74(2), 245–254.

Moberg, G.P., Mench, J.A. 2000. *The Biology of Animal Stress. Basic Principles and Implications for Animal Welfare.* CABI Publishing, Wallingford, UK.

Mohr, E. 1971. *The Asiatic Wild Horse*. Allen & Co Ltd, London.

Monkemoller, S., Keel, R., Hambsch, D., Muller, J., Kalpen, A. *et al.* 2005. Pliance Mobile-16HE: A study about pressure measurements under the saddle after the adjustment of the saddle fit. *Pferdeheilkunde*, 21, 102 *et seq.*

Moore, B.R., Reed, S.M., Biller, D.S., Kohn, C.W., Weisbrode, S.E. 1994. Assessment of vertebral canal diameter and bony malformations of the cervical part of the spine in horses with cervical stenotic myelopathy. *American Journal of Veterinary Research*, 55(1), 5–13.

Morris, D. 1988. *Horsewatching*. Jonathan Cape, London.

Morris, R. 2007. Stress and the hippocampus. In: Eds: Andersen, P., Morris, R., Amaral, D., Bliss, T., O'Keefe, J. *The Hippocampus Book*. New York, Oxford University Press, 751–768.

Münz, A., Eckardt, F., Witte, K. 2014. Horse-rider interaction in dressage riding. *Human Movement Science*, 33, 227–237.

Murphey, R.M., Moura Duarte, F.A., Torres Penendo, M.C. 1981. Response of cattle to humans in open spaces: breed comparisons and approach–avoidance relationships. *Behaviour Genetics*, 2, 37–47.

Murphy, J. 2007. An innovative approach to equitation foundation training (backing the horse) within an automated horse walker may reduce conflict behavior in the horse. In: Proceedings of the 3rd International Equitation Science Symposium, Michigan. Eds: D. Goodwin, C. Heleski, P. McGreevy, A. McLean, H. Randle, C. *et al.* MSU, Michigan, 13.

Murphy, J., Arkins, S. 2007. Equine learning behaviour. *Behavioural Processes*, 76, 1–13.

Murphy, J., Sutherland, A., Arkins, S. 2005. Idiosyncratic motor laterality in the horse. *Applied Animal Behaviour Science*, 91, 297–310.

Myers, R.D., Mesker, D.C. 1960. Operant responding in a horse under several schedules of reinforcement. *Journal of Experimental Animal Behaviour*, 3, 161–164.

Nadeau, J.A., Andrews, F.M., Mathew, A.G., Argenzio, R.A., Blackford, J.T. *et al.* 2000. Evaluation of diet as a cause of gastric ulcers in horses. *American Journal of Veterinary Research*, 61, 784–790.

Nangalama, A.W., Moberg, G.P. 1991. Interaction between cortisol and arachidonic acid on the secretion of LH from ovine pituitary tissue. *Journal of Endocrinology*, 131, 87–94.

Nestadt, C., Davies, H. 2014. Effects of thoracic posture on the nuchal ligament in foetal foals. *Equine Veterinary Journal* Supplement, 46, 44.

Neveu, P.H., Moya, S. 1997. In the mouse, the corticoid stress response depends on lateralisation. *Brain Research*, 749, 344–346.

Nevison, C.M., Hughes, A., Cole, M.D. 2011. Variability in lower leg aids used to achieve gait transitions on a Dressage Simulator. *Journal of Veterinary Behavior*, 6, 294.

Nevison, C.M., Timmis, M.A. 2013. The effect of physiotherapy intervention to the pelvic region of experienced riders on seated postural stability and the symmetry of pressure distribution to the saddle: A preliminary study. *Journal of Veterinary Behavior*, 8, 261–264.

Nicol, C.J. 1996. Farm animal cognition. *Journal of Animal Science*, 62, 375–391.

Nicol, C.J. 2002. Equine learning: progress and suggestions for future research. *Applied Animal Behaviour Science*, 78, 193–208.

Nicol, C.J. 2006. How animals learn from each other. *Applied Animal Behaviour Science*, 100, 58–63.

Nicol, C.J., Badnell-Waters, A.J., Bice, R., Kelland, A., Wilson, A.D., Harris, P.A. 2005. The effects of diet and weaning method on the behaviour of young horses. *Applied Animal Behaviour Science*, 95, 205–221.

Nielsen, B.L., Jezierski, T., Bolhuis, J.E., Amo, L., Rosell, F. *et al.* 2015. Olfaction: An overlooked sensory modality in applied ethology and animal welfare. *Frontiers in Veterinary Science*, 2, 69.

Nierobisch, K. 2016. Form des Kehlenprofils als potentieller Indikator für tierwohlrelevante Kopf-Hals-Positionen beim Pferd – Zusammenhänge zwischen

Kehlenprofil, Gliedmaßen- und Kopf-Hals-Winkelung. BSc thesis, University of Goettingen, Germany. 31 pp.

Noble, G.K., Li, Z., Zhang, D., Sillence, M.N. 2016. Randomised clinical trial on the effect of a single oral administration of L-tryptophan, at three dose rates, on reaction speed, plasma concentration and haemolysis in horses. *The Veterinary Journal*, 213, 84–86.

ICVGAN 2012. Nomina Anatomica Veterinaria. Prepared by the International Committee on Veterinary Gross Anatomical Nomenclature ICVGAN. Authorized by the General Assembly of the World Association of Veterinary Anatomists WAVA in Knoxville. http://www.wava-amav.org/nav_nev.htm [Accessed 18 July 2012].

Nordendorf, E.S., Hekele, P. 1997. *Österreichische Militärgeschichte – Österreichische Kavallerie von den Anfängen bis zur Gegenwart. (In German) „ Austrian Military History – Austrian Cavalry from its Beginnings to the Present.* Verlagsbuchhandlung Stöhr, Vienna, Austria. 127 pp.

Normando, S., Haverbeke, A., Meers, L., Ödberg, F.O., Talegon, M.I., Bono, G. 2003. Effect of manual imitation of grooming on riding horses' heart rate in different environmental situations. *Veterinary Research Communications*, 27, 615–617.

Nyikos, S., Werner, D., Muller, J.A., Buess, C., Keel, R. *et al.* 2005. Measurements of saddle pressure in conjunction with back problems in horses. *Pferdeheilkunde*, 21, 187–198.

O'Brien, J.K., Heffernan, S., Thomson, P.C., McGreevy, P.D. 2008. Effect of positive reinforcement training on physiological and behavioural stress responses in the Hamadryas baboon (*Papio hamadryas*). *Animal Welfare*, 17(2), 125–138.

Ödberg, F.O. 1987. Chronic stress in riding horses. *Equine Veterinary Journal*, 18, 268–269.

Ödberg, F.O., Bouissou, M-F. 1999. The development of equestrianism from the Baroque period to the present day and its consequences for the welfare of horses.

The role of the horse in Europe. *Equine Veterinary Journal Supplement*, 28, 26–30.

Odendaal, J.S.J., Meintjes R.A. 2003. Neurophysiological correlates of affiliative behaviour between humans and dogs. *The Veterinary Journal*, 165(3), 296–301.

Ogden, C.L., Carroll, M.D., Kit, B.K., Flegal, K.M. 2014. Prevalence of childhood and adult obesity in the United States, 2011–2012. *JAMA*, 311(8), 806–814.

Oka, T., Oka, K., Hori, T. 2001. Mechanisms and mediators of psychological stress-induced rise in core temperature. *Psychosomatic Medicine*, 63, 476–486.

Oki, H., Kusunose, R., Nakaoka, H., Nishiura, A., Miyake, T., Sasaki, Y. 2007. Estimation of heritability and genetic correlation for behavioural responses by Gibbs sampling in the Thoroughbred racehorse. *Journal of Animal Breeding and Genetics*, 124(4), 185–191.

Olsen, S.L. 1996. Horse hunters of the Ice Age. In: *Horses Through Time*, 35–56. Ed: S.L. Olsen. Robert Rinehart Publishers, Boulder, CO, USA.

Parelli, P. 1995. *Natural Horsemanship*. Western Horseman, Colorado Springs, CO, USA.

Parker, M., Redhead, E.S., Goodwin, D., McBride, S.D. 2008. Impaired instrumental choice in crib-biting horses (*Equus caballus*). *Behavioural Brain Research*, 191, 137–140.

Paul, E.S., Harding, E.J., Mendl, M. 2005. Measuring emotional processes in animal: The utility of a cognitive approach. *Neuroscience and Biobehavioral Reviews*, 29, 469–491.

Pavlov, I.P. 1927. *Conditioned Reflexes*. Oxford University Press, Oxford, UK.

Pavlov, I.P. 1941. *Lectures on Conditioned Reflexes*. International Publishers, New York.

Payne, E., Boot, M., Starling, M., Henshall, C., McLean, A. *et al.* 2015. The evidence for horsemanship and dogmanship in veterinary contexts. *The Veterinary Journal*. 204(3), 247–254.

Peeters, M., Sulon, J., Beckers, J.F., Ledoux, D., Vandenheede, M., 2011. Comparison between blood serum and salivary cortisol concentrations in horses using an adrenocorticotropic hormone challenge. *Equine Veterinary Journal*, 43, 487–493.

Peham, C. 2008. Forces acting on the horse's back and the stability of the rider in sitting and rising trot – a comparison. *Pferdeheilkunde*, 24(3), 337–342.

Peham, C., Licka, T., Schobesberger, H., Meschan, E. 2004. Influence of the rider on the variability of the equine gait. *Human Movement Science*, 23, 663–671.

Peloso, J.G., Mundy, G.D., Cohen, N.D. 1996. Prevalence of, and factors associated with, musculoskeletal racing injuries of Thoroughbreds. *Journal of the American Veterinary Medical Association*, 204(4), 620–626.

Perone, M. 2003. Negative effects of positive reinforcement. *Behaviour Analysis*, 26, 1–14.

Pfungst, O. 1965. *Clever Hans: (The horse of Mr von Osten)*. Holt, Rinehard and Winston, Inc., New York.

Physick-Sheard, P.W., Marlin, D.J., Thornhill, R., Schroter, R.C. 2000. Frequency domain analysis of heart rate variability in horses at rest and during exercise. *Equine Veterinary Journal*, 32, 253–262.

Pilliner, S., Elmhurst, S., Davies, Z. 2002. *The Horse in Motion*, 65, 150. Blackwell, Oxford, UK.

Pinchbeck, G.L., Clegg, P.D., Proudman, C.J., Morgan, K.L., French, N.P. 2004. Whip use and race progress are associated with horse falls in hurdle and steeplechase racing in the UK. *Equine Veterinary Journal*, 36, 384–389.

Podhajsky, A. 1966. *The Complete Training of Horse and Rider in the Principles of Classical Horsemanship*. Translated by E. Podhajsky and V.D.S. Williams. Doubleday, Bantam Doubleday Dell, New York.

Powell, D.M., Bennett-Wimbush, K., Peeples, A., Duthie, M. 2008. Evaluation of indicators of weight-carrying ability of light riding horses. *Journal of Equine Veterinary Science*, 28(1), 28–33.

Pratt, D. 1980. *Alternatives to Pain in Experiments on Animals*. Pratt, Dallas, USA.

Premack, D. 2007. Human and animal cognition: continuity and discontinuity.

Proceedings of the National Academy of Sciences, 104(35), 13861–13867.

Prokasy, W.F., Whaley, F.L. 1963. Inter-trial interval range shift in classical eyelid conditioning. *Psychological Reports*, 12, 55–58.

Promerova, M., Andersson, L.S., Juras, R., Penedo, M.C., Reissmann, M. *et al.* 2014. Worldwide frequency distribution of the 'Gait keeper' mutation in the DMRT3 gene. *Animal Genetics*, 45, 274–282.

Proops, L., McComb, K. 2010. Attributing attention: the use of human-given cues by domestic horses (*Equus caballus*). *Animal Cognition*, 13, 197–205.

Proops, L., McComb, K. 2012. Cross-modal individual recognition in domestic horses (*Equus caballus*) extends to familiar humans. *Proceedings of the Royal Society B: Biological Sciences*, 279, 3131–3138.

Proops, L., McComb, K., Reby, D. 2009. Cross-modal individual recognition in domestic horses (*Equus caballus*). *Proceedings of the National Academy of Sciences*, 106, 947–951.

Proops, L., Rayner, J., Taylor, A.M., McComb, K. 2013. The responses of young domestic horses to human-given cues. *PLoS ONE*, 8(6), e67000.

Proops, L., Walton, M., McComb, K. 2010. The use of human-given cues by domestic horses, *Equus caballus*, during an object choice task. *Animal Behaviour*, 79, 1205–1209.

Puers, R. 1993. Capacitive sensors – when and how to use them. *Sensor. Actuator. A-Phys.* 37–8, 93–105.

Pullin, J.G., Collier, M.A., Durham, C.M., Miller, R.K. 1996. Use of force-sensing-array technology in the development of a new equine saddle pad: Static and dynamic evaluations and technical considerations. *Journal of Science*, 16, 207–216.

Ragozzino, M.E. 2007. The contribution of the medial prefrontal cortex, orbitofrontal cortex, and dorsomedial striatum to behavioral flexibility. *Annals of the New York Academy of Science*, 1121, 355–375.

Ramseier, L.C., Waldern, N.M., Wiestner, T., Geser-von Peinen, K., Weishaupt, M.A. 2013. Saddle pressure distributions of three saddles used for Icelandic horses and their effects on ground reaction forces, limb movements and rider positions at walk and trot. *The Veterinary Journal*, 198, Supplement 1.

Randle, H., McGreevy, P.D. 2011. The effect of noseband tightness on rein tension in the ridden horse. Proceedings of the 7th International Equitation Science Conference, 84. Eds: M.C van Dierendonck, P. de Cocq, K. Visser. Wageningen Academic Publishers, Wageningen.

Rankin, C.H., Abrams, T., Barry, R.J., Bhatnagar, S., Clayton, D.F. *et al.* 2009. Habituation revisited: An updated and revised description of the behavioral characteristics of habituation. *Neurobiology of Learning and Memory*, 92, 135–138.

Rees, L. 1977. *The Horse's Mind*. Ebury Press, London.

Regan, T. 1983. *The Case for Animal Rights*. University of California Press, Berkeley, Los Angeles, USA.

Reilly, S.M., McElroy, E.J., Biknevicius, A.R. 2007. Posture, gait and the ecological relevance of locomotor costs and energy-saving mechanisms in tetrapods. *Zoology*, 110, 271–289.

Rhodin, M., Gomez Alvarez, C.B., Bystrom, A., Johnston, C., van Weeren, P.R. *et al.* 2009. The effect of different head and neck positions on the caudal back and hindlimb kinematics in the elite dressage horse at trot. *Equine Veterinary Journal*, 41, 274–279.

Rhodin, M., Johnston, C., Holm, K.R., Wennerstrand, J., Drevemo, S. 2005. The influence of head and neck position on kinematics of the back in riding horses at the walk and trot. *Equine Veterinary Journal*, 37, 7–11.

Rivera, E., Benjamin, S., Nielsen, B., Shelle, J., Zanella, A.J. 2002. Behavioral and physiological responses of horses to initial training: the comparison between pastured versus stalled horses. *Applied Animal Behaviour Science*, 78(2–4), 235–252.

Roberts, J.M., Browning, B.A. 1998. Proximity and threats in highland ponies. *Social Networks*, 20(3), 227–238.

Roberts, K., Hemmings, A., Moore-Colyer, M., Hale, C. 2015. Cognitive differences in horses performing locomotor versus oral stereotypic behaviour. *Applied Animal Behaviour Science*, 168, 37–44.

Roberts, M. 1997. *The Man Who Listens to Horses*. Arrow Books, London.

Roberts, M. 2000. *Join-Up – Horse Sense for People*. Harper Collins, London.

Roberts, T. 1992. *Equestrian Technique*. J.A. Allen & Co Ltd, London.

Rochais, C., Henry, S., Fureix, C., Hausberger, M. 2016. Investigating attentional processes in depressive-like domestic horses (*Equus caballus*). *Behavioural Processes*, 124, 93–96.

Rochais, C., Henry, S., Sankey, C., Nassur, F., Góracka-Bruzda, A., Hausberger, M. 2014. Visual attention, an indicator of human–animal relationships? A study of domestic horses (*Equus caballus*). *Frontiers in Psychology*, 5, 108.

Rollin, B.E. 2000. Equine welfare and emerging social ethics. Animal Welfare Forum: Equine Welfare. (*Journal of the American Veterinary Medical Association*, 216(8), 1234–1237.

Rolls, E.T. 2000. Précis of the brain and emotion. *Behavioral and Brain Sciences*, 23, 177–234.

Rørvang, M.V., Ahrendt, L.P., Christensen, J.W. 2015a. A trained demonstrator has a calming effect on naïve horses when crossing a novel surface. *Applied Animal Behaviour Science*, 171, 117–120.

Rørvang, M.V., Ahrendt, L.P., Christensen, J.W. 2015b. Horses fail to use social learning when solving spatial detour tasks. *Animal Cognition*, 18, 847–854.

Rose, R.J., Hodgson, D.R. 1993. *Manual of Equine Practice*. W.B. Saunders, Edinburgh, UK.

Rothman, K.J. 1990. No adjustments are needed for multiple comparisons. *Epidemiology*, 1, 43–46.

Ruis, M.A., te Brake, J.H., Buwalda, B., De Boer, S.F., Meerlo, P. *et al.* 1999. Housing familiar male wild-type rats together reduces the long-term adverse behavioural and physiological effects of social defeat. *Psychoneuroendocrinology*, 24, 285–300.

Sankey, C., Henry, S., André, N., Richard-Yris, M-A., Hausberger, M. 2011. Do horses have a concept of person? *PLoS ONE*, 6(3), e18331.

Sankey, C., Henry, S., Górecka-Bruzda, A., Richard-Yris, M-A., Hausberger, M. 2010a. The way to a man's heart is through his stomach: What about horses? *PLoS ONE*, 5(11), e15446.

Sankey, C., Richard-Yris, M-A., Henry, S., Fureix, C., Nassur, F., Hausberger, M. 2010b. Reinforcement as a mediator of the perception of humans by horses (*Equus caballus*). *Animal Cognition*, 13, 753–764.

Sankey, C., Richard-Yris, M-A., Leroy, H., Henry, S., Hausberger, M. 2010c. Positive interactions lead to lasting positive memories in horses, *Equus caballus*. *Animal Behaviour*, 79, 869–875.

Sapolsky, R.M. 2002. The Endocrinology of the Stress-Response. In: Becker, J.B., Breedlove, S.M., Crews, D., McCarthy, M.M., *Behavioral Endocrinology*, 2nd Ed., Massachusetts Institute of Technology, 409–450.

Sapolsky, R.M. 2004. *Why Zebras don't get Ulcers*. The acclaimed guide to stress, stress-related diseases, and coping, 3rd edn. St Martin's Griffin, New York.

Sappington, B.F., Goldman, L. 1994. Discrimination learning and concept formation in the Arabian horse. *Journal of Animal Science*, 72, 3080–3087.

Sappington, B.K.F., McCall, C.A., Coleman, D.A., Kuhlers, D.L., Lishak, R.S. 1997. A preliminary study of the relationship between discrimination reversal learning and performance tasks in yearling and 2-year-old horses. *Applied Animal Behaviour Science*, 53, 157–166.

Saslow, C.A. 2002. Understanding the perceptual world of horses. *Applied Animal Behaviour Science*, 78, 235–252.

Schaefer, A.L., Stewart, M., Webster, J.R., Cook, N.J., Colyn, J.J. *et al.* 2006. Objective measurement of pain and fear in cattle using infrared thermography. Proceedings of the International Society of Applied Ethology, North American Regional Meeting. Vancouver, Canada: The University of British Columbia, 55. [http://www. Applied ethology.org/isaemeetings_files/2006%20 Canada-USA%20Regions%20ISAE%20 Proceedings.pdf].

Schilder, M.B.H., van der Borg, J.A.M. 2004. Training dogs with help of the shock collar: Short and long term behavioural effects. *Applied Animal Behaviour Science*, 85, 319–334.

Schmid, S., Wilson, D.A., Rankin, C.H. 2015. Habituation mechanisms and their importance for cognitive function. *Frontiers in Integrative Neuroscience*, 8, Article 97.

Schmidt, A., Möstl, E., Aurich, J., Neuhauser, S., Aurich, C. 2009. Comparison of cortisol and cortisone levels in blood plasma and saliva and cortisol metabolite concentrations in faeces for stress analysis in horses. In: 5th International Equitation Science Conference, Sydney, 53. Eds: P. McGreevy, A. Warren-Smith, C. Oddie.

Schmidt, A., Biau, S., Möstl, E., Becker-Birck, M., Morillon, B. *et al.* 2010a. Changes in cortisol release and heart rate variability in sport horses during long-distance road transport. *Domestic Animal Endocrinology*, 38, 179–189.

Schmidt, A., Möstl, E., Wehnert, C., Aurich, J., Müller, J., Aurich, C. 2010b. Cortisol release and heart rate variability in horses during road transport. *Hormones and Behavior*, 57, 209–215.

Schmidt, A., Aurich, J., Möstl, E., Müller, J., Aurich, C. 2010c. Changes in cortisol release and heart rate and heart rate variability during the initial training of 3-year-old sport horses. *Hormones and Behavior*, 58, 628–636.

Schonholtz, C.M. 2000. Animals in rodeo – a closer look. Animal Welfare Forum: Equine Welfare. *Journal of the American Veterinary Medical Association*, 216(8), 1246–1249.

Schramm, U. 1986. *The Undisciplined Horse – Causes and Corrections*. J.A. Allen & Co. Ltd, London.

Scofield, R., Randle, H. 2013. Preliminary comparison of behaviors exhibited by horses ridden in bitted and bitless bridles. *Journal of Veterinary Behavior: Clinical Applications and Research*, 8(2), e20–e21.

Le Scolan, N., Hausberger, M., Wolff, A. 1997. Stability over situations in temperamental traits of horses as revealed by experimental and scoring approaches. *Behavioural Processes*, 41, 257–266.

Seaman, S.C., Davidson, H.P.B., Waran, N.K. 2002. How reliable is temperament assessment in the domestic horse (*Equus caballus*)? *Applied Animal Behaviour Science*, 78, 175–191.

Segal, E.F. 1969. The interactions of psychogenic polydipsia with wheel running in rats. *Psychonomic Science*, 14, 141–144.

Segal, E.F. 1972. Induction and the provenance of operants. In: *Reinforcement: Behavioral analysis*, Eds: Gilbert, R.M., Millenson, J.R. Academic Press, New York.

Seligman, M.E.P. 1970. On the generality of the laws of learning. *Psychological Review*, 77, 406–408.

Seligman, M.E.P. 1971. Phobias and preparedness. *Behaviour Therapy*, 2, 307–320.

Seligman, M.E.P. 1975. *Helplessness: On Depression, Development and Death*. W.H. Freeman & Co, San Francisco, USA.

Seligman, M.E.P., Altenor, A., Weinraub, M., Schulman, A. 1980. Coping behavior: Learned helplessness, physiological change and learned inactivity. *Behavioural Research and Therapy*, 18, 459–512.

Seligman, M.E.P., Maier, S.F. 1967. Failure to escape traumatic shock. *Journal of Experimental Psychology*, 74, 1–9.

Selye, H. 1979. *The Stress of my Life: A scientist's memoirs*. New York, Van Nostrand.

Sewell, A. 1877. *Black Beauty*. Penguin Classics.

Shettleworth, S.J. 2001. Animal cognition and animal behaviour. *Animal Behaviour*, 61(2), 277–286.

Sidman, M. 2006. The distinction between positive and negative reinforcement: Some additional considerations. *The Behavior Analyst*, 29, 135–139.

Sighieri, C., Tedeschi, D., De Andreis, C., Petri, L., Baragli, P. 2003. Behaviour patterns of horses can be used to establish a dominant–subordinate relationship between man and horse. *Animal Welfare*, 12(4), 705–708.

Sigurjonsdottir, H., Gunnarsson, V. 2002. *Controlled Study of Early Handling and Training of Icelandic Foals*. Eds: S. McDonnell, D. Mills. Dorothy Russell Havemeyer Workshop Horse Behavior and Welfare, Iceland, 13–16 June, 35–39.

Simpson, B. 2002. Neonatal foal handling. *Applied Animal Behaviour Science*, 78, 303–317.

Siqueira, L.O., Vieira, A.S., Ferrari, E.A.M. 2005. Time-of-day variation in the sensitization of the acoustic response in pigeons. *Biological Rhythm Research*, 36, 151–157.

Sivewright, M. 1984. *Thinking Riding, Book 2: In Good Form*. J.A. Allen & Co Ltd, London.

Skinner, B.F. 1938. *The Behavior of Organisms*. Appleton-Century-Crofts, New York.

Skinner, B.F. 1971. *Beyond Freedom and Dignity*. Hackett Publishing, Indianapolis, USA.

Skipper, L. 1999. *Inside Your Horse's Mind: A Study of Equine Intelligence and Human Prejudice*. J.A. Allen & Co Ltd, London.

Sleutjens, J., Smiet, E., van Weeren, R., van der Kolk, J., Back, W., Wijnberg, I.D. 2012. Effect of head and neck position on intrathoracic pressure and arterial blood gas values in Dutch Warmblood riding horses during moderate exercise. *American Journal of Veterinary Research*, 73, 522–528.

Sleutjens, J., Voorhout, G., Van Der Kolk, J.H., Wijnberg, I.D., Back, W. 2010. The effect of *ex vivo* flexion and extension on intervertebral foramina dimensions in the equine cervical spine. *Equine Veterinary Journal*, 42, 425–430.

Sloet van Oldruitenborgh-Oosterbaan, M.M., Barneveld, A., Schamhardt, H.C. 1995. Effects of weight and riding on workload and locomotion during treadmill exercise. *Equine Veterinary Journal Supplement*, 18(S18), 413–417.

Sloet van Oldruitenborgh-Oosterbaan, M.M., Blok, M.B., Begeman, L., Kamphuis, M.C.D., Lameris, M.C. *et al*. 2006. Workload and stress in horses: comparison in horses ridden deep and round ('Rollkur') with a draw rein and horses ridden in a natural frame with only light rein contact. *Tijdschrift voor Diergeneeskunde*, 131, 114–119.

Smiet, E., Van Dierendonck, M.C., Sleutjens, J., Menheere, P.P.C.A., van Breda, *et al.* 2014. Effect of different head and neck positions on behaviour, heart rate variability and cortisol levels in lunged Royal Dutch Sport Horses. *The Veterinary Journal*, 202, 26–32.

Smith, A.V., Proops, L., Grounds, K., Wathan, J., McComb, K. 2016. Functionally relevant responses to human facial expressions of emotion in the domestic horse (*Equus caballus*). *Biology Letters*, 12: 20150907.

Solomon, R.L. 1964. Punishment. *American Psychologist*, 19, 239–253.

Søndergaard, E., Halekoh, U. 2003. Young horses' reactions to humans in relation to handling and social environment. *Applied Animal Behaviour Science*, 84, 265–280.

Søndergaard, E., Jensen, M.B., Nicol, C.J. 2011. Motivation for social contact in horses measured by operant conditioning. *Applied Animal Behaviour Science*, 132, 131–137.

Søndergaard, E., Ladewig, J. 2004. Group housing exerts a positive effect on the behaviour of young horses during training. *Applied Animal Behaviour Science*, 87, 105–118.

Soproni, K., Miklósi, Á., Topál, J., Csányi, V. 2001. Comprehension of human communicative signs in pet dogs (*Canis familiaris*). *Journal of Comparative Psychology*, 115, 122–126.

Spalding, D. 1873. Instinct: With observations on young animals. *Macmillan's* magazine, 27, 283–293. (Reprinted in the *British Journal of Animal Behaviour*, 2, 1–11.)

Spier, S.J., Pusterla, J.B., Villarroel, A., Pusterla, N. 2004. Outcome of tactile conditioning of neonates, or 'imprint training' on selected handling measures in foals. *The Veterinary Journal*, 168, 252–258.

Stacey, R., Messinger, D., Dye, G., Komar, W., McGee, J. *et al.* 1999. Passive restraint training in *Tursiops truncatus*. In: *Animal Training: Successful Animal Management Through Positive Reinforcement*, Ed: Ramirez, K.. John G. Shedd Aquarium, Chicago.

Staddon, J.E.R., Simmelhag, V.L. 1971. The 'superstition' experiment: A re-examination of its implications for the principles of adaptive behavior. *Psychological Review*, 78, 3–43.

Staddon, J.E.R. 1977. Schedule-induced behavior, 125–152. In: *Handbook of Operant Behavior*, Eds: Honig, W.K., Staddon, J.E.R. Prentice-Hall, Englewood Cliffs NJ.

Staller, L. 2005. Understanding analog to digital converter specifications. Embedded Systems Design. embedded.com. [Accessed 20 September 2013.] http://www.embedded.com/design/embedded/4025078/Understanding-analog-to-digital-converter-specifications

Starke, S.D., Willems, E., May, S.A., Pfau, T. 2012. Vertical head and trunk movement adaptations of sound horses trotting in a circle on a hard surface. *The Veterinary Journal*, 193(1), 73–80.

Starling, M.J., Branson, N., Cody, D., McGreevy, P.D. 2013. Conceptualising the impact of arousal and affective state on training outcomes of operant conditioning. *Animals*, 3, 300–317.

Steiner, G.Z., Barry, R.J. 2014. The mechanism of dishabituation. *Frontiers in Integrative Neuroscience*, 8, Article 14.

Stewart, M., Stafford, K.J., Dowling, S.K., Schaefer, A.L., Webster, J.R. 2008. Eye temperature and heart rate variability of calves disbudded with or without local anaesthetic. *Physiology & Behavior*, 93, 789–797.

Stewart, M., Webster, J., Verkerk, G., Colyn, J., Schaefer, A. 2007. Non-invasive measurement of stress in dairy cows using infrared thermography. *Physiology & Behavior*, 92, 520–525.

Stoffel-Willame, M., Stoffel-Willame, Y. 1999. Horses of the Namib. *Africa, Environment & Wildlife*, 7(1), 58–67.

Stolba, A., Baker, N., Wood-Gush, D.G.M. 1983. The characterization of stereotyped behavior in stalled sows by information redundancy. *Behavior*, 8(7), 157–182.

Suwala, M., Jezierski, T., Gorecka-Bruzda, A. 2012. Localisation of artefacts in two models of equine heart rate monitors – a pilot study, 68. Annual Meeting of the International Society for Equitation Science, Edinburgh, UK.

Swann, W.J. 2006. Improving the welfare of working equine animals in developing countries. *Applied Animal Behaviour Science*, 100, 148–151.

Task Force of the European Society of Cardiology, t.N.A.S.o.P.E. 1996. Heart rate variability: standards of measurement, physiological interpretation, and clinical use. *Circulation*, 93, 1043–1065.

Taylor, K. 2010. Counter-conditioning. In: *The Encyclopedia of Applied Animal Behaviour and Welfare*, Eds: Mills, D.S., Marchant-Forde, J.N., McGreevy, P.D., Morton, D.B., Nicol, *et al.* CAB International, UK, 145.

Terada, K. 2000. Comparison of head movement and EMG activity of muscles between advanced and novice horseback riders at different gaits. *Journal of Equine Science*, 11, 83–90.

Terada, K., Mullineaux, D.R., Lanovaz, J., Kato, K., Clayton, H.M. 2004. Electromyographic analysis of the rider's muscles at trot. *Equine and Comparative Exercise Physiology*, 1(3), 193–198.

The Norwegian Harness Racing Association (Det Norske Travselskap) 2015. DNTs Lopsreglement (In Norwegian) 'DNTs racecourse regulations'). Online available: http://www.travsport.no/PageFiles/7662/DNTs%20L%c3%b8psreglement%202015.pdf [Accessed 15 November 2016.]

Thivierge, M., Leger, L. 1989. Critical review of heart rate monitors. *CAHPER J.*, 55(3), 26–31.

Thomas, K.E., Annest, J.L., Gilchrist, J., Bixby-Hammett, D.M. 2006. Non-fatal horse-related injuries treated in emergency departments in the United States, 2001–2003. *British Journal of Sports Medicine*, 40, 619–626.

Thomas, R.K. 1986. Vertebrate intelligence: A review of the laboratory research. In: *Animal Intelligence: Insights into the animal mind*, 37–56. Eds: R.J. Hoage, L. Goldman. Smithsonian Institution Press, Washington, DC.

Thompson, K., McGreevy, P., McManus, P. 2015. A critical review of horse-related risk: A research agenda for safer mounts, riders and equestrian cultures. *Animals*, 5, 561–575.

Thorbergson, Z.W., Nielsen, S.G., Beaulieu, R.J., Doyle, R.E. 2016. Physiological and behavioral responses of horses to wither scratching and patting the neck when under-saddle. *Journal of Applied Animal Welfare Science*, 19, 245–259.

Thorndike, E.L. 1911. *Animal Intelligence*. Macmillan, New York.

Thorne, J.B., Goodwin, D., Kennedy, M.J., Davidson, H.P.B., Harris, P. 2005. Foraging enrichment for individually housed horses: practicality and effects on behaviour. *Applied Animal Behaviour Science*, 94, 149–164.

Thorpe, W.H. 1963. *Learning and Instinct in Animals*, 2nd edn. Methuen, UK.

Tobin, T. 1978. A review of the pharmacology of reserpine in the horse. *Journal of Equine Medical Surgery*, 2(10), 433–438.

Tolman, E.C. 1948. Cognitive map in rats and men. *Psychological Review*, 55, 189–209.

Trut, L., Oskina, I., Kharlamova, A. 2009. Animal evolution during domestication: the domesticated fox as a model. *BioEssays*, 31, 349–360.

Tyler, S.J. 1972. The behaviour and social organization of the New Forest ponies. *Animal Behaviour Monograph*, 5, 85–196.

Ueda, Y., Yoshida, K., Oikawa, M. 1993. Analyses of race accident conditions through use of patrol videos. *Journal of Equine Veterinary Science*, 13, 707–710.

USDF, 2002. *Glossary of Dressage Judging Terms*. Compiled by United States Dressage Federation Council of Judges. Lincoln, USA.

Valenchon, M., Lévy, F., Fortin, M., Leterrier, C., Lansade, L. 2013a. Stress and temperament affect working memory performance for disappearing food in horses, *Equus caballus*. *Animal Behaviour*, 86, 1233–1240.

Valenchon, M., Lévy, F., Prunier, A., Moussu, C., Calandreau, L., Lansade, L. 2013b. Stress modulates instrumental learning performances in horses (*Equus caballus*) in interaction with temperament. *PLoS ONE*, 8(4), e62324.

Valentine, B.A., Hintz, H.F., Freels, K.M., Reynolds, A.J., Thompson, K.N. 1998. Dietary control of exertional rhabdomyolysis in horses. *Journal of the American Veterinary Association*, 212(10), 1588–1593.

Valera, M., Bartolomé, E., Sánchez, M.J., Molina, A., Cook, N., Schaefer, A. 2012. Changes in eye temperature and stress assessment in horses during show-jumping competitions. *Journal of Equine Veterinary Science*, 32, 827–830.

van Breda, E. 2006. A non-natural head-neck position (Rollkur) during training results in less acute stress in elite, trained, dressage horses. *Journal of Applied Animal Welfare Science*, 9(1), 59–64.

van Dierendonck, M.C. 2006. Assessment of ethological methods as a diagnostic tool to determine early overtraining in horses, 13. In: Proceedings of the 2nd International Equitation Science Symposium, Milan. Eds: M. Minero, E. Canali, A. Warren-Smith, A. McLean, D. Goodwin, *et al.* University of Milan, Milan.

van Dierendonck, M.C., Devries, H., Schilder, M.B.H. 1995. An analysis of dominance, its behavioural parameters and possible determinants in a herd of Icelandic horses in captivity. *Netherlands Journal of Zoology*, 45(3–4), 362–385.

van Erck-Westergren, E. 2011. Dynamic respiratory videoendoscopy in ridden sport horses: Effect of head flexion, riding and airway inflammation in 129 cases. *Equine Veterinary Journal*, 43, 18–24.

van Heel, M.C.V., Kroekenstoel, A.M., Van Dierendonck, M.C., van Weeren, P.R., Back, W. 2006. Uneven feet in a foal may develop as a consequence of lateral grazing behaviour induced by conformational traits. *Equine Veterinary Journal*, 38(7), 646–651.

van Weeren, P.R., Meyer, H., Johnston, C., Roepstorff, L., Weishaupt, M.A. 2006. The effect of different head and neck positions on the thoracolumbar kinematics in the unridden horse. In: Report of the FEI Veterinary and Dressage Committee's Workshop. The use of over-bending ('Rollkur') in FEI Competition, 31 January, during the FEI Veterinary Committee meeting at the Olympic Museum, Lausanne, 8.

Visser, E.K. 2002. Horsonality: A study on the personality of the horse. PhD thesis, Wageningen University and Research Center Publications (The Netherlands).

Visser, E.K., Ellis, A.D., van Reenen, C.G. 2008. The effect of two different housing conditions on the welfare of young horses stabled for the first time. *Applied Animal Behaviour Science*, 114, 521–533.

Visser, E.K., van Reenen, C.G., Hopster, H., Schilder, M.B.H., Knaap, J.H. *et al.* 2001. Quantifying aspects of a young horse's temperament: Consistency of behavioural variables. *Applied Animal Behaviour Science*, 74(4), 241–258.

Visser, E.K., van Reenen, C.G., Schilder, M.B.H., Barneveld, A., Blokhuis, H.J. 2003. Learning performances in young horses using two different learning tests. *Applied Animal Behaviour Science*, 80, 311–326.

von Borstel, U.U., Keeling, L.J., Duncan, I.J.H. 2005. Transfer of nervousness from the rider to the horse. 39th International Congress of the International Society of Applied Ethology, Sagamihara, Japan, 84.

von Borstel, U.U., Duncan, I.J.H., Shoveller, A.K., Millman, S.T., Keeling, L.J. 2007. Transfer of nervousness from competition rider to the horse. In: Proceedings of the 3rd International Society for Equitation Science, Michigan, 17. Eds: D. Goodwin, C. Heleski, P. McGreevy, A. McLean, H. Randle, *et al.* MSU, Michigan, USA., p. 17.

von Borstel, U. 2008. *Fear in Horses and Riders: Two Hearts Living in just One Mind – The Influence of Rider, Training and Genetics on horses' fear*. Verlag Dr. Müller, Saarbrücken. 132 pages.

von Borstel, U., Duncan, I., Shoveller, A., Merkies, K., Keeling, L., Millman, S. 2009. Impact of riding in a coercively obtained Rollkur posture on welfare and fear of performance horses. *Applied Animal Behaviour Science*, 116, 228–236.

von Lewinski, M., Biau, S., Erber, S., Ille, N., Aurich, J. *et al.* 2013. Cortisol release, heart rate and heart rate variability in the horse and its rider: Different responses to training and performance. *The Veterinary Journal*, 197, 229–232.

von Peinen, K., Wiestner, T., Bogisch, S., Roepstorff, L., van Weeren, P.R., Weishaupt, M.A. 2009. Relationship between the forces acting on the horse's back and the movements of rider and horse while walking on a treadmill. *Equine Veterinary Journal*, 41(3), 285–291.

von Peinen, K., Wiestner, T., von Rechenberg, B., Weishaupt, M.A. 2010. Relationship between saddle-pressure measurements and clinical signs of saddle soreness at the withers. *Equine Veterinary Journal*, 42, 650–653.

von Uexküll, J. 1957. A stroll through the worlds of animals and men: a picture book of invisible worlds. In: *Instinctive Behavior: The Development of a Modern Concept*, 5–80. Ed. and trans. Claire H. Schiller. International Universities Press, Inc., New York.

Waldern, N.M., Wiestner, T., von Peinen, K., Álvarez, C.G.G., Roepstorff, L. *et al.* 2009. Influence of different head-neck positions on vertical ground reaction forces, linear and time parameters in the unridden horse walking and trotting on a treadmill. *Equine Veterinary Journal*, 41, 268–273.

Walker, W.F., Liem, K.F. 1994. *Functional Anatomy of the Vertebrates: An evolutional perspective*. Saunders College, New York.

Waran, N.K., Clarke, N., Farnworth, M. 2008. The effects of weaning on the domestic horse (*Equus caballus*). *Applied Animal Behaviour Science*, 110, 42–57.

Waran, N., McGreevy, P., Casey, R.A. 2002. Training methods and horse welfare. In: *The Welfare of Horses*, 151–180. Ed: N. Waran. Kluwer Academic Publishers, Dordrecht, The Netherlands.

Waring, G.H. 2003. *Horse Behavior*. 2nd edn. Noyes/William Andrew, New York.

Warren-Smith, A.K., McLean, A.N., Nicol, H.I., McGreevy, P.D. 2005a. Variations in the timing of reinforcement as a training technique for foals. *Anthrozoös*, 18(3), 255–272

Warren-Smith, A.K., Curtis, R.A., McGreevy, P.D. 2005b. A low-cost device for measuring the pressures exerted on domestic horses by riders and handlers. In: Proceedings of the 1st International Equitation Science Symposium, Broadford, Victoria, 44–55. Eds: P. McGreevy, A. McLean, N. Waran, D. Goodwin, A. Warren-Smith. Post-Graduate Foundation in Veterinary Science, Sydney.

Warren-Smith, A.K., Greetham, L., McGreevy, P.D. 2007a. Behavioral and physiological responses of horses (*Equus caballus*) undergoing head lowering. *Journal of Veterinary Behavior: Clinical Applications and Research*, 2–3, 59–67.

Warren-Smith, A.K., Curtis, R.A., Greetham, L., McGreevy, P.D. 2007b. Rein contact between horse and handler during specific equitation movements. *Applied Animal Behaviour Science*, 108, 157–169.

Warren-Smith, A.K., McGreevy, P.D. 2006. An audit of the application of the principles of equitation science by qualified equestrian instructors in Australia. In: Proceedings of the 2nd International Equitation Science Symposium, Milan, 12. Eds: M. Minero, E. Canali, A. Warren-Smith, A. McLean, D. Goodwin, *et al.* University of Milan.

Warren-Smith, A.K., McGreevy, P.D. 2007c. The use of blended positive and negative reinforcement in shaping the halt response of horses *(Equus caballus)*. *Animal Welfare*, 16, 481–488.

Warren-Smith, A.K., McGreevy, P.D. 2008a. Equestrian coaches' understanding and application of learning theory in horse training. *Anthrozoös*, 21(2), 153–162.

Warren-Smith, A.K., McGreevy, P.D. 2008b. Preliminary investigations into the ethological relevance of roundpen (round-yard) training of horses. *Journal of Applied Animal Welfare Science*, 11(3), 285–298.

Wasilewski, A. 2005. 'Friendship' in ungulates? Sociopositive relationships between non-related herd members of the same species. http://www.staff.unimarburg.de/~z-phylog/wisstaff/waso-sum.htm. [Accessed 16 March 2007.]

Waters, A.J., Nicol, C.J., French, N.P. 2002. Factors influencing the development of stereotypic and redirected behaviours in young horses: findings of a four-year prospective epidemiological study. *Equine Veterinary Journal*, 34(6), 572–579.

Watt, L.M., McDonnell, S.M. 2001. Demonstration of concept formation in the horse. Equine Behavior Laboratory, University of Pennsylvania School of Veterinary Medicine, August 2001, Interim Report.

Webster, A.J.F. 1994. *Animal Welfare: A Cool Eye towards Eden*. Blackwell Science, London.

Weeks, J.W., Crowell-Davis, S.L., Caudle, A.B., Heusner, G.L. 2000. Aggression and social spacing in light horse (*Equus caballus*) mares and foals. *Applied Animal Behaviour Science*, 68(4), 319–337.

Weiler, H. 2002. *Insertionsdesmopathien beim Pferd*. FN-Verlag, Warendorf, Germany. 168 pp.

Weinraub, M., Schulman, A. 1980. Coping behavior: Learned helplessness, physiological change and learned inactivity. *Behavioural Research and Therapy*, 18, 459–512.

Weishaupt, M.A., Bystrom, A., von Peinen, K., Wiestner, T., Meyers, H. *et al.* 2009. Kinetics and kinematics of the passage. *Equine Veterinary Journal*, 41(3), 263–267. Epub 2009/05/28 ISES, 2016 position statement.

Weishaupt, M.A., Wiestner, T., von Peinen, K., Waldern, N., Roepstorff, L. *et al.* 2006. Effect of head and neck position on vertical ground reaction forces and interlimb coordination in the dressage horse ridden at walk and trot on a treadmill. *Equine Veterinary Journal*, 38, 387–392.

Weiss, J.M. 1972. Psychological factors in stress and disease. *Scientific American*, 226, 104–113.

Weiss, J.M., Glazer, H.I., Pohorecky, L.A., Brick, J., Miller, N.E. 1975. Effects of chronic exposure to stressors on avoidance–escape behavior and on brain norepinephrine. *Psychosomatic Medicine*, 37, 522–534.

Wells, S.M., von Goldschmidt-Rothschild, B. 1997. Social behaviour and relationships in a herd of Camargue horses. *Z Tierpsychol.* 49, 363–380.

Wergard, E.M., Temrin, H., Forkman, B., Spangberg, M., Fredlund, H., Westlund, K. 2015. Training pair-housed Rhesus macaques (*Macaca mulatta*) using a combination of negative and positive reinforcement. *Behavioural Processes*, 113, 51–59.

dem Sattel: Eine Studie mit einem elektronischen Sattel-Messsystem (Novel GmbH). *Pferdeheilkunde*, 18, 125–140.

Wickens, C.L., Heleski, C.R. 2010. Crib-biting behaviour in horses: a review. *Applied Animal Behaviour Science*, 128, 1–9.

Wickler, S.J., Hoyt, D.F., Cogger, E.A., Hall, K.M. 2001. Effect of load on preferred speed and cost of transport. *Journal of Applied Physiology*, 90, 1548–1551.

Wickler, S.J., Hoyt, D.F., Cogger, E.A., Myers, G. 2003. The energetics of the trot-gallop transition. *Journal of Experimental Biology*, 206, 1557–1564.

Wiepkema, P.R. 1987. Behavioural aspects of stress. In: *Biology of Stress in Farm Animals: An Integrative Approach*, 113–133. Eds: P.R. Wiepkema, P.W.M. van Adrichem. Martinus Nijhoff, Leiden, The Netherlands.

Wijnberg, I.D., Sleutjens, J., Van Der Kolk, J.H., Back, W. 2010. Effect of head and neck position on outcome of quantitative neuromuscular diagnostic techniques in Warmblood riding horses directly following moderate exercise. *Equine Veterinary Journal*, 42, 261–267.

Wilewski, K.A., Rubin, L. 1999. Bit seats: A dental procedure for enhancing performance of show horses. *Equine Practice*, 21(4), 16–20.

Williams, D.E., Norris, B.J. 2007. Laterality in stride pattern preferences in racehorses. *Animal Behaviour*, 74, 941–950.

Williams, J.L., Friend, T.H., Collins, M.N., Toscano, M.J., Sisto-Burt, A., Nevill, C.H. 2002. The effects of early training sessions on the reactions of foals at 1, 2 and 3 months of age. *Applied Animal Behaviour Science*, 77, 105–114.

Williams, J.L., Friend, T.H., Collins, M.N., Toscano, M.J., Sisto-Burt, A., Nevill, C.H. 2003. Effects of imprint training procedure at birth on the reactions of foals at age six months. *Equine Veterinary Journal*, 35, 127–132.

Winkelmayr, B., Peham, C., Frühwirth, B., Licka, T., Scheidl, M. 2006. Evaluation of the forces acting on the back of the horse with an English saddle and a side saddle at walk, trot and canter. *Equine Veterinary Journal Supplement*, 36, 406–410.

Wittling, W., Roschmann, R. 1993. Emotion-related hemisphere asymmetry: subjective emotional responses to laterally presented films. *Cortex*, 29, 431–448.

Wolff, A., Hausberger, M. 1996. Learning and memorisation of two different tasks in horses: The effects of age, sex and sire. *Applied Animal Behaviour Science*, 46, 137–143.

Wolff, A., Hausberger, M., Scolan, N.L. 1997. Experimental tests to assess emotionality in horses. *Behavioural Processes*, 40, 209–221.

Woolf, C.J., Ma, Q. 2007. Nociceptors – noxious stimulus detectors. *Neuron*, 55, 353–364.

Wolpe, J., Lazarus, A.A. 1969. *The Practice of Behaviour Therapy*. Pergamon, New York.

Woodward, A.L. 1999. Infants' ability to distinguish between purposeful and non-purposeful behaviors. *Infant Behavior and Development*, 22, 145–160.

Wouters, L., De Moor, A. 1979. Ultrastructure of the pigment epithelium and the photoreceptors in the retina of the horse. *American Journal of Veterinary Research*, 40, 1066–1071.

Wright, M. 1973. *The Jeffery Method of Horse Handling. An Introduction to a New Approach to the Handling of Horses*. R.M. Williams, Prospect, South Australia.

Wutke, S., Andersson, L., Benecke, N., Sandoval-Castellanos, E., Gonzalez, J. *et al.* 2016. The origin of ambling horses. *Current Biology*, 8(26), 15, R697–R699.

Xenophon. 1962. *The Art of Horsemanship*. Translated by M.H. Morgan. J.A. Allen & Co Ltd, London.

Yarnell, K. 2012. An investigation into the use of infrared thermography as a tool to assess the physiological stress response in the horse. PhD thesis. Nottingham Trent University.

Yarnell, K., Hall, C., Billett, E. 2013. An assessment of the aversive nature of animal management procedures using behavioral and physiological measures. *Physiology and Behavior*, 118, 32–39.

Yerkes, R.M., Dodson, J.D. 1908. The relation of strength to stimulus to rapidity of habituation. *Journal of Comparative Neurology and Psychology*, 18, 459–482.

Zebisch, A., May, A., Reese, S., Gehlen, H. 2014a. Effect of different head-neck positions on physical and psychological stress parameters in the ridden horse. *Journal of Animal Physiology and Animal Nutrition*, 98, 901–907.

Zebisch, A., May, A., Reese, S., Gehlen, H. 2014b. Effects of different head-neck positions on the larynges of ridden horses. *Journal of Animal Physiology and Animal Nutrition*, 98, 894–900.

Zeitler-Feicht, M. 2004. *Horse Behaviour Explained. Origins, Treatment and Prevention of Problems*. Manson Publishing, London.

Index

Note: Page numbers in *italic* denote figures, those in **bold** denote tables.

Equitation Science, Second Edition. Paul McGreevy, Janne Winther Christensen,
Uta König von Borstel and Andrew McLean.
© 2018 John Wiley & Sons Ltd. Published 2018 by John Wiley & Sons Ltd.
Companion website: www.wiley.com/go/mcgreevy/equitation

Printed and bound by CPI Group (UK) Ltd, Croydon, CR0 4YY

16/12/2024

14612675-0001